Topics in Environmental Physiology and Medicine

Edited by Karl E. Schaefer

Alain Reinberg
Michael H. Smolensky

Biological Rhythms and Medicine

Cellular, Metabolic, Physiopathologic, and Pharmacologic Aspects

With Contributions by H. von Mayersbach,
J. E. Pauly, L. A. Scheving, L. E. Scheving, and T. H. Tsai

With 148 Illustrations

Springer-Verlag New York Berlin Heidelberg Tokyo

Alain Reinberg, M.D., Ph.D.
Director de Recherches au CNRS
Fondation A. de Rothschild
Laboratoire de Physiologie
29 Rue Manin
75940 Paris Cedex 19
France

Michael H. Smolensky, Ph.D.
Associate Professor of
  Environmental Sciences
University of Texas Health
  Sciences Center at Houston
School for Public Health
Graduate School of Biomedical
  Sciences
Houston, Texas 77025
U.S.A.

Library of Congress Cataloging in Publication Data
Reinberg, Alain.
  Biological rhythms and medicine.
  (Topics in environmental physiology and medicine)
  Includes index.
  1. Biological rhythms. 2. Metabolism. I. Smolensky,
Michael H. II. Title. III. Series.
[DNLM: 1. Biological clocks. QT 167 R364b]
QP84.6.R44 1983   599′.01882   82-19675

Typeset by Bi-Comp Incorporated, York, Pennsylvania.
Printed and bound by Halliday Lithograph, West Hanover, Massachusetts.
Printed in the United States of America.

9 8 7 6 5 4 3 2 1   **110000**

ISBN 0-387-**90791**-2 Springer-Verlag New York Berlin Heidelberg Tokyo
ISBN 3-540-**90791**-2 Springer-Verlag Berlin Heidelberg New York Tokyo

Contents

Dedication

This book is dedicated to Heinz von Mayersbach for very simple reasons—his prominence as a leading expert on biological rhythms of mammalian cells and our heart-felt warmth for him as one of our dearest friends. In recalling our fond memories of this man, we find it difficult to disassociate Heinz the scientist from Heinz our friend. In 1978, when traveling together in the United States from Florida to Texas, we discussed the outline and organization of this book. Heinz knew he had cancer. We remember him at the airport experiencing pain but nonetheless smiling and expressing apologies for not being a better travel companion. Such lessons of courage and gentleness were presented in Hannover, Federal Republic of Germany, in July 1979 when he hosted the XIV Meeting of the International Society for Chronobiology (ISC). Although suffering badly, his major concern was the success of the meeting, not only from a scientific point of view but also for the sake of each attendant.

Heinz was gifted and accomplished in several scientific disciplines. As a researcher, he was untiringly inquisitive, inventive, and rigorous. He was a prominent figure in his field of scientific specialization—cellular and subcellular physiology, chemistry, and morphology—as well as in chronobiology. One of Heinz's greatest talents was his ability to communicate and stimulate discussion. Heinz was a fantastic lecturer. He utilized his depth of experience and knowledge, well organized into precise concepts and thoughts, to explain with simplicity difficult and complex matters. And this was necessary to successfully convince his peers of his findings that a cell possesses not only an anatomy in space but an anatomy in time programed to conduct different metabolic activities at different times. This was not an easy task. His concepts and experimental findings had to be clear and indisputable. The reader will once more experience these qualities in this volume (Chap. 3). Heinz had hoped also to contribute a second chapter on animal chronotoxicology. Unfortunately, illness prevented the completion of this task.

Even though a hard-working scientist, Heinz gave of himself. He was personable and well liked even by his academic adversaries; he enjoyed socializing with his international peers and searched for means of better understanding between them. At a time when many persons, including scientists in countries of the old continent, were just beginning to recognize the need to reach better accord, Heinz's achievements already were outstanding. Perhaps this was the motivation for his multiple endeavors to organize scientific meetings on chronobiology. Apart from the ISC meetings in Hannover in 1973 and 1979, he was responsible for the first meeting on "The Cellular Aspects of Biorhythms" in 1967, the first symposium on "Chronotoxicology and Chronopharmacology" in Mainz in 1976, and the meeting on chronobiology for the German Academy of Sciences (Leopoldina Deutsche Akademie der Naturforscher) in 1976.

Heinz was of Austrian origin, but was born in Italy. He graduated in Austria with his Medical Doctorate and attended the Royal Postgraduate Medical School in London. Thereafter he was Assistant Professor at the University of Graz, Austria; Associate Professor at the University of Lausanne, Switzerland; and full Professor at the University of Nijmegen, The Netherlands, and finally at the University of Hannover. Heinz had mastered several languages and was able to teach in most of them except in Latin, despite the fact that he was supposed to do so at the University of Nijmegen. (He used to tell us funny tales about this and many other situations, for he had a highly developed sense of humor.) From 1966 until his death, Heinz von Mayersbach was full Professor and Head of the Department of Anatomy, Medical School of Hannover. He had served as President of the Histochemical Society (Federal Republic of Germany), Fellow of the Royal Microscopical Society (Oxford), and Honorary President of the ISC. When composing the final version of this book, we fully realized how much we missed Heinz's help; usually it was given in the form of friendly but firm criticisms and suggestions interspersed during times of relaxation with humorous stories and anecdotes. This book is dedicated to our friend Heinz with fond memories and respect. We convey also to Dietlinde von Mayersbach our warmest thoughts.

Preface

During the past decade many review papers and books have been devoted to descriptions and analyses of biological rhythms (chronobiology) in plants and animals. These contributed greatly to demonstrating the importance of bioperiodicities in living beings in general. However, the practical aspects of chronobiology with regard to human health and improving the treatment of disease have not yet been a major focus of publication.

One of our aims is to establish the relevance of biological rhythms to the practice of medicine. Another is to organize and convey in a simple fashion information pertinent to health- and life-science professionals so that students, researchers, and practitioners can achieve a clear and precise understanding of chronobiology. We have limited scientific jargon to unavoidable basic and well-defined terms and we have emphasized illustrative examples of facts and concepts rather than theories or hypothetical mechanisms.

This volume is divided into seven chapters, each of which is comprehensive in its treatment and includes an extensive bibliography. The book is organized to serve as a textbook and/or reference handbook of modern applied chronobiology. Chapter 1 describes the historical development of chronobiology and reviews why, when, and how major concepts were introduced, accepted, and transformed. The chapter covers, for example, human temporal structure and its genetic origin, the existence and role of periodic environmental signals in resetting biological clocks, and the value of biological rhythmicity as an adaptive phenomenon for coping with cyclic, and thus predictable, environmental changes for individuals and, presumably, species.

Chapter 2 discusses the major considerations of human chronobiologic investigations in terms of subjects, materials, and methods. Particular attention is given to the standardization of subjects for chronobiologic study. Suggestions for solving often-encountered problems in analyzing time series by special techniques, especially when data are collected at unequal intervals, are presented in a straightforward and clear manner.

Chapter 3 constitutes the last scientific contribution of Heinz von Mayersbach. His works on biological rhythmicity in cell morphology are classic. One of Heinz's major findings was the demonstration that sequences of metabolic processes in cells, such as those of the liver, are programed precisely in time, for example along the 24-hr scale. This chapter, which was completed just before his death, has been updated and represents the current state of knowledge on this topic.

Larry Scheving and his colleagues were invited to contribute Chap. 4. These authors are renowned for their research on biological rhythms of mitosis as well as toxic effects (chronotoxicology) at the cellular level— information that is critical for understanding major aspects of cancer and its treatment.

Chapter 5 presents a comprehensive review on aspects of human chronopathology—time-dependent variations in the exacerbation or occurrence of illness and symptoms. For example, the occurrence and worsening of allergic, cardiovascular, seizure, and inflammatory diseases are not random, but vary predictably as rhythms over 24 hr, the menstrual cycle, and the year. Knowledge of human chronopathologies, representing the interactions of cyclic ambient events and bioperiodic physiochemical component functions, is indispensable for understanding the etiology of diseases as well as their treatment and prevention.

Chapter 6 is devoted to clinical chronopharmacology, defined as rhythmic changes in drug effectiveness, with reference to both laboratory and human investigations. The presentation is based on new concepts, such as bioperiodic changes in drug disposition (chronopharmacokinetics), target biosystem susceptibility (chronesthesy), and the overall effects of medicines (both chronoeffectiveness and chronotolerance). Illustrative examples of the clinical optimization of several classes of medicines using these concepts are given.

Chapter 7 is devoted to biological rhythms and nutrition. The topic is organized with consideration of four complementary aspects: food intake as a rhythmic phenomenon, persistence of biological rhythms during fasting, circadian and other periodicities in metabolic processes, and the significance of timed food intakes as an entrainer of circadian rhythms. A special section is devoted to chronobiologic studies of nutrition in shift workers.

Acknowledgments

The authors benefited from the assistance of many dedicated persons during the preparation of this volume. We are unable to thank everyone; however, we wish to express our gratitude to Annonciade Nicolaï and Gay Robertson, who in typing and editing the many redrafts worked numerous days, evenings, and weekends untiringly and, yes, sometimes tiringly; and also to our many academic colleagues: Israel Ashkenazi (University of Tel Aviv), Ivan Assenmacher (Université de Montpellier), Jean De Prins (Université Libre de Bruxelles), Pierre Gervais (Université de Paris, VII), Jean Ghata (Université de Genève), Erhard Haus (University of Minnesota), Gaston Labrecque (Université Laval, Quebec), Francis Lévi (CNRS, Paris, France), Jack P. McGovern (McGovern Allergy Clinic, Houston, Texas), Lawrence E. Scheving (University of Arkansas, Little Rock), Thérèse Vanden Driessche (Université Libre de Bruxelles), and Yvan Touitou (Université de Paris VI), who provided critical reviews and useful suggestions. We, in addition, are indebted to Dietlinde Von Mayersbach whose input was very much appreciated and to Karl Schaefer who until his death served as editor of the series *Topics In Environmental Physiology and Medicine* for Springer-Verlag and who made it possible for us to express our findings and philosophies herein. Our work was facilitated by the skillful contributions of the Medical Arts personnel (Fran Holden, Connie Harris, and Bett Oaks) of the University of Texas School of Public Health, Health Sciences Center at Houston, and librarians of both the School of Public Health and the Houston Academy of Medicine Texas Medical Library, especially Marlene Caldwell. Finally, we acknowledge the patience of our wives—Marie-Anne and Nita Beth—our children—Agnès and André Laszlo, Anne-Christine, and Olivier Reinberg, as well as Melissa and Susan Smolensky and Brian Burroughs—while we exhibited weak social synchronization and displayed free-running tendencies when extending our activity late into the night and early morning.

Contributors

Heinz von Mayersbach, M.D. (deceased), Professor and Head, Department of Anatomy, Medical School of Hannover, D-3000 Hannover 61, Federal Republic of Germany

John E. Pauly, Ph.D., Professor and Chairman, Department of Anatomy, University of Arkansas College of Medicine, Little Rock, Arkansas 72205, U.S.A.

Lawrence A. Scheving, B.A., Department of Anatomy, University of Arkansas College of Medicine, Little Rock, Arkansas 72205, U.S.A.

Lawrence E. Scheving, Ph.D., Rebsamen Professor of Anatomical Sciences, Department of Anatomy, University of Arkansas College of Medicine, Little Rock, Arkansas 72205, U.S.A.

T. H. Tsai, Ph.D., Department of Anatomy, University of Arkansas College of Medicine, Little Rock, Arkansas 72205, U.S.A.

1

Introduction to Chronobiology

Alain Reinberg and Michael H. Smolensky

Recorded recognition of the importance of biological rhythms in plants and animals dates back at least to 5000 B.C. Over the years, the understanding of rhythmic phenomena has grown, but the acceptance of chronobiology as a science has been slow nonetheless. This chapter reviews the development of modern chronobiology by recounting the milestone events that have contributed to the current knowledge in this field, and discusses why chronobiology has developed slowly as a science.

Acquisition of Facts and Concepts in Chronobiology

Chronobiology is the study of mechanisms and alterations of each organism's temporal structure under various situations (Halberg et al. 1977). Such a definition, while clear and useful for chronobiologists, requires amplification for those unfamiliar with the concept of biological time structure. In actuality, this concept is not new. It is stated in Genesis that the first task of God was to create light and then the alternation of light

and darkness. Today, it is well recognized that the light–dark cycle of the ambient and laboratory environments serves to synchronize the phasing of 24-hr and perhaps yearly physiochemical rhythms of organisms. Direct evidence that the importance of temporal factors was recognized by mankind even in biblical times comes from Ecclesiastes: "To every thing there is a season and a time to every purpose under the heaven: a time to be born and a time to die; a time to plant, and a time to pluck up that which is planted. . . ." Apart from the obvious wisdom of this recommendation, the precise reference to time of year conveys the early knowledge of the critical importance of cyclical environmental changes for the survival of species. Such a recognition also is present in the aphorisms of Hippocrates (1961) with specific reference to seasonal differences in the occurrence of human diseases.

As a matter of fact, biological systems possess a very prominent temporal structure. Major periodic components of biological rhythms are found around 24 hr and 1 year.* Other bioperiodicities (τ) such as those less than 24 hr (termed ultradian rhythms) or approximately equaling 7 days, 20 days, 30 days, etc. (called infradian rhythms), are exhibited by certain biological functions of many species. However, circadian† ($\tau \cong 24$ hr) and circannual ($\tau \cong 1$ year) biological rhythms, having been widely documented for a multitude of physiological variables of both plant and animal species, including ours, are most familiar to scientists. Obviously, with respect to evolution, circadian rhythms appear to be related to the rotation of the Earth around its axis (Fig. 1); similarly, circannual rhythms appear to be related to the rotation of the Earth around the Sun.

It is likely that circannual rhythms represent an adaptive phenomenon from the perspective of the reproduction and survival of species. Man learned rapidly that nutrients were not continually available in quality and quantity; this is true of prehistoric man—the hunter, fisherman, and gatherer—and thereafter of modern man—the farmer, peasant, and animal breeder. There was, and remains, a time to plant and a time to harvest. This cannot be ignored nor altered appreciably.

In connection with this, it is widely accepted that astronomical clocks were built long ago in Carnac (Brittany), in Stonehenge (near London), in Chichén Itzá (Yucatán), etc., serving both religious and practical agricultural purposes. The answers to the critical questions such as when to plant and when to harvest domesticated plant species were obtained by consulting astronomical clocks as well as other "signs" (signals), such as the precise timing of matings of many animal species, the flowering of certain plants growing in the wild, and bird migrations, among others. Seasons of planting and harvesting were of such importance that they often were celebrated as religious feasts. Thus, even early man monitored time, at least on a yearly basis, with regard to predictable annual changes in the reproduction of both edible animals and plants. With this in mind, it is not surprising that a set of bioperiodic phenomena were reported by several Greek and Roman scholars including Aristotle, Pliny, and Galen in connection with the reproductive patterns of sea animals, among others (Aschoff 1974; Fox 1923).

For centuries it was believed that cyclic changes in organisms represented exclusively the simultaneous effects of cyclic changes in environmental factors, such as the alternation of light with darkness and/or of heat with cold over periods of both 24 hr and 1 year. In ancient times, the Sun was given the status of an omnipresent and omnipotent God: the Egyptian Ra, the Greek Apollo, the Roman-Heliopolitan Jove, the Aztec Tonatiuh, etc. Not until 1729 was the accepted tenet of an "exclusively exogenous origin" of circadian rhythms in plants questioned. The French astronomer J. J. de Mairan reported in 1729 that the circadian changes in the position of appendages of the heliotrope persisted in constant darkness. This was the beginning of a wide variety of research. However, as far as plants are concerned, it was not until the work of Pfeffer (1875, 1915) started at the end of the nineteenth century that convincing experimental evidence was produced indicating that circadian rhythms persist in complete and constant darkness. Using a set of specially designed devices enabling the continuous mechanical recording of changes in plant limb and leaf positions, Pfeffer tested the hypothesis that the light–dark (LD) alternation over 24 hr plays

---

* The term "biorhythm" is used infrequently by chronobiologists, since it has been given a completely invalid and unacceptable definition by proponents of the astrological forecasting business. Among many scientifically valid objections, it is not possible to predict attributes of biologic time structure by one datum only, i.e., date of birth. A thorough and unbiased review of many scientific investigations of the popularized concept reveals a clear lack of support for biorhythm forecasting (Klein and Wegmann 1979, AGARD Lecture Series 105:2.10–2.12).

† The use of the Latin root *circa* (about) in the term "circadian" (about 24 hr) was proposed by Halberg et al. (1977) to specify with respect to both statistical and biological considerations that the period is not necessarily exactly 24 hr.

Eine Blumen-Uhr

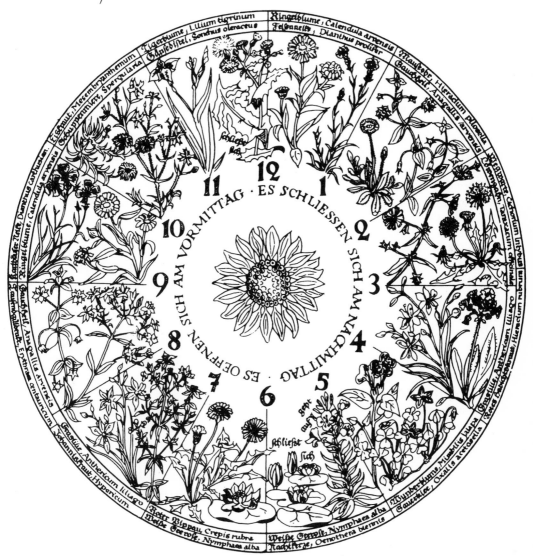

Fig. 1. The "Flower-Clock," designed by K. Linné in 1745, relies on the knowledge that at relatively precise (sun-related) clock hours flowers of certain plant species are open while those of others are closed. The half-circle to the left presents those plant species for which the flower openings occur between 0600 and 1200; the half-circle to the right shows plants for which the flower closing occurs in the afternoon, between 1300 and 1800. According to Linné, a trained botanist walking through the country without a watch should be able to estimate the time by noting the pattern of flower closings and openings of selected plants. For example, the water lily opens between 0600 and 0700; the St. John's wort opens between 0700 and 0800; the scarlet pimpernel opens between 0800 and 0900 and closes between 1300 and 1400; the oenothera, or evening primrose, closes between 1700 and 1800. (Drawing by U. Schleicher-Benz in *Lindauer Bilderbogen*. Published by Friedrich Boër and J. Thorbecke, Lindau, Badensee, West Germany. Reproduced with permission of the publishers.)

the major role in inducing plant movement.
Despite the experimental attempts of Pfeffer, the hypothesis that leaf and limb movements are caused by the LD alternation
never fitted the data. Instead, the pioneer
work of Pfeffer demonstrated the endogenous origin of circadian changes; the persistence of biological rhythms in organisms
maintained in constant environmental conditions has been widely confirmed for many
species, from the eukaryote to man (Aschoff 1963; Boissin and Assenmacher 1969;
Bünning 1963; Halberg 1960b; Halberg and
Reinberg 1967; Mills 1964, 1966; Pittendrigh 1960; Reinberg 1974; Schweiger et al.
1964; Sweeny 1969; Vanden Driessche
1973; Weitzman et al. 1979).

It was not until many years later, around
1950, that Pfeffer's findings were clearly
understood and appreciated. Yet results of
investigations on temporal factors in the organization of biological functions were, in
general, slow to be recognized by the scientific community. Several other examples of
the long latency in the development of scientific interest in biological rhythms follow;
these were selected from experimental
studies that emphasize reported data and
findings, rather than from philosophical
considerations of the "cyclicity of time"
without supporting data, as is the case for
ancient Chinese medicine (Reinberg 1974)
or as presented in *The Art of Prolonging
Life* (Hufeland 1789) at the end of the eighteenth century.

As a first example, we cite the work of
Sanctorius, who in 1657 constructed a mon-
umental balance with a huge tray on which
a completely furnished room was set. Sanctorius resided for several consecutive
months on his balance tray (Fig. 2). A ser-
vant provided food and assistance and
made readings on the balance scale. By
means of this self study, Sanctorius was the
first to design a "laboratory for chronobiology" and to use an "autorhythmometric method"—repeated self-measurements
of physiological variables as a function of
time—to document bioperiodic phenomena
(Halberg et al. 1977). Sanctorius reported a

monthly rhythm (circamensual variation
with period, $\tau \cong 30$ days) both in his body
weight and in the turbidity of his urine.
Later Seguin and Lavoisier (1790, 1797)
reported a circadian rhythm in the body
weight of the healthy human male. In fact,
they state in their paper that the period was
about 24 hr (". . . *a peu près de* 24 *heures
. . .*") and that a subject who does not exhibit a circadian rhythm in his body weight
should be suspected to be ill.

The Briton J. Davy (1845) was the first
to report the existence of both circadian
and circannual rhythms in his own body
core temperature. Previously, in 1773, Martin reported some "effects of sleep on the
body heat" (Martin 1773). Again, the use of
an autorhythmometric procedure allowed
Davy to demonstrate that these bioperiodicities were closely related neither to physical activity, for example the riding of a
horse or running, nor to environmental
temperature, which was actually measured
and compared with that of Davy's body
temperature. The fact that the same variable could undergo rhythms of different periods was demonstrated later by Halberg
and his colleagues (1965) through reanalyz-
ing data collected by Hamburger (1954).
Hamburger collected each of his daily urine
voidings for 16 years, measuring the volume and 17-ketosteroid concentration. The
statistical technique of spectral analysis
clearly revealed prominent periods approximately equaling 24 hr, 7 days, 30 days, and
1 year. As a result of these findings, emphasis must be given to two facts thus discovered: (1) the existence of both a circadian
and a circannual periodicity, among others,
in the same variable, for example, in body
temperature as well as in the urinary volume and 17-ketosteroid concentration and
(2) the persistence of biological rhythms independent of internal (exercise) or external
(environmental temperature) factors.

During the nineteenth century, additional data were accumulated to evaluate
the nature and origin of biological rhythms.
Some experiments were designed so that
measurements of phenomena were done at

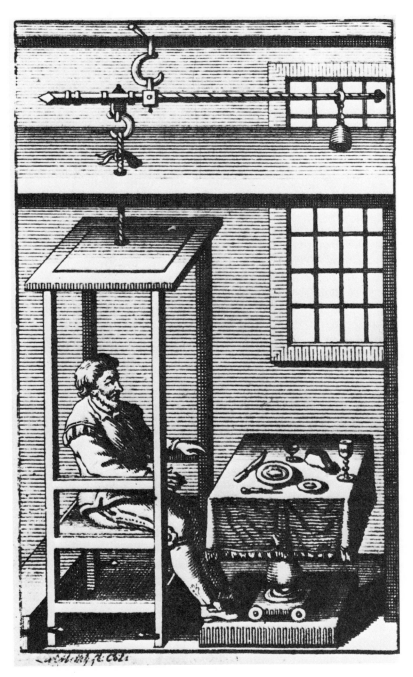

Fig. 2. Sanctorius is depicted sitting upon the tray of his room-scale balance. This scientist, an original pioneer of experimental chronobiology, was by 1711 already performing self-measurements several times daily—a method which is now termed "autorhythmometry." Sanctorius found evidence for a circadian rhythm of body weight related to perspiration. In addition, he reported the existence of 30-day rhythms in body weight in the human adult male. (From Kayser 1952, reproduced with permission.)

regular intervals while the organism—animal or plant—was maintained under constant laboratory conditions. Other research involved investigations conducted under circumstances allowing for random changes in the experimental environment. Results of these types of investigations provided important new information about the role of environmental influences upon bioperiodicities. For example, the fact that circadian rhythms persist in constant conditions with a period differing from 24 hr was first reported by de Candolle (1832). According to this Genevan plant physiologist, the leaf movements of *Mimosa pudica* persist in darkness with a period of 22–23 hr. This is precisely the type of result Pfeffer obtained, although he thought this was due to light leaks in the darkroom until he confirmed the persistence of the rhythm and change in period length in leaf and limb movement under constant conditions.

Two additional major breakthroughs in chronobiology were derived from the research of Bünning before 1950. The first, in 1935, was the direct demonstration of the genetic origin of circadian rhythm characteristics in the beanplant *Phaseolus* (Bünning 1935). For example, the circadian rhythm of stem and leaf movements in this plant differs between two genetically distinct stocks exhibiting periodicities of about 23 and 27 hr, respectively. Hybridization experiments produced plants with hybrid circadian rhythm characteristics ($\tau \cong 25$ hr). Thus, Bünning demonstrated that biological periodicities, i.e., circadian rhythms, are transmitted from generation to generation according to genetic rules. Evidence exists to support the theory that the controlling elements which transcribe the circadian rhythms reside in the nuclear genetic material. Recent work on *Drosophila* has identified several genes responsible for certain biological rhythm characteristics. Using circadian rhythm mutants of *Drosophila* to build a genetic mosaic of mutant and nonmutant parts, Konopka and Benzer (1971) showed the rhythm of the composite flies resembled the genotype of

the head. This is also the case, for example, when circadian rhythm patterns of a female Drosophila (XX) differ from that of the male (XY) (Rensing 1973).

The second major finding of Bünning (1963) was that an organism, such as a plant, is able to "measure" time. A sophisticated manipulation of the lighting regimen over 24-hr durations allowed Bünning to demonstrate that a time-restricted short exposure to light induced flowering when given at a critical clock hour for several days. Bünning found the same quantity and quality of light when given at other clock hours to be ineffective in inducing flowering. In other words, light serves not only as a source of energy but also as a signal. Whether or not a light signal is effective in inducing a biological response, in this case flowering, varies according to the (biological) time it is presented. Further research by Bünning contributed to developing the concept of the "biological clock." The message was that organisms possess built-in and inborn mechanisms enabling the measurement of time, at least over 24 hr and 1 year. This message is still valid (Ehret 1974; Queiroz 1974), although it is presented in a different manner. Modern chronobiologists (Ehret 1974; von Mayersbach 1978; von Mayersbach and Leske 1961) consider a cell to be genetically programed for performance of a given task at a specific biological time, or to reach the maximum of a certain activity at a precise circadian phase. When organisms are synchronized to environmental conditions (see Chap. 2), the biological times and phases coincide with specified clock hours in the 24-hr scale.

The concept of how organisms use biosystems to measure time has changed in complexity and in the depth of understanding from the initial one posed by Bünning in the thirties. The photofraction (duration of light in each 24-hr span) or the scotofraction (duration of darkness in each 24-hr span) varies with the time of year. Because of their precise predictability, photoperiodic phenomena appear to be "the most appropriate references for precisely measuring time" for an organism (Queiroz 1974). In fact, the appropriate photoperiod is strictly delineated for each species with regard to programing activities such as reproduction, migration, diapause, dormancy, etc., in plants and animals. For example, according to Bünning, over the 24-hr span there is an "external coincidence" between the external alternation of light and darkness and the alternation of phase during which a plant is either sensitive or insensitive to light with regard to the induction of flowering. Taking into consideration experimental data obtained later by Aschoff (1960, 1963), Hamner and Takimoto (1964), and Pittendrigh (1960, 1961), the complementary hypothesis of an "internal coincidence" among temporal patterns in both the internal and external environments was derived. This newer concept takes into consideration the existence of several circadian oscillators driven either by a signal such as sunrise (light-on) and/or sunset (light-off). Therefore with regard to the photofraction, the interval of time between the two signals—the phase relationship of sunrise and sunset—determines whether or not the phenomenon, flowering, occurs. In addition, as Pittendrigh (1960, 1961) emphasized the light signals can be replaced by a system capable of shifting the phase of the oscillators, e.g., by causing change in the crest time of the 24-hr cycle of external temperature, hormonal secretions, or other biological functions. The capabilities of biological systems to measure time or to program activities represent two sides of the same coin. For instance, a biological system's ability to respond and the efficiency of its response to a signal can depend upon the phase of the bioperiod.

The concept of biological clocks developed by Bünning represented a significant step forward. Unfortunately, the expression "biological clock" has been and continues to be misused. It is tempting, especially for some animal biologists, to search for a master clock somewhere within the body. Initially, the proposed master clock

was envisioned as being located within the pituitary, although many experiments showed this not to be the case (Reinberg 1974). Then, the search for the home of the wandering master clock was relocated t the hypothalamus. Again, dissection a inspection of this structure proved fruitl As was the case for the legendary phc the master clock reborn from exper ashes tries to find a place today in docrine structures, either the epiphysis o the suprachiasmatic nucleus (SCN). The latter is likely to be the circadian oscillator system which drives certain neuroendocrine circadian rhythms such as those of adrenocorticotrophic hormone (ACTH), thyroid stimulating hormone (TSH), and prolactin (PRL). Physical destruction or neurotoxic inhibition of the SCN results in the cessation of these neurohormonal circadian rhythms. However, their ultradian rhythms continue to persist, as do circadian rhythms in other physiochemical functions of the body including rest and activity, eating and drinking, body temperature, and corticosterone hormone secretion from the adrenal cortex (Fuller et al. 1981; Moore-Ede et al. 1980; Moore 1980; Krieger 1979; Mornex and Jordan 1980; Suda et al. 1979; Szafarczyk et al. 1981).

With evidence for an endogenous, i.e., genetic, basis of biological rhythms, the role of exogenous factors upon rhythmic systems was not immediately understood. It was not until 1954 that Halberg et al. (1954) and Aschoff (1954) almost simultaneously developed the idea that cyclic variations in environmental factors are capable of influencing the expression of circadian rhythms. Aschoff (1954) coined the word "Zeitgeber" (time giver); Halberg et al. (1967) coined the word "synchronizer," and Pittendrigh (1960) proposed "entraining agent." Despite the fact that the exact definitions of the terms given by these three scientists differ, there is general consensus among chronobiologists that "synchronizer," "Zeitgeber," and "entraining agent" are synonymous. One of the most powerful synchronizers for a large variety of plants and animals is the LD alternation over 24 hr. But other cyclic changes in environmental factors, such as temperature, noise, social interaction, etc., also must be considered as having synchronizer potential. The respective strength of each one as an influence upon biological rhythms depends upon the experimental circumstances and the investigated species. What must be kept in mind is that *a synchronizer does not create a rhythm;* it is capable only of influencing its expression, for example, by forcing an alteration in period length and/or timing of the circadian crest with respect to clock hour. It was Jürgen Aschoff and his group in Erling-Andechs, Germany (1959, 1960, 1974) who demonstrated that the circadian period can be manipulated or entrained by the period of the Zeitgeber only within certain narrow limits (e.g., 24 ± 2 hr).* Beyond these limits the organism's circadian rhythms resist entrainment and instead become free-running; they oscillate, exhibiting their spontaneous period as is the case when known synchronizers are suppressed, for example, when constant laboratory conditions are experimentally instituted. Aschoff (1960, 1974) also demonstrated that without time clue and cue the period of free-running circadian rhythms is shorter than 24 hr for nocturnally active species (e.g., rodents), while it is longer than 24 hr for diurnally active species (e.g., man). Another important basic contribution from the Erling-Andechs group was the demonstration that newborn lizards (Hoffman 1957) and chickens (Aschoff and Meyer-Lohmann 1954) exhibit circadian rhythms even if the mother and, thereafter, the eggs during incubation are maintained in constant environmental conditions (for example, continuous darkness and fixed temperature and humidity).

With regard to human beings, Halberg

* This is generally the case. However, some exceptions have been demonstrated, e.g., the Japanese quail. J. Boissin and I. Assenmacher (1970) demonstrated that the period of activity/rest as well as of adrenal activity can be entrained by a LD schedule quite different from 24 hr, e.g., LD = 16 hr or LD = 36 hr.

and his group in Minnesota (Halberg et al. 1959a) demonstrated that the most powerful synchronizer of circadian rhythms is cyclic changes in socioecological factors. For our species this means that the alternation of rest and activity related to our social interactions constitutes the major synchronizer for most functions. Usually we are active during the daytime, the span associated with natural or artificial light. Yet this time span coincides also with relatively higher levels of light, temperature, noise, and odors among others in our ecological niche. Chronobiologists recognize that the mere consideration or statement of clock hours, per se, need have no meaning relative to biological time, especially in modern society in which millions of persons worldwide are involved in night or shift work and transmeridian flight (Klein and Wegmann 1979). Specifically, the hours given by the clock have no synchronizing effect if there is no obligation for adherence to a given rest–activity routine defined by the specific scheduling of work, rest, and social interaction. This was clearly demonstrated by Mills (1964, 1966) in an underground cave experiment during which an isolated subject was found to disregard time cues provided by his own wrist watch. The subject exhibited so called free-running (non-24-hr) circadian rhythms.

Although interest in biological time structure increased during the first half of the twentieth century, it was not until 1960 that an objective, statistical approach for detecting and quantifying such was fully appreciated. In 1960 Colin Pittendrigh organized at Cold Spring Harbor in Massachusetts a meeting during which two major topics were addressed (Aschoff 1960; Halberg 1960b; Pittendrigh 1960). The first topic was practical as well as critical for the subsequent development of the field and dealt with the requirements for modern chronobiology as a quantitative biological science, i.e. the utilization of rigorous methods for data sampling, gathering, and statistical analysis. The second topic emphasized at this meeting dealt with the findings of specially designed experiments relying upon specific and accurate physical and chemical measurements (see Chap. 2) by Aschoff (1959, 1960), Halberg (1960a, b), and Pittendrigh (1960) producing evidence for the temporal structure of organisms.

Circadian rhythms in a large variety of physiological functions and biological phenomena have now been demonstrated. The respective peaks and troughs of such rhythms are not randomly distributed over 24 hr. On the contrary, their timings represent a morphology, an anatomy in time, with more or less strict temporal relationships among processes.

Knowledge about the temporal organization of biological functions, especially in mammals, has developed since 1960 (Bartter et al. 1962). Thus, new and obviously well-documented illustrative examples can be given (Bartter et al. 1962; Halberg and Reinberg 1967; Halberg et al. 1967; Krieger 1974; Reinberg 1974; Weitzman 1974). Let us consider (Fig. 3) a healthy human adult synchronized with diurnal activity and nocturnal rest. The peak time of plasma ACTH occurs during nightly sleep. At this time, there is almost no adrenal hormone secretion. Subsequently, after a certain phase delay with reference to the ACTH circadian peak, the plasma cortisol level rises to its peak around the time of awakening. The crest time of the urinary 17-OHCS rhythm occurs approximately 4 hr later with reference to the plasma cortisol peak. Plasma cortisol as well as other corticosteroids influence certain circadian patterns of other physiological variables such as the urinary excretion of potassium, grip strength, and airway patency. The peak of these variables usually occurs 4 to 6 hr after that of plasma cortisol (Fig. 3). The concept of biological time structure is so important to the field of chronobiology that it is included in the definition of chronobiology given at the beginning of this chapter.

Returning to the historical perspective and the acquisition of new concepts in chronobiology, it is not surprising that ultradian rhythms, with τ ranging from a fraction of a second to a fraction of a day, were not discovered until the development of appropriate monitoring equipment and analytical techniques. The discovery of ultradian rhythms enhanced the understanding of biological time structure. In connection with this, the continuous recording of electric potentials (EEG, eye movements, etc.) during sleep enabled Kleitman (1963) to describe electrical stages of sleep associated with the ultradian periodicity of rapid eye movement (REM). New methods for hormone determinations in plasma samples as small as 0.1 ml enabled the withdrawal of blood at intervals of a few minutes, instead of a few hours, and led to the detection of both ultradian and circadian rhythms in endocrine activity (Weitzman 1974; Krieger 1974). Ultradian rhythms in neural and muscular activity had already been explored in the 1930's by neurophysiologists using electrophysiological methods, among others. Both Fessard (1936) and Cardot (1933) were experimentally justified in stating that ". . . rhythmic activity is a basic property of excitable systems." (*"L'activite rythmique est une propriété fondamentale des systèmes excitables."*) However, these authors were concerned with ultradian rhythms of only neuromuscular and related systems. Reinberg and Ghata (1957) generalized this concept to other biological systems and to circadian and infradian (rhythms with period lengths greater than 28 hr) spectral domains. It is now well accepted that rhythmic activity is a fundamental property of living matter (Halberg et al. 1977; Halberg and Reinberg 1967; Reinberg 1974).

In retrospect, the Sixties can be considered the golden age of molecular biology. It was of mutual interest for both molecular biologists and chronobiologists to study cellular bioperiodicities. The major question was and remains: What are the basic mechanisms underlying circadian and other biological rhythms in the cell? Barnum (Barnum and Halberg 1953; Barnum et al. 1958), Hastings (Hastings 1959; Hastings and Keyman 1965), Sweeney (1969), Ehret

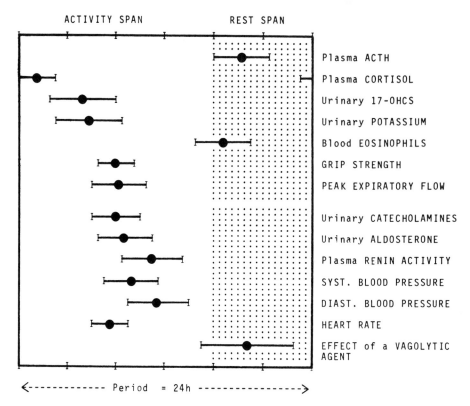

ACTIVITY SPAN   REST SPAN

Plasma ACTH
Plasma CORTISOL
Urinary 17-OHCS
Urinary POTASSIUM
Blood EOSINOPHILS
GRIP STRENGTH
PEAK EXPIRATORY FLOW
Urinary CATECHOLAMINES
Urinary ALDOSTERONE
Plasma RENIN ACTIVITY
SYST. BLOOD PRESSURE
DIAST. BLOOD PRESSURE
HEART RATE
EFFECT of a VAGOLYTIC AGENT

←------------ Period = 24h ------------------→

Fig. 3. Aspects of the human temporal structure. The acrophase, ϕ (crest time of the best-fitting cosine function approximating all data as determined by the least squares method, see Chap. 2) is given for each variable with 95% confidence limits. Subjects' synchronization was approximately 16 hr of diurnal activity and 8 hr of nocturnal rest. ϕ's are not randomly distributed over the 24-hr scale. On the contrary, they represent physiologically validated temporal relationships. The circadian ϕ of plasma ACTH leads that of plasma cortisol in phase. The ϕ of blood eosinophils coincides roughly in phase opposition with that of cortisol. This latter leads in phase the ϕ's of physiologically related variables such as urinary 17-OHCS and K^+, grip strength, and peak expiratory flow (bronchial patency). The ϕ both for systolic and diastolic blood pressure as well as that for heart rate are roughly in phase with the ϕ of urinary catecholamine and aldosterone concentration as well as plasma renin activity. A larger dose of a vagolytic agent—SCH1000 (iapropium bromide)—is required during the rest than during the activity span to be effective on bronchial tone. The temporal organization of these and other variables can be viewed as representative of adaptative phenomena. Since man is a diurnally active animal, it is not surprising that both the activity of his adrenal glands and sympathetic nervous system predominate during the day. (This chart utilizes data gathered from studies of F. Bartter, C. Gaultier, J. Ghata, F. Halberg, M. Lagoguey, A. Reinberg, L. Scheving, M. Smolensky, and E. Weitzman.)

(1974), Schweiger (Schwieger et al. 1964), Queiroz (1974), Vanden Driessche (1973, 1975), and Ashkenazi (Ashkenazi et al. 1973) were pioneers who initially contributed to the current understanding of the temporal organization of molecular activi- ties. This topic is treated in detail from the point of view of cellular morphology and mitosis in Chaps. 3 and 4 of this book.

Those aspects of chronobiology presently applied to medicine—which include chronopathology, chronotoxicology, chronopharmacology, chrononutrition, and chronotherapy (Halberg et al. 1977; Halberg and Reinberg 1967; Reinberg 1974; Reinberg and Halberg 1971)—also have historical background. Although circadian and/or circannual changes in physiological and pathological phenomena were considered many centuries ago by Hippocrates (1961), such rhythms have been studied rigorously only since the nineteenth century (Beau 1836; Féré 1888). For example, a circannual rhythm in human birth was reported by Quetelet in 1826. Circadian rhythms in epileptic seizures were reported by Beau in 1836 and by Féré in 1888. Manson in 1880 reported the circadian rhythm of microfilaria. The circannual rhythmicity of suicide in 1897, with a crest in spring, was reported by Durkheim (1952). Pincus (1943) reported a diurnal rhythm in the excretion of urinary ketosteroids by young men. It has to be emphasized that the *existence* and the *importance* of endogenous bioperiodicities were either ignored or underestimated until the birth of modern chronoepidemiology (Ghata and Reinberg 1954; Reinberg et al. 1973; Smolensky et al. 1972; Smolensky 1980). In human beings, among other animal species, there is an alternation in one's tolerance and susceptibility to potentially noxious agents as a function of the time of day, month, and/or year (Halberg 1960a,b; Halberg et al. 1960; Reinberg et al. 1973; Reinberg and Halberg 1971; Smolensky et al. 1972, 1980). In other words, there must be an appreciation for an old tenet dating back to Hippocrates—the organism's temporal structure has to be taken into consideration to better understand circadian and circannual changes in the incidence of disease as mirrored by both morbidity and mortality statistics. This topic is discussed further in Chap. 5.

In 1814, Virey in earning his Doctor of Medicine degree from the University of Paris devoted his entire thesis to chronobiology and chronopharmacology. The first to gain his medical diploma by researching chronobiology, Virey considered the signifi-

cance of human circadian rhythms in relation to both the risk and treatment of disease. According to Thomas Sydenham, as quoted by Virey, laudanum (opium) must be taken in the evening while purgatives and enema must be administered in the morning to be fully effective. In the conclusion of his thesis, Virey suggested that priority be given to researching the importance of timing in therapeutic intervention. Yet Virey's recommendations were not heeded until a century later when reports were published by other pioneers such as Möllerström (1953), Jöres (1935a,b), and Menzel (1944, 1958). The experimental attempt to determine at what time insulin must be given to a diabetic (Möllerström 1953) or to escape from the "stupidity of a three times a day" drug administration (Jöres 1935a,b) has still to receive appropriate attention by the medical community.

The dramatic experiments of Halberg (Halberg 1960a,b; Halberg et al. 1959b, 1960) on the "hours of changing resistance of mice" were the beginning of modern chronotoxicology (Fig. 4). A fixed dose of a potentially noxious agent (*E. coli* endotoxin or ouabain, for example) might kill 80% of the mice treated at a certain clock hour but only 20% of the mice treated 12 hr earlier or later. Other investigations performed on laboratory animals by Halberg et al. (1959b, 1960), Scheving et al. (1974), Pauly and Scheving (1964), and von Mayersbach (1978) further demonstrated that the effect(s) of a drug varies as a function of the biological time of administration. These same studies also showed that the timing of medications can alter the characteristics of rhythms (Chap. 6). Systematic investigations of human chronopharmacology actually commenced with the studies of Reinberg et al. (Reinberg 1965; Reinberg and Sidi 1966; Reinberg et al. 1964, 1965, 1967), Halberg et al. (1967), and Rutenfranz and Singer (1967). Aspects of these as well as other chronopharmacologic studies are provided in Chap. 6.

Finally, it must be recognized that the

HOURS OF DIMINISHED RESISTANCE

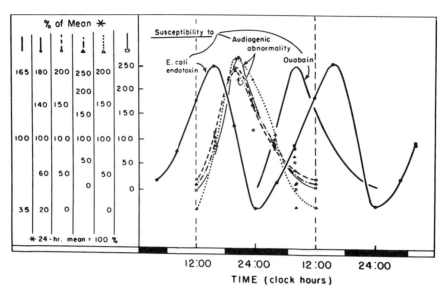

Fig. 4. Chronotoxicology was first considered as the hours of diminished resistance. Experimental results reported by Halberg (1960b) demonstrated the existence of circadian rhythms in the susceptibility of mice exposed to various potentially noxious agents, for example, a fixed "dose" of *E. coli* endotoxin, ouabain, or white noise. The end point of response in the studies on mice herein summarized was the number of deaths per treatment group per time of testing. In addition to circadian variability, susceptibility rhythms of about 7 days, 30 days, and 1 year, using other indices, are now known for a large variety of agents, animals, and plant species (see text). (From Halberg 1960b, reproduced with permission.)

current motivation for chronobiologic studies of nutrient metabolism dates back to Charles Chossat in 1832. Chossat demonstrated that the circadian rhythm of the cloacal temperature of pigeons that had been deprived of food and water persisted with a large amplitude even until death. The circadian rhythm in temperature was independent of 24-hr changes in the environmental temperature. This phenomenon was redemonstrated in mice 130 years later by Galicich et al. (1963) for other physiological variables. The persistence of circadian rhythms during fasting conditions is, therefore, known today as Chossat's phenomenon and, of course, pertains to chrononutrition, which is presented in Chap. 7.

Let us consider now, still from an historical point of view, an interesting question which constitutes the second part of this introductory chapter.

Why the Importance of Chronobiology Was Not Recognized Earlier

To understand why the importance of chronobiology was not recognized earlier, it is necessary to consider the environmental and educational milieu of early scientists, including their educational background, exposure to misleading hypotheses, and limited access to research tools, techniques, and methods for investigating biological rhythms.

Inadequate Educational Background

Most scientists since the seventeenth century grew up and resided in cities. Childhood and youth were spent far from a rural environment. The experiences of children raised in an urban setting differed widely from those of children raised in a rural setting. Most of the knowledge that inhabitants of cities possessed about plant and animal life was acquired from school lessons and readings. The personal experiences of rural children, especially with regard to the behavior of wild and domesticated animals, plant cycles, etc., were replaced for urban children by second-hand information, with the possibility of numerous distortions. During the nineteenth and the first half of the twentieth centuries, circadian and circannual changes were either ignored or regarded as a "curiosity of nature" by city-bred scientists. To recognize the crucial importance and the major interest of bioperiodic phenomena, the student would have had to experience as a young person how widespread and generalized they are among observable species.

In addition to this common lack of personal experience with the manifestations of overt biological rhythms, the education of young students of western countries provided an exclusively linear representation of time. The Western model of time as the sand clock (or the candle-clock) with its continuous and constant flow envisions life as a simple and constant addition of hours, days, and years from birth until death. In opposition to this model, the oriental (Chinese, Indian, etc.) representation of time is more subtle, since cyclic and periodic changes are taken into consideration. A spiral representation of time results from the combination of both linear and nonlinear changes. From one morning to another we are neither exactly the same person, nor a very different one. An understanding of this point of view is trivial for the oriental culture. On the other hand for the occidental culture of western scientists, which takes for granted that time is linear, consideration of the significance of time from any other point of view—in terms of period, phase, and waveform—requires reorientation.

Yet another related set of circumstances helps to explain why chronobiology did not develop at a faster pace. Medical disci-plines advance through teaching and research. The discipline of chronobiology has been rather slow to advance for a variety of practical reasons.

First, none of the currently active chronobiologists entered undergraduate, graduate, or medical school with the primary intent of biological rhythm study. As a matter of fact, until very recently chronobiology was not taught in colleges or medical schools, since no chairs or departments of chronobiology existed. Many became aware of biological rhythms only by accident, discovering them through repeated trials of their research protocols at different clock hours. It is in this manner that most scientists were introduced to chronobiology; it is these experimenters who discovered for themselves the practical significance of the temporal organization of physiochemical processes; it is they—those strictly schooled in "homeostatic" theory—who are responsible for the current advances in chronobiology.

Second, for any new philosophy to gain attention and be influential, there must exist a large enough nucleus of academically well-respected and well-organized individuals to make an impact on scientific thought. Until the last decade, the number of active and well-trained chronobiologists was quite small. A review of the quantity of citations dealing with chronobiology in *Index Medicus* under the entries of "Periodicity," "Diurnal," or "Circadian" reveals only a moderate number, even until 1955–1960. In 1983, several pages of citations are devoted to publications of chronobiologic research. This reflects the elevated prominence of the field and the increased number of scientists conducting research on biological rhythms.

Third, a scientific society serves as a catalyst for the development of a field of specialization. The International Society for the Study of Biological Rhythms was initiated in 1939. Among the founders were Hjalmar Holmgren, Jacob Möllerström, and Arthur Jöres. After World War II the Society formally resumed its international activities in 1953. In 1970, the Society became known as the International Society for Chronobiology.

Fourth, findings are communicated primarily through the publication of research. Earlier, it was not easy to publish findings dealing with biological rhythms, since without the availability of a convenient methodology and appropriate quantitative statistical procedures for time series analysis (Chap. 2), editors were reluctant to accept manuscripts. This is no longer the case, with improvements in both experimental design and statistical techniques for time series analyses. Let us point out that many classically trained scientists—editors of respected journals—viewed biological rhythms more as a scientific curiosity than as an important and undeniable component of biology. Prior to 1970, no journal was devoted solely to the field of chronobiology. Now there are two: *The International Journal of Chronobiology/Biological Rhythm Research* and *Chronobiologia*.

In summary, from the perspective of education the slow progress of chronobiology as a science resulted from a lack of (1) appropriate numbers of adequately trained chronobiologists to teach its methods, (2) departments or chairs in academic institutions dedicated to developing and teaching this science, (3) national and international societies to transfer findings and methods, (4) communication through the publication of relevant manuscripts, and (5) research grants and long-term research programs for chronobiology.

Misleading Hypotheses

In addition to the existence of inadequate educational opportunities, prevailing theory slowed or inhibited the advance of chronobiologic hypotheses and concepts. Several generations of students, including ours, have been taught that a set of regulatory mechanisms maintain the constancy of biological systems and physiological functions in a "homeostatic" manner. The constancy of the internal milieu (*milieu inté-rieur*) is presented as law. Tables of so-called biological constants are given in many medical textbooks for reference. Regulatory mechanisms are usually considered exclusively as feedback processes. A change in biological function is supposed to be immediately counteracted or balanced in such a way that the so-called "equilibrium," "steady-state," or "constant level" is maintained. Change is interpreted as resulting from stress, an explanation which is usually well accepted even if the term stress has *never* been defined adequately.

One has to realize that at the end of the nineteenth century, during the time of Claude Bernard (Bernard 1926), and through the time of Cannon (Cannon 1929) in the 1920's, the quality of biological measurements and determinations as well as the quantity of experimental data were very limited. Although the homeostatic *theory* (Cannon 1929) represented a considerable step forward in biology and medicine, it unfortunately has been overlooked that Claude Bernard himself emphasized the existence and importance of biological variability in the internal milieu (see Halberg 1967). It also has been forgotten that even for Cannon homeostatic regulation represented no more than a theory, certainly not a law. As advocated by Bernard, the theory must be changed when it no longer fits experimental facts.

In conventional biological tables, the value of a variable is given as a mean ($\bar{x}$) ± 95% according to sex, age, and health status. The margin of error, which is typically quite large, includes all types of "noise" such as (1) instrumental noise related to the imprecision of experimental laboratory techniques, (2) methodological noise related to difficulties in standardizing individuals and experimental conditions, and (3) biological noise related to interindividual variability. But the margin of error also includes predictable variabilities related to biological rhythms. With the homeostatic approach, these latter are simply included as additional sources of noise, even if the amplitudes of the rhythms create an unacceptably large range of values, as is the case for such variables as plasma cortisol and testosterone, circulating lymphocytes, and blood pressure, to mention a few.

The homeostatic "law" is associated with a set of misleading concepts such as "biological equilibrium" (the only state of equilibrium in biology is death, since exchanges are the rule), "steady state," etc. The feedback model was put forth to explain fluctuations around a proposed "constant level" of function. According to this argument, biological rhythms thus represent a non-meaningful and insignificant component of such fluctuations. By 1957 (Reinberg and Ghata 1957), it was obvious that this model could not explain why the fluctuation in a variable exhibits a precise period in a given species (e.g., the period of the ovulatory cycle in mammals) and why the fluctuation persists when environmental factors are kept constant. The feedback model, proposed as an explanation of biological rhythms in order to fit homeostatic theory, represented nothing more than a kind of intellectual regression, a blindfold. It inhibited both deeper discussion of existing experimental evidence as well as detailed research on mechanisms of biological rhythms (Halberg and Reinberg 1967).

The homeostatic theory fails to fit the experimental findings that a fixed dose of a potentially noxious agent will kill 100% of a group of mice at one phase of a circadian rhythm, while 100% of a comparable group of mice treated identically 12 hr earlier or later will survive. The "stress" in these experiments is rigorously standardized. While a given toxicant is totally inefficient when presented at one time, it leads to the complete destruction of a sample of animals when presented at another. These effects are both predictable and reproducible. Moreover, the homeostatic theory does not fit the fact that in persons adhering to diurnal activity and nocturnal rest, the plasma cortisol concentration can be as high as 20 μg/100 ml in the morning just before arising from sleep, and be nearly undetectable ($\cong 0$ μg/1) during a 6-hr span of time during

nightly rest (Krieger 1974; Weitzman 1974). The homeostatic theory cannot explain why in the same patient who has been rigidly standardized for chronobiologic study a glucose tolerance test yields different responses depending upon whether it is performed in the morning or in the evening (Jarrett and Keen 1969), or in April or in September (Méjean et al. 1977).

Obviously, the concept of homeostasis has been both overgeneralized and misused in biology and medicine by the epigones of Bernard and Cannon. Predictable cyclic variations with *several homeostases* can be considered (e.g., from a theoretical point of view as a circadian rhythm of "set points"). It has to be emphasized again that precise end points or limits must be interpreted as being variable in time due to periodic fluctuations (biological rhythms). Even if one wishes to explain why plasma potassium or blood glucose are almost constant (in fact they exhibit small-amplitude circadian rhythms), one must take into consideration large-amplitude circadian rhythms in the involved control systems (e.g., secretions of insulin, glucagon, and cortisol).

In actuality, the relative constancy of variables (for example, plasma glucose, electrolytes, hormones, proteins, and water, blood pressure, and body temperature, among others) appears to be critical for survival. Organisms are confronted with both periodic (predictable) and aperiodic (nonpredictable and random) changes in their environments. Regulatory mechanisms, presumably involving feedback loops, are responsive to aperiodic changes in the environment over the time domain of seconds, minutes, and hours. On the other hand, genetically programed biological rhythms constitute the basis for which organisms respond to periodic environmental changes having prominent τs of approximately 24 hr, 7 days, 30 days, and 1 year. For example, large-amplitude circadian rhythms of both neuroendocrine and endocrine secretions control the variables of plasma glucose, electrolytes, proteins, etc., so that only small-amplitude circadian changes result even though the environmental inputs, prominently exemplified by the intake of food, vary randomly in time, quality, and quantity. Short-term regulatory mechanisms also are subject to influence by circadian and other bioperiodicities.

One must admit that the homeostatic theory was a powerful braking force in the development of chronobiology, slowing the appreciation and understanding of clean experimental evidence documenting periodicity. In the name of the scientifically canonized "Saint Homeostasia" (Reinberg 1974), objective demonstrations of chronobiologic facts either were simply ignored or denied. In addition, papers submitted for publication in journals of high regard were rejected unanimously by "experts" (up to now, only some of them have offered their *mea culpa*). The homeostatic theory was a dogma, an article of faith. As it happened chronobiologists were asked: "Do you really *believe* in biological rhythms?" with a touch of condescending irony. (Fortunately, there was no witch-hunt of chronobiologists, despite the fact they are often working at the "witching time of night": *Hamlet,* III, ii). With respect to scientific discovery and advancement, some scientists behave as if they were blind and deaf when confronted with facts that are incompatible with their education.

The best manner of overcoming the retarding effects of obsolete theoretical considerations is to gather a critical mass of experimental evidence. This was the task of chronobiologists in the Sixties. One of the present tasks, as far as medicine is concerned, is to evaluate whether or not the chronobiologic approach for diagnosing and treating disease is more accurate, more effective, and more powerful than the homeostatic one. Since physiological variables such as blood pressure (Halberg and Reinberg 1967; Halberg et al. 1967), plasma cortisol (Krieger 1974; Weitzman 1974), and plasma testosterone (Dray et al. 1965), vary as a function of both the time of day and year, the definitions of hyper- or hypo-

tension, hyper- or hypocorticism, etc., require revision. Similarly, the experimental treatment of certain diseases such as cancer based upon an animal model (see Chap. 4) shows that the *chronobiologic approach* proposed by Scheving and Halberg (sinusoidal change in the administration of carcinostatic agents with the highest dose given at the circadian time of best drug tolerance) is both *less dangerous* (lower risk of injury or death due to drug toxicity) and more effective (up to 10 times greater survival at a given time) *than the homeostatic approach* (same amount of agent given in equal doses at equidistant time intervals).

Inadequate Tools, Techniques, and Investigative Methods

In order to collect data for the study and description of biological rhythms, special equipment and methods of investigation are necessary. Relatively precise instruments are needed to record biological events with regard to month, day, hour, minute, and second. Earlier in this chapter it was mentioned that astronomical clocks and related calendars were constructed during the stone age to serve both religious and practical purposes. The critical chronobiologic answers to questions such as when to plant, when to hunt, and when to harvest were given by astronomical clocks and calendars as well as natural signals from bird migrations, plant flowering, etc. Although primitive measures of the time of day (solar clocks) and time of night (water clocks) were used in ancient Egypt (the water clock of Ramses II), reliable mechanical clocks did not become available until the seventeenth and eighteenth centuries due to the genius of Huyghens and Harrison, who developed the pendulum spring, and marine clocks. Obviously, precise reference to time of day for biological events could only be provided when accurate, reliable, and inexpensive time pieces were widely marketed.

Chronobiologic studies of body weight and body temperature became possible only with the availability of accurate balances and thermometers (Sanctorius 1711; Davy 1845). Blood glucose levels can now be determined every minute continuously during 24-hr spans by entirely automated instruments, while Claude Bernard had to be satisfied with only a single (nonspecific) glucose determination per day, requiring a large amount of blood.

The development of modern chronobiology is closely related to the development of tools, instruments, and techniques permitting study of variables over relatively long spans of time (Kayser and Heusner 1967). Precision, reliability, and reproducibility are required, as is miniaturization. It is not surprising that radioimmunoassay methods enabled a step forward in chronoendocrinology (Krieger 1974; Weitzman 1974). Nowadays plasma cortisol can be determined every minute during 24 hr using only minute quantities of blood. When Pincus first demonstrated in 1943 a circadian rhythm in the urinary excretion of 17-ketosteroids, he utilized only 3 samples per 24 hr. Today measurements of physiological variables such as EKG, EEG, rectal temperature, wrist movements, and respiratory movements can be recorded continuously for many days from normally ambulatory subjects using portable and miniaturized instruments.

Just as histology and pathology enable separation of anatomical components into spatial serial sections, with careful planning and adequate experimental protocols and sampling procedures chronobiology enables separation of biological variables into temporal serial sections (Reinberg 1974). Chronobiologic methodology involving a minimal set of requirements is needed to design and conduct meaningful experiments. Reducing the "thickness" of the "slices of time" does not solve the problems related to rhythm detection, quantification, and interpretation. It is necessary to know how the subjects were synchronized and how they were standardized for chronobiologic research. In addition to these particulars, other pertinent information such as time of year, nutritional status and regimen, age, sex, and weight is required as well. When these minimal methodological requirements are neglected, rhythms may not be detectable, as was the case when some authors reported an absence of circadian rhythmicity in plasma calcium in healthy adult men, while others reported its existence (Halberg and Reinberg 1967). Moreover, when a proper chronobiologic methodology is not used, authors studying the same rhythm may report different peak times and amplitudes (Halberg and Reinberg 1967). This apparent lack of reproducibility of periodicity in, for example, calcium and some other studied variables, did not favor the scientific credibility of chronobiology.

Today it is also well recognized that the appropriate statistical analysis of time series comprises an indispensible aspect of chronobiologic methodology. Problems of data gathering and analysis are closely related in chronobiology. When specific methods of statistical analyses were not available, the quantification of rhythms constituted a problem that was not easily solved, especially when the temporal variations were of small amplitude. Discussion of methods pertinent to all aspects of chronobiology—chronopharmacology, chrononutrition, chronopathology, chronotoxicology, etc.—is presented in great detail in the following chapters. With rare exception, it is no longer appropriate to subjectively evaluate the parameters of rhythms through the use of chronograms (graphs of data over time) alone. Several appropriate, objective statistical techniques specifically designed for chronobiologic experimentation are readily available.

References

Aschoff, J (1954) Zeitgeber der tierischen Tagesperiodik. Naturwissenschaften 41:49–56.

Aschoff, J (1959) Zeitliche Strukturen biologischer Vorgänge. Nova Acta Leopoldina 21:147–177.

Aschoff, J (1960) Exogenous and endogenous

components in circadian rhythms. Cold Spring Harbor Symp Quant Biol 25:11–28.

Aschoff, J (1963) Comparative physiology; diurnal rhythms. Ann Rev Physiol 25:581–600.

Aschoff, J (1974) Speech after dinner. Chronobiological aspects of endocrinology. In: Aschoff, J, Ceresa, F, and Halberg F. *Chronobiological Aspects of Endocrinology*. Chronobiologia, Suppl. 1, 1:483–495.

Aschoff, J, and Meyer-Lohmann, J (1954) Angeborne 24-Stunden-Periodik beim Kücken. Pflüg Arch 260:170–176.

Ashkenazi, YE, Ramot, B, Brok-Simoni, F, and Holtzman, FJ (1973) Blood leucocyte enzyme activities. I. Diurnal rhythm in normal individuals. Interdiscipl Cycle Res 4(3):193–203.

Barnum, CP, and Halberg, F (1953). A 24-hour periodicity in relative specific activity of phosphorus fractions from liver microsomes of mice. Metabolism 2:271–275.

Barnum, CP, Jardetsky, CD, and Halberg, F (1958) Time relations among metabolic and morphologic 24-hour changes in mouse liver. Amer J Physiol 195:301–310.

Bartter, FC, Delea, CS, and Halberg, F (1962) A map of blood and urinary changes related to circadian variations in adrenal cortical function in normal subjects. Ann New York Acad Sci 98:969–983.

Beau, M (1836) Recherches statistiques pour servir à l'histoire de l'épilepsie et de l'hystérie. Arch Gen Med 11:328–352.

Bernard, C (1926) Introduction à l'étude de la médecine expérimentale. Paris: Lafuma.

Boissin, J, and Assenmacher, I (1970) Circadian rhythms in adrenal cortical activity in the quail. J Interdiscipl Cycle Res 1:251–265.

Bünning, E (1935) Zur Kenntnis der erblichen Tagesperiodizität bei den Primärblättern von *Phaseolus multiflorus*. Jahrb wiss Botan 81:411–418.

Bünning, E (1963) *Die physiologische Uhr*. Berlin: Springer-Verlag (2nd Ed).

Candolle de, AP (1832) *Physiologie Végétale*. Paris: Béchet Jeune.

Cannon, WB (1929) Organization for physiological homeostasis. Physiol Rev 9:399–431.

Cardot, H (1933) *L'automatisme cardiaque des invertébrés*. (Assoc des Physiologistes, Liége) Paris: Doin.

Chossat, C (1843) Recherches expérimentales sur l'inanition. Mémoires présentés par divers savants à l'Académie Royale des Sciences de l'Institut de France 8:438–640 (cf., in particular, pp. 532–566).

Davy, J (1845) On the temperature of man. Phil Trans Royal Soc London, 319–333.

Dray, F, Reinberg, A, and Sebaoun, J (1965). Rythme biologique de la testostérone libre du plasma chez l'Homme adulte sain: existence d'une variation circadienne. CR Acad Sci, Paris 261:573–576.

Durkheim, DE (1952) *Le Suicide*. Translated as Suicide: A Study in Sociology by JA Spaulding and Simpson. London: Routledge and Kegan Paul.

Ehret, CF (1974) The sense of time: evidence for its molecular basis in the Eukariotic gene-action system. In: *Advances in Biological and Medical Physics,* Vol. 15. New York: Academic Press, pp. 47–77.

Féré, C (1888) De la fréquence des accés d'épilepsie suivant les heures. CR Soc Biol, Paris 40:740–742.

Fessard, A (1936) *Propriétés rythmiques de la matiére vivante*. Paris: Hermann.

Fox, HM (1923) Lunar periodicity in reproduction. Proc Roy Soc B 95:523–550.

Fuller, CA, Lydic, R, Sulzman, FM, Albers, HE, Tepper, B, and Moore-Ede, MC (1981) Circadian rhythm of body temperature persists after suprachiasmatic lesions in the squirrel monkey. Amer J Physiol 241:R385–R391.

Galicich, JH, Halberg, F, and French, LA (1963). Circadian adrenal cycle in C mice kept without food and water for a day and a half. Nature 197:811–813.

Ghata, J, and Reinberg, A (1954) Variations nycthémérales, saisonniéres et géographiques de l'élimination urinaire du potassium et de l'eau chez l'homme adulte sain. CR Acad Sci, Paris 239:1680–1682.

Goodwin, BC (1963) *Temporal Organization in Cells*. New York: Academic Press.

Halberg, F (1960a) The 24-hour scale: a time dimension of adaptive functional organization. Per Biol Med 3:491–527.

Halberg, F (1960b) Temporal coordination of physiologic function. Cold Spring Harbor Symp Quant Biol 25:289–310.

Halberg, F (1967) Claude Bernard and the "Extreme variability of the internal milieu." In: Grande, F, and Visscher, MG, eds, *Claude Bernard and Experimental Medicine*. Cambridge, Mass.: Schenkman Publ. Company, pp. 193–210.

Halberg, F, and Reinberg, A (1967) Rythmes circadiens et rythmes de basses fréquences en physiologie humaine. J Physiol (Paris) 59:117–120.

Halberg, F, Visscher, MB, and Bittner, JJ (1954) Relation of visual factors to eosinophil rhythm in mice. Amer J Physiol 179:229–235.

Halberg, F, Halberg, E, Barnum, CP, and Bittner, JJ (1959a). Physiologic 24-hour periodicity in human beings and mice, the lighting regimen and daily routine, In: Withrow, RB, ed., *Photoperiodism and Related Phenomena in Plants and Animals*. Washington, D.C.: A.A.A.S. 55:803–878.

Halberg, F, Haus, E, and Stephens, A (1959b). Susceptibility to ouabain and physiologic 24-hour periodicity. Fed Proc 18:63.

Halberg, F, Johnson, EA, Brown, BW, and Bittner, JJ (1960). Susceptibility rhythm to *E. coli* endotoxin and bioassay. Proc Soc Exp Biol Med NY 103:142–144.

Halberg, F, Engeli, M, Hamburger, C, and Hillman, D (1965) Spectral resolution of low-frequency, small amplitude rhythms in excreted 17-ketosteroid; probable androgen-induced circaseptan desynchronization. Acta Endocrinol, Suppl. 103.

Halberg, F, Tong, YL, and Johnson, EA (1967) Circadian system phase: an aspect of temporal morphology; procedures and illustrative examples. In: von Mayersbach, H, ed, *The Cellular Aspects of Biorhythms* Symp. on Rhythmic Research, 8th Int. Cong. Anat. Berlin: Springer-Verlag, pp. 20–48.

Halberg, F, Carandente, F, Cornelissen, G, and Katinas, GS (1977) Glossary of chronobiology. Chronobiologia 4, Suppl. 1.

Hamburger, C (1954) Six years' daily 17-ketosteroid determination on one subject. Seasonal variations and independence of volume of urine. Acta Endocrinol 17:116–127.

Hamner, KC, and Takimoto, A (1964) Circadian rhythms and plant photoperiodism. The American Naturalist 98:295–322.

Hastings, JW (1959) Unicellular clocks. Ann Rev Microbiol 13:297–312.

Hastings, JW, and Keyman, A (1965) Molecular aspects of circadian systems. In: Aschoff, J, ed, *Circadian Clocks*. Amsterdam: North Holland Publ. Co., pp. 167–182.

Hippocrates (1961) *Aphorismes*. Translated into French by C. Daremberg. Paris: Club du Libraire.

Hoffmann, K (1957) Angeborene Tagesperiodik bei Eidechsen. Naturwissenschaften 44:359–360.

Hufeland, CW (1789) *The Art of Prolonging Life*. London: J. Bell.

Jarett, RJ, and Keen, H (1969) Diurnal variations of oral glucose tolerance: a possible pointer to the evolution of diabetes mellitus. Brit Med J 2:341–344.

Jöres, A (1935a) Physiologie und Pathologie der 24-Stunden-Rhythmik des Menschen. Ergebn inn Med u Kinderheilk 48:574–629.

Jöres, A (1935b) Das Problem der Tagesperiodik in der Biologie. Med Klin 31:1139–1142.

Kayser, C (1952) Le rythme nycthéméral des mouvements d'energie. La Revue Scientifique 90:173–188.

Kayser, C, and Heusner, F (1967) Le rythme nycthéméral de la depense d'energie. J Physiol (Paris) 59:3–116.

Klein, KE, and Wegmann, Hans-M (1979) Circadian rhythms of human performance and resistance: operational aspects. In: Nicholson, AN, ed, *Sleep, Wakefulness and Circadian Rhythm*. AGARD Lecture Series 105: pp. 2.10–2.12.

Kleitman, N (1963) *Sleep and Wakefulness*. Chicago: Chicago Univ. Press.

Konopka, RJ, and Beuzer, S (1971) Clock mutants of Drosophila Melanogaster. Proc Nat Acad Sci 58:2112–2116.

Krieger, DT (1974) Factors influencing the circadian periodicity of plasma corticosteroid levels. Chronobiologia 1:125–126.

Krieger, DT (Ed) (1979) *Endocrine Rhythms*. New York: Raven Press.

Mairan de, JJ (1729) *Observation botanique*. Paris: Histoire de l'Académie Royale des Science, p. 35.

Manson, P (1880) Additional notes on filaria sanguinis hominis and filaria disease. China Imperial Customs Med Rep 18:31–52.

Martin, C (1773) Des effets du sommeil sur la chaleur de corps humain. J de Physique 2:292–294.

von Mayersbach, H (1978) Die Zeitstruktur des organismus. Arzneim Forsch/Drug Res 28:1824–1836.

von Mayersbach, H and Leske, R (1961) Tageszyklinische Untersuchungen an Rattenlebern. II. Symp Histol Internat, Lausanne, 1961. Acta Anta (Basel) 48:182.

Méjean, L, Reinberg, A, and Debry, G (1977) Circannual changes in the plasma insulin response to glucose tolerance test of healthy young human males. Proc Int Union Physiol Sci, Vol 13, Paris, 1475:498 (abstract).

Menzel, W (1944) Der Tagesrhythmus in seiner Bedeutung für Pathologie und Klinik. In Klinische Fortbildung. Neue Dtsche Klin 8:406–436.

Menzel, W (1958) Krankheit und biologische Rhythmen. Arzt Mitteilungen Dtsches Arztebl 41:1201–1219.

Mills, JN (1964) Circadian rhythms during and after three months in solitude underground. J Physiol (Lond) 174:217–231.

Mills, JN (1966) Human circadian rhythms. Physiol Rev 46:128–171.

Möllerström, K (1953) Rhythmus, Diabetes und Behandlung. 3d Conf Int Soc Biological Rhythms, Hamburg, 1949. Acta Med Scand (Stockh) Suppl. 278.

Moore, R (1980) Suprachiasmatic nucleus, secondary synchronizing stimuli and the central neural control of circadian rhythms. Brain Research 183:13–28.

Moore-Ede, MC, Lydic, R, Czeisler, CA, Fuller, CA, and Albers, HE (1980) Structure and function of suprachiasmatic nuclei (SCN) in human and non-human primates. Neuroscience Abstracts 6:708.

Mornex, R, and Jordan, D (1980) Serotonin and endocrine rhythms. Biomedicine 32:163–165.

Pauly, JE, and Scheving, LE (1964) Temporal variations in the susceptibility of white rats to pentobarbital sodium and tremorine. Int J Neuropharmacol 3:651–658.

Pfeffer, W (1875) Die periodischen Bewegungen der Blattorgane. Leipzig: W Engelmann.

Pfeffer, W (1915) Beiträge zur Kenntnis der Entstehung der Schlafbewegungen. Abhandl Math Phys Kl Königl Sächs Ges d Wissensch 34:1–154.

Pincus, G (1943) A diurnal rhythm in the excretion of urinary ketosteroids by young men. J Clin Endocrinol 3:195–201.

Pittendrigh, CS (1960) Circadian rhythms and the circadian organization of living systems. Cold Spring Harbor Symp Quant Biol 25:159–182.

Pittendrigh, CS (1961) On temporal organization in living systems. Harvey Lect Ser 56:93–125.

Queiroz, O (1974) Circadian rhythms and metabolic patterns. Ann Rev Plant Physiol 25:115–134.

Quetelet, LAJ (1826) Mémoire sur les lois des naissances et de la mortalité à Bruxelles. Nouveaux mémories de l'Académie Royale des Sciences et Belles Lettres de Bruxelles 3:495–512.

Reinberg, A (1965) Hours of changing responsiveness in relation to allergy and the circadian adrenal cycle. In: Aschoff, J, ed, Circadian Clocks. Amsterdam: North-Holland Publ. Co., pp. 214–218.

Reinberg, A (1974) Des Rythmes Biologiques à la Chronobiologie. Paris: Gaultier-Villars. (3rd. ed, 1979)

Reinberg, A, and Ghata, J (1957) Les Rythmes Biologiques. Paris: Presse Universitaire de France, 3rd. Ed, 1978. English translation: Biological Rhythms. New York: Walker (1964).

Reinberg, A, and Halberg, F (1971) Circadian chronopharmacology. Ann Rev Pharmacol 11:455–492.

Reinberg, A, and Sidi, E (1966) Circadian changes in the inhibitory effects of an antihistaminic drug in man. J Invest Der 46:415–419.

Reinberg, A, Ghata, J, and Sidi, E (1964) Les variations circadiennes (environ 24 h) des réactions cutanées à l'histamine et le ryhthme cortico-surrénalien. Ann Endocrinol 25:670–674.

Reinberg, A, Sidi, E, and Ghata, J (1965) Circadian reactivity rhythms of human skin to histamine or allergen and the adrenal cycle. J Allergy 36:273–283.

Reinberg, A, Zagulla-Mally, Z, Ghata, J, and Halberg, F (1967) Circadian rhythm in duration of salicylate excretion referred to phase of excretory rhythms and routine. Proc Soc Exp Biol Med NY 124:826–832.

Reinberg, A, Gervais, P, Halberg, F, Gaultier, M, Roynette, N, Abulker, C, and Dupont, J (1973) Mortalité des adultes: rythmes circadiens et circannuels. Nouvelle Presse Médicale 2:289–294.

Rensing, L (1973) Biologische Rhythmen und Regulation. Stuttgart: Gustav Fischer Verlag.

Rietveld, WJ, and Groos, GA (1980) The central neural regulation of circadian rhythms. In: Scheving, LE, and Halberg, F, eds, Chronobiology: Principles and Applications to Shifts in Schedules. The Netherlands: Sijthoff and Noordhoff, Alphen aan den Rijn, pp. 189–204.

Rutenfranz, J, and Singer, R (1967) Untersuchungen zur Frage einer Abhängigkeit der Alkoholwirkung von der Tageszeit. Int Z angew Physiol 24:1–17.

Sanctorius, CI (1711) De Statica Medicina Aphorismi. Hagae-Comitis, ex. typographia A Vlaco. Text in Latin (1722). Translation into

French: *Science de la transpiration ou méde-cine statique. C'est-à-dire manière ingénieuse de se peser et rétablir la santé par la connais-sance du poids de l'insensible transpiration.* Paris: Dans l'édition de Le Breton, chez Claude Jombert.

Scheving, LE, von Mayersbach, H, and Pauly, JE (1974) An overview of chronopharmaco-logy. Europ J Toxicol 7:203–227.

Schweiger, E, Wallraff, HG, and Schweiger, HG (1964) Endogenous circadian rhythm in cytoplasma of acetabularia. Influence of the nucleus. Science 146:658–659.

Seguin, A, and Lavoisier, AL (1797) Sur la tran-spiration des animaux. Mémoires de l'Acade-mie des Sciences présenté le 14 avril 1790, publié en 1797 (an V de la République), 601–612.

Smolensky, MH (1980) Chronobiological as-pects of the epidemiology of human reproduc-tion and fertility. In: Ortavant, R, and Rein-berg, A, eds, *Rythmes et Reproduction.* Paris: Masson, pp. 210–242.

Smolensky, M, Halberg, F, and Sargent, F II (1972) Chronobiology of the life sequence. In: Ito, S, Ogata, K, and Yoshimura, H, eds, *Ad-vances in Climatic Physiology.* Tokyo: Igaku Shoin, pp. 281–318.

Smolensky, MH, Reinberg, A, Prevost, RJ, McGovern, JP, Sargent, F, II, and Gervais, P (1980) The application of chronobiological finding and methods to the epidemiological in-vestigation of the health effects of air pollu-tants on sentinel organisms. In: Smolensky, MH, Reinberg, A, and McGovern, JP, eds, *Recent Advances in the Chronobiology of Al-lergy and Immunology.* Oxford: Pergamon Press, Ltd., pp. 211–236.

Suda, M, Hayaishi, O, and Nakagawa, H (eds) (1979) *Biological Rhythms and their Central Mechanism.* Amsterdam: Elsevier/North Hol-land, Biomedical Press.

Sweeney, BM (1969) *Rhythmic Phenomena in Plants.* New York: Academic Press.

Szafarczyk, A, Ixart, G, Alonso, G, Mlaval, F, Nouguier-Soule, J, and Assenmacher, I (1981) Effects of raphé lesions on circadian ACTH, corticosterone and motor activity rhythms in free-running blinded rats. Neuroscience Let-ters 23:87–92.

Vanden Driessche, T (1973) A population of os-cillators: a working hypothesis and its com-patibility with experimental evidence. Int J Chronobiol 1:253–258.

Vanden Driessche, T (1975) Circadian rhythms and molecular biology. Biosystems 6:188–201.

Virey, JJ (1814) Ephémérides de la vie humaine ou recherches sur la révolution journalière et la périodicité de ses phénomènes dans la santé et les maladies. Paris: Thèse Fac Méd, 23 April 1814.

Weitzman, ED (1974) Temporal patterns of neuro-endocrine secretion in man: Rela-tionship to the 24 h sleep waking cycle. In: Aschoff, J, Ceresa, F, and Halberg, F, eds, *Chronobiological Aspects of Endocri-nology.* Stuttgart: FK Schattauer Verlag, pp. 169–184.

Weitzman, ED, Czeisler, CA, and Moore-Ede, MC (1979) Sleep-wake, neuroendocrine and body temperature circadian rhythm under en-trained and non-entrained (free-running) con-ditions in man. In: Suda, M, Hayaishi, O, and Nakagawa, H, eds, *Biological Rhythms and Their Central Mechanism.* Amsterdam: Else-vier/North Holland, Biomedical Press.

Wever, RA (1979) *The circadian system of man. Results of experiments under temporal isola-tion.* Heildelberg: Springer-Verlag.

2

Investigative Methodology for Chronobiology

Alain Reinberg and Michael H. Smolensky

Progress in the developing science of chronobiology has closely paralleled the emergence of new and improved research methodologies. Methodological requirements for biological rhythm study have been reviewed previously (Halberg et al. 1972, 1977; Reinberg 1971, 1974; Smolensky et al. 1974). This chapter outlines a minimum set of conditions and procedures necessary for conducting sound chronobiologic investigations. The recommendations which are put forward should be regarded as proposals and/or suggestions rather than rules or criteria for judging the quality of experimentation. It is obvious that each study dictates a specific methodology depending upon, among other things, the goals of the investigation and the state of knowledge. The contents of this chapter provide necessary information for designing chronobiologic research protocols and for minimizing the occurrence of those types of mistakes typically experienced in earlier chronobiologic investigations.

Types of Synchronizers and the Synchronization of Biological Rhythms

Common to all biological research, particulars related to species, sex, age, weight, height, food intake, state of health or disease, etc., must be stated. These general requirements are mentioned here as a reminder, only, despite the fact they are critical.

With respect to chronobiologic methods, when experimenting on laboratory animals, it is mandatory that the timing of the natural or artificial light (L)–dark (D) cycle be monitored, recorded, and reported since the LD cycle is recognized as a primary synchronizer of circadian and possibly other rhythms. The LD cycle influences the period length and peak time of rhythms of many species, such as birds, rodents, and monkeys.* Other potential synchronizers,

* The term synchronizer refers to an environmental periodicity capable of determining the temporal staging, with respect to clock hour or calendar date, of a given endogenous rhythmicity.

such as cyclic changes in temperature, noise, odors, humidity, and food availability, should be maintained at more or less constant levels. In so doing, only *one* (known) synchronizer is operational, whether or not it is manipulated. The concurrent influence of several synchronizers may lead to a complex situation which may be difficult to analyze. Even with one synchronizer, such as the LD alternation, the duration, intensity, and quality (wavelength) of the light as well as the abruptness of change from L to D can influence the findings (Aschoff 1960; Boissin and Assenmacher 1971; Halberg et al. 1959). Therefore each must be well defined.

Many authors prefer using the LD:12/12 lighting regimen in which 12 hr of light alternate with 12 hr of darkness.* With regard to animal models involving typically nocturnally active rodents (rats and mice), some authors (Halberg 1973; von Mayersbach 1978) recommend a LD:8/16 schedule, since it seems to better simulate human synchronization, i.e., 16 hr of activity alternating with 8 hr of rest.

Selection of appropriate LD schedules constitutes one of the most fundamentally important steps in conducting animal research, whether or not one is involved in chronobiologic studies, for many reasons as discussed below. Some experimenters are unaware of, or choose to ignore, the significance of the LD schedule as a synchronizer of animal rhythms. Oftentimes, animals are maintained under constant illumination. The assumption made in housing rodents and other species under such conditions is that the absence of alternating LD cyclicity attenuates or obliterates biological rhythmicity. Some investigators, even if a LD schedule is provided, attempt to "con-

trol" for rhythm effects by restricting research procedures to one or two particular clock hours. The experimenter by adhering to this type of sampling schedule does a disservice to his research and to science for several reasons. With respect to research on rodents, a vast number of chronobiologic investigations conducted during the past two to three decades utilizing comparable LD synchronizer schedules (usually LD:12/12) have enabled the "mapping" of a multitude of circadian rhythmicities. The term mapping refers to aspects of the rhythm's form over time, for example, the peak and trough times, with respect to the stated LD schedule. When the LD schedule is known, it is possible to predict rather precisely when either high, low, or average levels of a constituent of tissue, blood, urine, etc., will occur. Thus, the maximum of the circadian rhythm in serum corticosterone (the major adrenal corticosteroid hormone in mice) is expected to coincide with the timing of the transition of light to darkness in the animal room. It is also predictable that reduced levels of corticosterone will occur approximately 12 hr earlier or later, around the transition of darkness to light (Fig. 1) (Smolensky et al. 1978). In other words, different—early, middle, or late—stages of the light or dark span are coincident with particular features, such as the peak values (also referred to as the acrophase, discussed later in this chapter) of various circadian rhythmicities (Fig. 2). Relating the LD schedule to local time enables the determination of the clock hour of the aforementioned rhythmic features, since animals synchronized to fixed LD cycles display periodicities of almost precisely 24.0 hr. Under such highly standardized research conditions, clock hour thus is representative of circadian stage.

When animals are housed under constant light or darkness, i.e., without a LD synchronizer, the phenomenon of "free-running" often results—the occurrence of differing non-24-hr circadian cycles which vary in periodicity (τ) between biological functions in the same animal and/or be-

---

* Chronobiologists rely upon certain abbreviations to convey pertinent information about synchronizer type and schedule. LD:12/12 designates the synchronizer to be the Light (L)-dark (D) cycle with L and D each having a 12-hr duration. LD:8/16 conveys that the synchronizer is the light–dark cycle with the duration of the former being 8 hr and the latter 16 hr. Time or clock hour is expressed using the international designation, e.g., 1:00 P.M. is referred to as 1300.

tween animals for the same function. Under free-running conditions, it is possible, for example, that a given variable in one rodent might exhibit a 23.8-hr rhythm, while in a litter mate in another cage in the same animal room it may exhibit a 23.4-hr rhythm (Apfelbaum et al. 1969). The existence of free-running rhythms in the absence of synchronizers results in the clock hour being predictive of neither a particular circadian phase in one nor an identical circadian phase in all of the animals in the colony. For example, for the 0.4-hr difference in period duration for the theoretical condition raised above (one animal had a period of 23.8 hr and the other 23.4 hr), there would exist after 10 days a 4-hr (0.4 hr/day × 10 day) difference in phasing of this rhythmic function between the two animals. One can envision a large colony of animals, hundreds for example, under constant light or darkness with each animal being desynchronized at least to some extent with respect to the others. Under such experimental conditions, a clock hour would not correspond to or predict a given circadian stage in any one animal, nor in the colony as a whole (Scheving et al. 1977).

Research restricted only to certain clock hours in an assumed attempt either to "take into account" or "control for" rhythms should also be considered. Even when the animal colony is LD synchronized, the quantity and quality of data obtained are likely to be compromised when single-time-point samplings are done, since the responsiveness of animals is typically circadian-stage-dependent. For example, when conducting bioassays for potency, the injection of methylprednisolone (MP), a synthetic corticosteroid widely used to treat various human inflammatory disorders, is expected to produce a dose-dependent increase in liver glycogen deposition, as has been found so often in single-time-point experiments with this and many other synthetic corticosteroids. Yet as Fig. 3 shows, in singly caged, 5-week-old male Balb-C mice housed with food and water available *ad libitum,* ambient conditions of

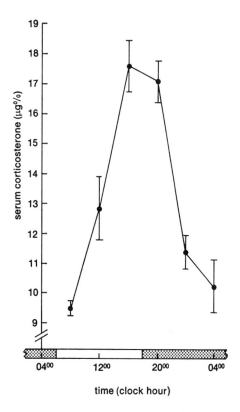

Fig. 1. Circadian rhythm of serum corticosterone in more than 240 ~12-week-old male Balb-C mice (40–44 mice killed at each of the 6 indicated time points over the 24-hr scale). For at least 2 weeks prior to investigation, animals were standardized for chronobiologic study of this adrenocortical rhythm by housing 1 per cage with food and water available *ad libitum,* in rooms constructed of sound-retarding materials with temperature 23° ± 1°C, humidity ≅ 50%, and light (L) from 0600–1800 alternating with darkness (D) from 1800–0600. The peak in adrenal corticosterone occurs between 1600 and 2000, or around the transition from inactivity to activity and as the environmental conditions change from light to dark. (From Smolensky et al. 1978.)

L(0600–1800):D(1800–0600), and constant temperature and relative humidity, the response to MP varies according to the circadian stage of treatment. Intraperitoneal injections of MP—4 mg daily or 8 mg on alternate days per 20 g body weight—only at 1600 (around the validated crest of the

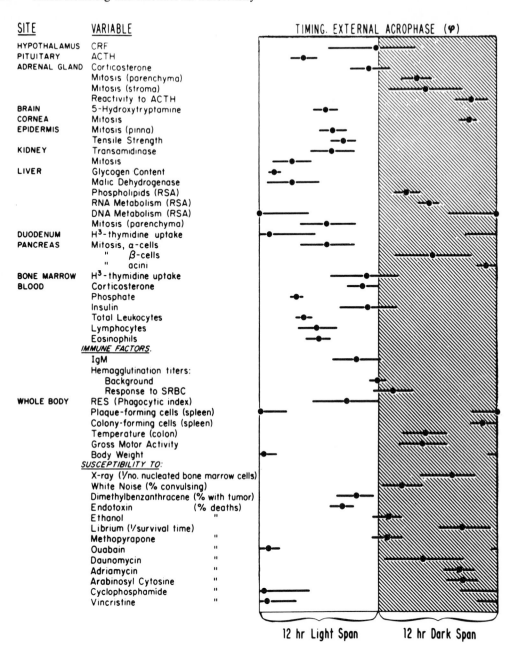

Fig. 2. The circadian temporal structure of the mouse is shown by a so-called acrophase map—a display by graphic means of the circadian acrophase (designated by φ for a phase reference corresponding to midlight), the time of the crest, of different biological functions. The acrophase, *black dot,* and the 95% confidence limits, *lateral extensions,* depict the timing of highest expected values for the designated function. By knowing the LD schedule, one can determine with confidence the biological time structure at a given clock hour of sampling or experimentation. (From Halberg and Nelson 1978, reproduced with permission.)

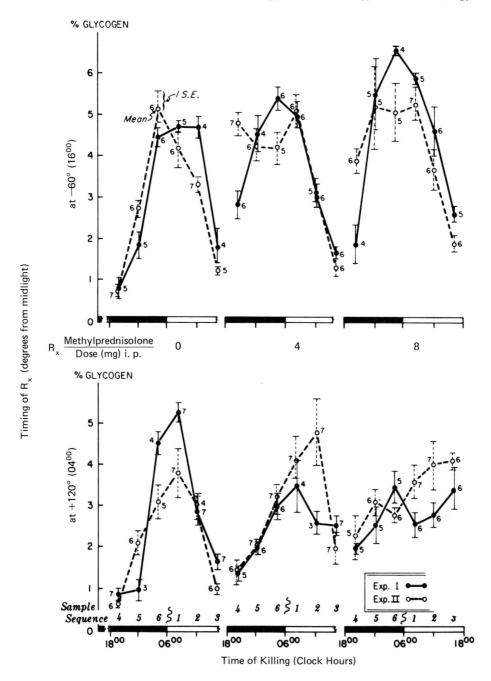

Fig. 3. Temporal changes in liver glycogen based on data from 2 experiments of 7 and 8 days duration, respectively. For groups of mice given the vehicle for MP, greatest glycogen content occurred during the commencement of the diurnal span of inactivity, around 0400–0800. In general, MP given daily or on alternate days (AD) did not appreciably alter the waveform of this rhythm except for the "1600–4 mg" daily and "0400–8 mg" AD groups of Experiment II. For mice given MP at 1600, glycogen content increased with dosage. Although the "0400–8 mg" glycogen content increased over control values, the change was very slight and less than that observed for groups administered MP at 1600 on alternate days. (From Smolensky et al. 1980a.)

circadian rhythm of serum corticosterone in rodents kept under the aforementioned synchronization) for either 7 or 8 days produces the expected increased liver glycogen deposition relative to vehicle-injected (0 mg MP) controls. Litter mates of these same mice injected with MP 12 hr earlier, at 0400, fail to respond with a statistically significant elevation in liver glycogen in comparison to vehicle-injected controls. Obviously, the circadian (biological) timing of MP has an effect on the bioassay. The extent to which failure to utilize appropriate chronobiologic research protocols, including animal synchronization and multiple-time-point samplings, has led to incorrect characterizations of potentially useful pharmacologic agents in the past and present is unknown. Similarly, the extent to which failure to use chronobiologic methods had led to different findings among alledgedly competent investigators working in the same or different laboratories because of an inadvertent selection of different circadian stages for experimentation, even in standardized animals, also is not known.

With respect to methodological procedures for chronobiologic research on rodents, it is pertinent to discuss here some of the ramifications of the all too common practice of conducting studies on mice or rats only during the light span of the LD synchronizer schedule. Quite often the investigator finds it least troublesome to conduct research during the daytime, when the laboratory is well lighted. Even though work during the light instead of the dark span is more convenient, let us point out that rodents, being nocturnally active animals, are physiologically at rest when studied during their light span. A priori it seems illogical to predict human responses to different agents—chemical, bacterial, or physical—utilizing data obtained from animals awakened from rest rather than utilizing data obtained from animals during their usual activity span, since human exposure to potentially hazardous materials is most likely during the span of activity. Actually, data from both the rest and activity spans

are required to best describe the overall susceptibility/resistance of a species to a given agent. To facilitate the gathering of data from rodents, it is possible to alter the LD schedule of an animal colony in such a manner that the rodents' activity (dark) span coincides with the experimenter's activity span. By carefully manipulating the LD synchronizer schedule in the animal colony rooms so that in some it is opposite that of the ambient surroundings, animals removed from the different colonies at the same clock hour will differ in circadian staging. This type of experimental methodology enables the study of biological rhythms during the normal diurnal activity span of the researcher. However, it should be recognized that a sufficiently long standardization span (at least 2 to 3 weeks) is required for the animals' biological rhythms to become synchronized to the altered LD schedule (see below).

Also related to laboratory animal synchronization is the important problem of biological samplings and data collections during the experimenter's usual rest span, i.e., when sampling cannot be automated or involves the removal of organs, tissues, or blood or necessitates carrying out manmade measurements. To better standardize an experiment as well as to avoid night work, it has been proposed that two to six isolation facilities be utilized in which comparable subsets of animals, usually rats and mice, can be maintained under the same fixed duration of light and dark. In each of the isolation facilities all conditions are maintained identically except for the particular clock hours of light-on and light-off, which varies between the isolation facilities. With this methodology diurnal samplings during the usual working hours of the laboratory personnel are sufficient to evaluate responses at several different circadian stages. (This is the methodology used in the chronobiology laboratories in L'Aquila, Italy, and Little Rock, Arkansas, among other places.) Thus, one can detect and characterize circadian rhythms, at least for chronopharmacologic studies. However, it is necessary that a set of control experiments be performed to demonstrate that the animals are actually synchronized to each one of the programed LD cycles. Some circadian rhythms—for example, body core temperature and locomotor activity—can be adjusted to a new schedule rather rapidly, in about 1 week; others—for example, the mitotic rhythm of the digestive tract (Scheving, Chap. 4)—require more time and may not be completely synchronized to the new LD schedule even 1 month following the LD change. This explains why many chronobiologists still prefer experimental protocols involving data gathering at equal intervals, every 2 or 4 hr around the clock, even if work must be done at night and sleep foregone.

Research on human beings in both the laboratory and field requires special attention to the subjects' synchronization. The suppression of known synchronizers, as demonstrated by isolation experiments conducted in caves where time clues and cues are absent, raises a set of practical considerations which sometimes are not fully understood (Apfelbaum et al. 1969; Halberg 1973; Wever 1979). Subtle synchronizers such as changes in the magnetic field (Wever 1979) as well as other possible influences, such as cosmic radiation, must be taken into account. As suggested by Brown (1965), the influence of the lunar day with a period of 24.8 hr must be examined when biological rhythms of such periods are detected in so-called free-running experiments (Apfelbaum et al. 1969).

In most research involving human subjects, socioecologic synchronizers are present even if they vary, for example, because of shift work or rapid travel across several time zones by transmeridian flight. Circadian changes in the clock hour of the sleep–wake schedule reveal the timing of the rest and activity cycle to be the most powerful synchronizer for man (Apfelbaum et al. 1969; Aschoff et al. 1971; Halberg et al. 1959). However, several components of man's socioecologic niche vary over 24 hr: light and darkness, heat and cold, noise and silence, and changes in psychological affect and stimulation resulting from social constraints related to work, activity, and interhuman relationships (Czeisler et al. 1981). Under certain circumstances these may have direct or indirect synchronizer action. Nonetheless, under usual situations, it seems that the timing of environmental factors associated with sleep and activity is the primary synchronizer of human circadian rhythms. Thus, in human research it is critical to ascertain and report the respective mean duration and timing of sleep and wakefulness or, at least, rest and activity during each 24 hr for either an individual or group under study. This information should be stated in terms of the clock hour of light-on and light-off with appropriate data from self-maintained diaries confirming the regularity and duration in days, weeks, and months of adherence to the given schedule.

Strict attention to synchronizer schedule is stressed for good reason. In chronobiologic investigations the timing, with regard to clock hour, of the synchronizer determines when the rhythm's crest, termed the acrophase, will occur. To locate the acrophase, ϕ, of a given circadian rhythm, for example, the phase reference, ϕ_0, must be known. The ϕ_0 may be midnight (0000) or another local time; both of these are obviously associated with the information related to light-on/light-off. Halberg and Simpson (1967) proposed that the midsleep (or midrest) span be used as the ϕ_0. When using this ϕ_0, comparison of acrophase values is possible between various populations adhering to different activity–rest routines or between those living at different geographic locations as well as between males and females, etc. Reference to the midrest span for ϕ_0 in animal experiments is recommended rather than midnight, since the former represents an index of the organism's internal time as synchronized by the imposed LD schedule. In certain experiments, the ϕ of one biological rhythm constitutes the best reference (ϕ_0) for the acrophase of another rhythmic function

studied concomitantly. This is the case, for
example, in the chronoradiotherapy of solid
tumors of the oral cavity investigated by
Gupta and Deka (1972). X-ray therapy appears to be more rapidly efficient when
given in phase with the ϕ of the tumor temperature. It is, therefore, of interest to consider this latter ϕ as the ϕ_0 for future research with this type of chronotherapy.

Besides synchronizer schedule, two
additional pieces of information—*geographic location* and *time of year* (even if
the research involves only circadian
rhythms) are of concern. With regard to the
latter, research on mice (Haus and
Halberg 1970), rats (von Mayersbach 1978),
frogs (Dupont et al. 1979), and man (Reinberg 1974; Reinberg et al. 1975, 1978) reveals circannual alterations of parameters
characterizing a set of circadian rhythms,
such as the 24-hr time series mean M (referred to as the mesor), amplitude A, and
acrophase ϕ. Not only can the 24-hr M vary
as a function of the time of the year, but so
can the ϕ with reference to clock hour on
the 24-hr scale. Usually, but not necessarily,
small variation in the circadian M, A, and ϕ
may result because of differences between
the time of year experiments are conducted. Even the ability to detect circadian
rhythms may vary according to the time of
year the research is done. Certain rhythms
may be undetectable during certain months,
whereas they may be easily detectable and
found to be statistically highly significant
(with a large amplitude) during other
months (Dupont et al. 1979; Reinberg et al.
1975). The finding that the M, A, and ϕ of
circadian rhythms may be modulated over
the year is not totally unexpected since
rhythms of approximately one year represent an important facet of one's biological
time structure. Similarly, for women and
female rodents, as well as perhaps females
of other species, there appears to exist a
circamensual (about monthly) or circaes-
trual modulation of circadian rhythm characteristics—M, A, and ϕ (McGovern et al.
1977; Procacci et al. 1972; Simpson and
Halberg 1974; Simpson and Bohlen 1973;

Smolensky et al. 1974). The other variable,
geographic location, implicitly conveys
certain types of information, such as the
extent of change and timing of annual synchronizers that differ as a function of latitude (Aschoff 1981; Batchelet et al. 1973;
Ghata et al. 1977). Yet geographic location appears to have greater significance
than that directly ascribed to latitude,
alone, since it is closely related to the social
and eating habits, type of population, and
way of life of the studied sample (DuRuisseau 1965; Ghata et al. 1977; Reinberg et al.
1975). With respect to geographic location, certain chronobiologic questions remain to be answered. For example, what is
the nature of circannual synchronizers and
does adjustment of circannual rhythms occur when moving from the Northern to the
Southern Hemisphere, or in the reverse direction (Halberg et al, 1983)?

Chronobiologic Studies of Individuals

Many of the published findings and analyses from chronobiologic research deal with
data from groups of subjects. For the most
part, little attention has been given to the
existence of interindividual variations in
the rhythm characteristics between participants. Thus, although the definition of
chronobiology is the elucidation of *organismic* temporal structure based upon the
study of individuals, surprisingly few investigations pertain specifically to individual
rather than group rhythmic phenomena.
Yet interindividual differences of various
magnitude are known to chronobiologists
through their own research. The implication of these interindividual differences requires examination with at least the following two goals: (1) to obtain a realistic and
generally meaningful quantification of
rhythm parameters as a group phenomenon
for a given species, strain, or sample and (2)
to demarcate the range of features and alterations of rhythms which are usual and
representative of health as opposed to disease. Examination of interindividual differ-

ences in rhythmic phenomena provides a broader and deeper insight into conventional concepts such as the "homeostatically" derived one of "individual variability," which completely ignores the temporal dimension of biological organization. For the purpose of discussing the individuality of temporal structure, three illustrative examples are presented.

The first example deals with a comparison of circadian rhythmic patterns of monozygotic (MZ) and dizygotic (DZ) twins (Barcal et al. 1968). Since in this case the healthy MZ and DZ sibling reside in more or less the same physical and sociocultural environment, interindividual differences in rhythms imply a genetic origin. The findings indicate what might be expected. The patterns and waveforms of the circadian variables of core temperature, heart rate, and systolic blood pressure were quite similar for MZ siblings. There were greater qualitative and quantitative differences between DZ siblings.

The second example is intended not only to elucidate the existence of interindividual variability in rhythmic phenomena, but to show also the need for specific chronobiologic methods to detect and quantify such. Wever in 1979, analyzing results of many human experiments conducted under temporal isolation, demonstrated that, inter alia, the period of free-running circadian rhythms varied within certain limits from subject to subject. In addition, if in most subjects all the measured variables had the same period, some subjects exhibited an internal desynchronization; that is different variables oscillated with differing periods. The span of time needed to re-entrain the rhythms or to resynchronize the organism to an exact 24.0-hr periodicity, when effective synchronizers were reinstituted, varied also from subject to subject. These findings suggest the existence of interindividual differences in the tolerance to alterations in synchronizer schedule, such as that encountered in transmeridian flight ("jet lag") and shift work (Reinberg et al. 1979). There now exists sufficient evidence to consider certain persons, because of interindividual differences in their temporal anatomy, to be more fit for shift work than others. A question currently of interest is whether interindividual differences, for example, in the amplitude of the circadian rhythm of core temperature, is associated with interindividual differences in the ability of employees to tolerate shift work (Reinberg et al. 1979). To completely explore this possibility, autorhythmometry (self-monitoring of rhythms) is required to obtain sufficiently long time series both on large samples of employees who are tolerant and intolerant of shift work as well as large samples of other workers upon whom this hypothesis can be further explored.

The third example comes from studies by Bicakova-Rocher et al. (1980). Her results show that some subjects are prone to rhythmometric alterations, such as a reduction in amplitude or loss of rhythmicity, during control spans of research studies and also when confronted with certain atypical situations, such as when taking a placebo believed to be a tranquilizer. In her study, one-half of the subjects (six of twelve) exhibited such alterations.

From a methodological point of view these examples show the need for control(s) in both laboratory animal and clinical experiments. One of the issues, as far as man is concerned, is the design of protocols so that the subject serves as his own control. Rhythm patterns obtained for a set of variables during the control span may be used as a reference for a given individual in order to study changes resulting from various other situations, such as those observed in investigations on nutrition, transmeridian flight, physical training, aging, and disease. Methodological procedures for studying interindividual differences using longitudinal samplings as well as those for studying group phenomena are presented in detail in the next section. This section, referring to differences, should be kept in mind when considering the goals and limitations of the methods available for chronobiologic investigations.

Data Sampling and Gathering

Before initiating chronobiologic research and accumulating a time series, several decisions concerning sampling and design must be made: these are outlined below.

Δt: time interval between each datum—physical measurement, chemical determination, or other. Δt can be either fixed or varying, even random (unequal Δt's).

T: total duration of the sampling span.

Nos: number of samples during T.

A relationship exists between Δt, T, and Nos, as far as circadian, circamensual, and circannual rhythms are concerned. For both biological and statistical reasons, it is necessary to have, for example, as a minimum for circadian rhythms, $T \geq 24$ hr, $\Delta t \cong$ 4 hr, and Nos ≥ 36. This means that for a selected variable, measurements must be done every 4 hr (preferably at fixed clock times) either during *at least* 24 hr in 6 subjects or during at least 6 days in 1 subject.

Longitudinal sampling, for example, of one subject when T > 6 days and $\Delta t \cong 4$ hr is preferred for documenting rhythms in individual subjects. On the other hand, transverse sampling, for example of 6 subjects when $T \geq 24$ hr and $\Delta t \cong 4$ hr, is appropriate for documenting rhythms of small groups. Longitudinal and transverse sampling usually leads to similar results when comparable experimental conditions are maintained with respect to circadian and circannual synchronization as well as other criteria of experimental standardization (Halberg 1973).

In chronobiologic studies it must be decided whether data are to be acquired by serially dependent samplings provided by the same subject(s) over time, or by serially independent samplings provided by different but supposedly comparable subjects over time. When feasible, serially dependent data gathering is preferable. For example, similar circannual changes in urinary catecholamine excretion were found in persons residing in Paris with ϕ in January (T = 14 months; Δt = 1 month; serially dependent data of 5 subjects) and in those dwelling in Minneapolis with ϕ in December (T = 5 years; Δt = 1 day; serially dependent data of 1 subject). On the other hand, ϕ was found to be different in Milan (Descovich et al. 1974), occurring in June (serially independent data from various subjects). In certain circumstances, it is impossible to obtain more than a single datum from an organism. This is the case in chronotoxicology studies on mice when death is the monitored response. Obviously, only serially independent sampling is feasible. In this case, rigid standardization of experiments is required to "construct" the circadian or circannual curve (plexogram) (Halberg et al. 1977).

The choice of Δt, T, and Nos cannot be arbitrary. T must be equal to or preferably exceed the period (τ) for ultradian, circadian, circamensual, or circannual rhythms. If several τ's are evaluated simultaneously, Δt must be carefully selected. For example, the plasma cortisol circadian rhythm can be documented with $\Delta t = 4$ hr when $T \geq 24$ hr. However, some ultradian rhythms ($\tau < 4$ hr) cannot be examined. A Δt of 5–20 min makes possible the study of both circadian rhythms as well as so-called pulsatile secretory variations (Fig. 4) which may exhibit a specific "macroscopic" pattern over 24 hr (Weitzman et al. 1971).

When investigating circannual rhythms, transverse 24-hr samplings seem to offer several advantages, including the evaluation of both circadian and circannual periodicities (Reinberg 1974). At fixed time intervals, every month or every second or third month, transverse samplings with $\Delta t = 4$ hr and $T \geq 24$ hr should be conducted during a span of at least 1 year. Since the circadian M, A, and ϕ of a variable may differ circannually, study of circannual rhythms by sampling only once daily, even if the clock hour is fixed and subjects are rigidly synchronized, may provide erroneous information (Dupont et al. 1979; Haus and Halberg 1970; Reinberg et al. 1975, 1978). Similarly, the possibly significant influence of 28- to 30-day hormonal variations in women sug-

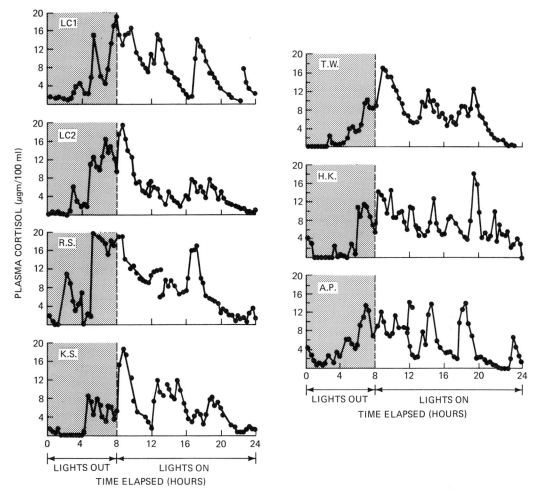

Fig. 4. Plasma cortisol values of normal subjects for 24-hr periods of study. Samples were obtained every 20 min. Period of time of lights out corresponds to sleep span. (From Weitzman et al. 1971, reproduced with permission.)

gests the transverse 24-hr sampling protocol to be the most efficient one for quantifying circadian as well as circamensual periodicities. In this case, a series of transverse samplings, each of 24-hr duration, is recommended at intervals of ≦7 days throughout one or more menstrual cycles (Smolensky et al. 1974).

Quality of Data

Not only the quantity but also the quality—the precision, specificity, and reproducibility with regard to methodology, instrumentation, and techniques—of data collection

are critical. This is true for each investigation in biology. Chronobiologists require instrumentation which enables precise measurements, yet just as importantly, the instrumentation must be small, portable, and lightweight. A set of tools for measuring and recording data on body temperature, airway patency, blood pressure, heart rate, EKG, EEG, and wrist movement is currently available for use in investigations on ambulatory rodents, monkeys, and man. However, the need for precision and specificity in data collection is even more important than it appears. Two examples illustrate this point.

It is necessary for both practical and theoretical reasons to measure the bronchial patency (bronchial diameter) of human subjects. Features of the circadian rhythm in bronchial patency are critical for evaluating, from a clinical point of view, the patient suffering from pulmonary disease, such as asthma, as well as for evaluating the effect of air pollutants on asthmatic and other types of patients (Gervais and Reinberg 1978; Prevost et al. 1980; Reinberg et al. 1971; Smolensky 1976; Smolensky et al. 1980a). The bronchial patency can be accurately measured in the laboratory with bulky, fragile, sophisticated, and expensive instruments. Although each datum obtained in this manner is very precise, it is ambiguous if the measurement is done without regard to time-qualified references (chronodesm, discussed later in this chapter) pertaining to time of day, week, month, and year (Gaultier et al. 1977; Tammeling et al. 1977). The bronchial patency can be measured adequately, although less accurately, by lightweight, portable, easy to carry, easy to check, and inexpensive instruments such as peak flow meters (Wright) or spirometers (Hildebrandt). The peak expiratory flow (PEF) thus measured is considered less precise and informative than that obtained by laboratory instruments, such as spirometry (for $FEV_{1.0}$) and plethysmography (for dynamic compliance and airways resistance), since PEF is representative only of the patency of bronchi up to the eighth dichotomy of the respiratory tree. In addition, PEF (and $FEV_{1.0}$) is an indicator of not only the bronchial diameter, but also the strength of the musculature of the chest (Brody et al. 1969). Despite these qualifications, with PEF measurements circadian and circannual changes in bronchial patency can be examined by the subject himself in different situations—at home, at work, or in environments having different levels of air pollution as well as before, during, and after transmeridian flights (Gervais and Reinberg 1976; Prevost et al. 1977; Reinberg et al. 1971; Smolensky 1976; Smolensky et al. 1980b). The high precision of one datum provided by sophisticated laboratory instrumentation is sufficiently compensated by the high precision resulting from a large series of meaningful PEF measurements appropriately quantified by time series analyses.

The significance of the quality of data also is exemplified by studies relying upon so-called "continuous" determination of blood variables. To examine both ultradian and circadian human hormonal rhythms, a large number of blood samples, each of 2 ml, is required. Using a venous catheter, it is possible to withdraw the 2 ml blood samples at 6-min intervals; however, over a single 24-hr span, a sizeable blood withdrawal of 480 ml would be necessary. To avoid the deleterious effects of such a large blood loss on the studied variables, new devices have been developed by Weitzman et al. (1971), among others, to replace the exact amount of blood withdrawn by saline via the same catheter.

Ethical Requirements

Obviously, for both healthy human beings and patients, experimental methods must fulfill certain ethical criteria. They must be safe, non-painful, non-disturbing, and preferably non-invasive. Moreover, the research must address meaningful hypotheses. These same considerations hold true for all patient and animal research.

Time Series Analysis

General Considerations

The problem of objectively evaluating collected time series data is among the most critical for chronobiology. The development of appropriate statistical procedures for analyzing time series was a major goal for chronobiologists in the Sixties. Despite great progress [spectral analyses and Cosinor methods (Halberg et al. 1965, 1967, 1972, 1977)], difficulties resulting from certain experimental circumstances have yet to be overcome.

Time series obtained by data gathering techniques serve as the basis for the *detection, description,* and *quantification* of rhythmicity. Quantitative methods for analysis of periodic phenomena were a primary concern of mathematicians and physicists during the nineteenth century. Chronobiologists, in developing more specific techniques of time series data analysis to fit their unique needs, nonetheless, use the same parameters and terminologies as physicists and mathematicians. A considerable amount of work has been devoted (Aschoff 1960; Aschoff et al. 1965; Halberg et al. 1977; Wever 1965; Winfree 1980) to the quantitative characterization of rhythms. Four major parameters are commonly utilized to achieve this objective. They are the period (τ), the time of the crest or acrophase (ϕ), the amplitude (A), and the rhythm-adjusted mean or mesor (M)—all determined through curve fitting techniques by the method of least squares (Halberg 1973; Halberg and Simpson 1967; Halberg et al. 1965, 1967, 1972, 1977; Nelson et al. 1979).

The period τ is the duration of one complete cycle of a rhythmic variation. It is customarily expressed in units of time, e.g., sec, min, hr, day, or year.

The acrophase ϕ is the estimated span of time to reach the crest of the validated rhythm for the τ under consideration. When using the Cosinor method (discussed later in this chapter), ϕ represents the crest time of the best-fitting mathematical function approximating the data. It is expressed as an interval from a designated phase reference (ϕ_0).

The amplitude A is the amount of variability due to a given rhythm. When the Cosinor method is used, it is numerically equal to one-half of the extent of rhythmic change for the considered τ. In other words, 2A is the crest-to-trough difference.

The mesor M is the rhythm-adjusted mean. When the interval of time between data sampling (Δt) is constant, M equals the arithmetic mean ($\bar{x}$).

Cosinor Methods

Halberg and coauthors (Halberg 1973; Halberg and Simpson 1967; Halberg et al. 1959, 1965, 1972, 1977; Nelson et al. 1979; Cornelissen et al. 1980) developed a computerized technique, the Cosinor, for the analysis of time series data. The least squares method serves to determine the best fitting function (usually a cosine) for approximating the data (Fig. 5). For this purpose one uses the following function:

$$y(t_i) = M + A \cos (\omega t_i + \phi)$$

in which: t_i = time; A = amplitude; ϕ = acrophase; ω = angular frequency ($\omega = 2\pi/\tau$, where τ = period and $1/\tau$ = frequency).

The cosine function was selected since the cosine of zero, being zero, is a handy phase reference, and since it provides a clockwise presentation (zero being midnight: 0000) when a polar plot is used to summarize ϕ and A estimates with confidence limits (Figs. 6 and 7). The Cosinor has been programed for use by large computers as well as for hand and pocket calculators. Estimation of τ with its confidence limits also can be achieved by this method. The Cosinor method can be used iteratively with different trial periods (e.g., τ = 12 hr, τ = 8 hr). Other techniques, such as fast Fourier transform and power spectrum, are also of great use for validating and quantifying prominent period(s) in time series. Thus, a spectral analysis can be obtained when values of T and Nos are large enough (Halberg et al. 1965; van Cauter 1974), making possible the detection of prominent periods in the ultradian, circadian, and infradian spectral domains.

When τ is known, either from data analysis or from the experimental conditions (as when subjects are standardized with a synchronizing period of $\cong$24 hr), other parameters such as ϕ, A, and M can be estimated. According to the type of data gathered, the Mean Cosinor or the Single Cosinor should be used (Halberg et al. 1977). The Mean Cosinor is the original procedure applicable to parameter (A, ϕ) estimation when deal-

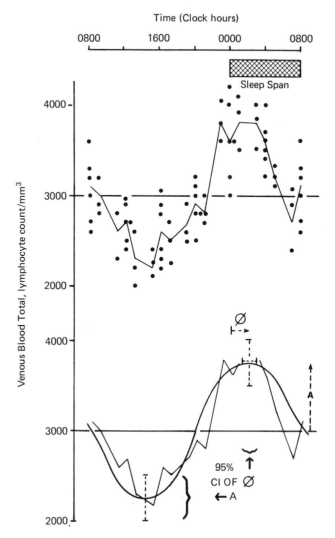

Fig. 5. A circadian rhythm in the total lymphocyte count/mm^3 of venous blood was substantiated in a sample of 12 healthy young adults (6 men, 20–28 years of age, and 6 women, 23–24 years of age) during December, 1974 in Paris, France. Subjects were synchronized with diurnal activity from 0800 to 0000 (midnight) and nocturnal rest (sleep). Blood samples were obtained every 4 hr ($\Delta t = 4$ hr) at fixed clock hours with the exact times of sampling differing between the three subgroups of subjects. **Top:** Chronogram. Raw data are displayed as a function of time (clock hours). The arithmetic mean of each of the time points (thin line) when connected appears to resemble a sine wave with small swings. **Bottom:** Single Cosinor analysis. The best-fitting cosine function approximating all data is presented. The least squares method is used; parameters characterizing the rhythm are given with their 95% confidence interval (CI). The acrophase ϕ, crest time with midnight as phase reference (ϕ_0) given in hours and minutes, is 0208 (95% CI = 0128–0248). ϕ also can be expressed in degrees ($\tau = 24$ hr = 360°) as a delay from the ϕ_0 (as a negative value with ϕ_0 being the midsleep span = $-60°$); in this case, $\phi = -332°$ [or $+28°$] (95% CI, $-304°$ to $-350°$). The amplitude A, equal to one-half of the total variability, is 756 lymphocytes/mm^3 (CI = 503–1009 lymphocytes/mm^3). The mesor M, the 24-hr rhythm-adjusted mean, is 3002 ± 39 (SE) lymphocytes/mm^3. A differs from zero with P < 0.0001. (Unpublished data from A. Reinberg and J. Clench.)

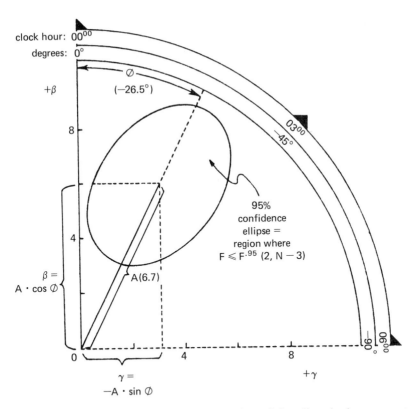

Fig. 6. Rectangular (β, γ) and polar (A, ϕ) representation of circadian rhythm parameter estimates with joint confidence region (single series). Estimates based on an abstract example with 24-hr cosine function. $(Y_{ti}) = M + A \cos (\omega t_i + \phi)$, fitted by least-squares to data collected at 2-hr intervals during the activity span. In this example, A = amplitude; ϕ = acrophase (degrees from 0000); M = mesor; $\omega = 15°/\text{hr}$; t = hours after 0000. (From Halberg et al. 1977, reproduced with permission.)

ing with three or more biological time series; this method is most often used for assessing the rhythm characteristics of a group or population. The Single Cosinor is applicable to a single biological time series composed of data from one individual (serially dependent data) or a group of individuals (serially independent data). When dealing with data from groups of subjects, individual time series are placed end-to-end with the option of adjusting the data into relative values first. For serially dependent data, both the Mean and Single Cosinor can be used. On the other hand, for serially independent data only the Single Cosinor is appropriate.

When rhythms are substantiated, estimates of A and ϕ are given with their re-

spective 95% confidence limits. When utilizing the Cosinor, it is assumed that the data are normally distributed around each of the sampled time points. This can be tested by examining the residuals resulting from the fitting of the approximating function (De Prins et al. 1976).

One of the major advantages of the Cosinor is that it permits objective testing of the hypothesis that the rhythm's amplitude differs from zero, in other words that a rhythm is validated for a considered τ. Usually evidence for rhythm detection is accepted when the probability (P) of A being zero is equal to or less than 0.05.

Estimates and end points from Cosinor analyses ordinarily are summarized in tables or by figures allowing the visualization

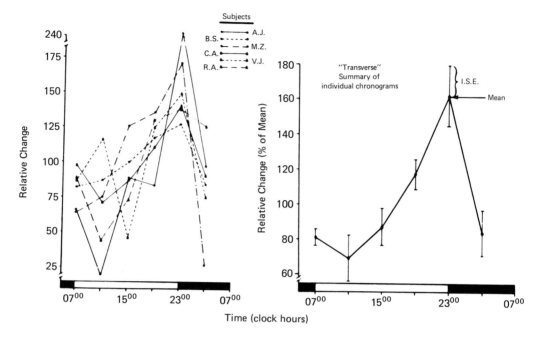

INDIVIDUAL CHRONOGRAMS

MEAN CHRONOGRAM

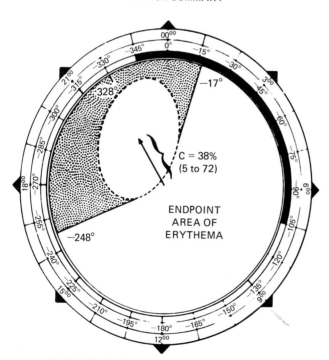

COSINOR SUMMARY

No Pole Overlap if Confidence Coefficient ≤ .968

of either the best-fitting cosine function along with plotted data (Fig. 5) or by means of a polar plot (Fig. 6). In the latter, confidence limits for A and ϕ are represented by an ellipse of error (Figs. 6 and 7). Estimates and end points of ϕ are depicted on the circular plot with regard to a phase reference, $\phi_0 = 0$. In this presentation, when $\tau = 24$ hr $= 360°$, then 1 hr $= 15°$ and $1° = 4$ min. The projection of a vector on the circle indicates the ϕ location; the tangents to the ellipse of error, drawn from the center of the polar plot, indicate the 95% confidence interval of ϕ. The length of the vector from the pole is proportional to the amplitude. Intersections of this vector with the error ellipse give the 95% confidence interval of A.

The Cosinor method also provides a "goodness of fit" approximation, i.e., the so-called percent of rhythm (PR). Most biological rhythms do not exactly resemble a cosine function. It is, therefore, important to determine the percentage of data included in the 95% confidence limits of the best-fitting cosine function. For example, a PR equal to 80% indicates that the proportion of variance accounted for by the approximation used, a single cosine curve, is rather good.

There are several major reasons why the Cosinor method is currently used widely by chronobiologists. It is useful for validating a rhythm and for quantifying the parameters of rhythms—τ, ϕ, A, and M. It is important to obtain these parameters as estimates and their respective confidence limits. The method can be used even if one deals with short time series as in the case

when T = 24 hr, $\Delta t = 4$ hr, number of subjects = 6, and the total number of data (Nos) = 36. Moreover with the Cosinor, Δt need not be fixed nor constant; this means that missing data as well as unequal sampling intervals are well tolerated. In other words, Cosinor methods are useful tools for validating, quantifying, and describing a rhythm. The Cosinor method can be used several times, utilizing different trial periods to detect harmonics. For example, in Figure 8 a better approximation of the overall time series is obtained when using $\tau = 12$ hr (1st harmonic) in addition to $\tau = 24$ hr, than when using only $\tau = 24$ hr for the fitting of the data. In other cases, several validated harmonics may be needed for the complete description of a rhythm's waveform.

Although the Cosinor method has proven valuable, there are some situations in which it is inadequate for rhythm description and quantification. This is the case when periodic phenomena are asymmetrical and therefore not amenable to fitting by a cosine function, even with the use of harmonics. In a case such as this, the computed acrophase (crest of the best-fitting cosine function) may not correspond well to the actual crest time (De Prins 1975; De Prins et al. 1976). To solve this problem, several other methods have been proposed, such as the computation of the *orthophase* or *paraphase* (De Prins et al. in press). These latter methods maintain the advantage of a rhythm detection and quantification while improving rhythm description relative to the "basic" Cosinor.

Fig. 7. Individual and mean chronograms and parameter estimations (Cosinor summary) for a circadian susceptibility rhythm of the skin (intradermal injections) to house dust extract: 6 allergic adult patients (2 women, 4 men). The direction of the arrow in the polar plot of the Cosinor and the adjacent shaded area depict the peak and 95% confidence range of greatest susceptibility, respectively; the length of the same arrow represents the extent of the predictable periodic change, i.e., the rhythm's amplitude. That a rhythm does indeed occur is indicated by the Cosinor method when the error ellipse, the white space within the shaded area, does not cover the middle of the center pole of the plot. (From Reinberg et al. 1969.)

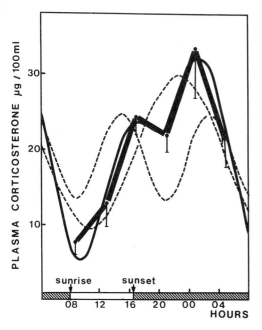

Fig. 8. Circadian rhythm in plasma corticosterone of intact male mature rats, synchronized with natural daylight (November), room temperature of 22° ± 1°C, and food and water available *ad libitum*. Sampling interval ≅ 4 hr (8–10 animals sampled at each time point). Raw data (chronogram) given with time point x̄ ± 1 SE in μg/100 ml (*heavy line*). Cosinor analyses by best-fitting cosine functions with τ's = 24 and 12 hr, respectively (*dashed lines*). Rhythm approximation with both component periods (24 and 12 hr) (*solid line*). The crest time of the latter is located at approximately 0015. The resultant curve thus obtained is closer to the chronogram form than that of the cosine function with τ = 24 hr. (From Guillemant et al. 1979, reproduced with permission.)

Display of Time Series as Chronograms and Plexograms

The description of a biological rhythm should first start with a simple display of the raw data as a function of time (Figs. 5 and 7). This elementary step provides an initial impression about the shape of the waveform of the time series and gives some idea of the already available method(s) that can be used to analyze the data (De Prins 1975; De Prins et al. 1976; Halberg et al. 1977; Reinberg 1971). A simple plot of the data usually provides information not available from more sophisticated methods. For example, plotting the raw data of plasma cortisol obtained by frequent blood sampling with Δt = 5 or 10 min throughout 24 hr reveals, according to Weitzman et al. (1971), that the waveform of this circadian rhythm in many subjects is asymmetrical. In diurnally active persons the curve (Fig. 4) shows a large peak in the morning and a total absence of hormone between 2100 and 0300. (Due to ultradian rhythms, averaging the data of several subjects may not reveal this important fact.) Yet generalization from a simple plot of raw data alone is not sufficiently informative in most cases to adequately describe the periodicity; nor does it lead to an unbiased, objective description or quantification of the time series.

Chronograms (and plexograms) constitute a second step in the analysis of time series data (Halberg et al. 1977). A *chronogram* is defined as an individual or averaged display of data as a function of time. A *plexogram* is defined as a display of data which were collected during a span longer than the period of the rhythm investigated (T > · τ) along the abscissa of a chosen single period (τ), only. Such a display may be presented irrespective of the (time) order of data collection, for example, as a function of a single conventional or other time unit, such as day, without regard for calendar date and/or subject. Since conventional statistical methods are used (means, variance analyses, t-test, etc.), parameters such as the mean (e.g., 24-hr mean), peak–trough difference, peak time location, and period of the rhythm can be estimated. In addition, the waveform of the curve can be visualized. If this latter appears to resemble a cosine function, it is of interest to use one of the Cosinor methods for the evaluation and quantification of rhythmicity. The chronogram, a plot of the data over time, proves to be very important in many circumstances. For example, in studies of shift-workers (Rutenfranz 1978) or of passengers or employees on transmeridian flights (Klein and Wegmann 1979), the chronogram indicates that the crest time of the body temperature rhythm shifts earlier (and faster) than the trough when the socioecologic (rest–activity) synchronizer is manipulated.

In many chronobiologic publications, both the raw data, in the form of chronograms, and the results of other data analyses (such as the Cosinor) are included. In so doing, several methods for the validation, description, and quantification of rhythms are presented.

Other Methods of Data Analysis

Many methods have been proposed for analyzing time series. Each offers certain advantages and disadvantages depending upon the type of experiment and the manner of data collection. All fulfill a specified purpose. The periodogram (van Cauter 1974), linear and nonlinear procedures (Batschelet et al. 1973), as well as methods such as those proposed by Wever (1965), Sollberger (1970), Del Pozo et al. (1979), Marotte (1979), De Prins (1975), De Prins et al. (1977), Martin (1981), and Winfree (1980) are available. The reader is encouraged to review the referenced works to obtain details about these complementary and/or alternate approaches.

It is not uncommon that nonmathematically inclined or inexperienced students and even accomplished scientists are confused when initially confronted with the practical problems of time series analysis. A large choice of methods, each having a set of advantages and limitations, compounds the problem. Perhaps the best approach in solving the problems of data analysis is to follow the advice of J. De Prins (De Prins 1975; De Prins et al. 1976, 1977, 1978): first consider the raw data displayed in the form of a chronogram or plexogram; then select several relevant methods of data analysis to determine which provides appropriate quantification of the considered time series. Today, the latter can be accomplished using a small computer equipped with a set of programs for the statistical analysis of time series. This approach allows one to visualize and screen the results to evaluate the respective advantages provided by the methods considered, including the display of data and the Cosinor.

The Chronodesm and the Problem of a Single Datum

Not only chronobiologists, but all biologists are troubled when trying to interpret the significance of a single datum. In the first chapter, it was mentioned that it is no longer acceptable to include as "noise" variations in biological values due to *predictable* circadian, circannual, and other rhythms. Inclusion of such rhythmic variability contributes to a widening of the limits or "range" of reference values. The influence of bioperiodic variabilities, especially ones of high amplitude, cannot be ignored. A special method for establishing and interpreting so-called physiochemical reference values has been suggested by Halberg et al. (1977). Conventionally (with the homeostatic approach), reference values are given as a mean ($\bar{x}$) ± confidence limits (SD or SE) ranging from 90% to 95%. A better and more appropriate representation is obtainable if time-qualified reference values are available for biological functions known to exhibit circadian and/or other rhythms. The time-qualified ranges for reference values can be presented in the form of a cosine function with confidence limits. Obviously the information must be defined with respect to sex, age, geographic location, subject's synchronization, etc. For circadian, circamensual, circannual, and other rhythms, such chronobiologically considered reference systems have been termed *chronodesms* (from the Greek, meaning "linked to time") by Halberg et al. (1977). For example, in considering circadian rhythms with only one datum, if both the time of sampling and the subject synchronization (e.g., light-on/light-off) are known it is possible to determine from the

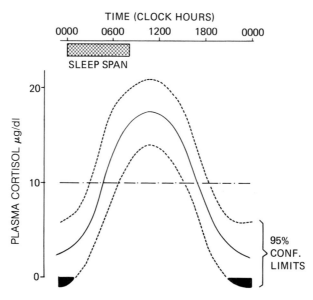

Fig. 9. Chronodesm of plasma cortisol of 8 healthy males, 20–30 years of age. Synchronization with light-on at 0800, light-off at 0000. Sampling interval is $\Delta t = 1$ hr; sampling span is $T = 24$ hr. Despite the fact that circadian changes in plasma cortisol do not exactly represent a cosine function, the latter can be used to derive a chronodesm. The conventional statistical analysis (without chronobiologic consideration) gives $\bar{x} = 10.0 \pm 9.2$ μg/100 ml (95% confidence limits). The chronodesm reveals that around 1100 in diurnally active persons plasma cortisol values of between 13.9 and 20.5 μg/100 ml (95% confidence limits) are within normal; while 12 hr later at 2300, plasma cortisol values between 0 and 5.7 μg/100 ml are within normal. If the subject's synchronization is known, the chronodesm allows the interpretation of one datum given with its sampling time. For example, 13 μg/100 ml at 0800 can be considered "normal," while at 2000 it would not be so for an adult subject with diurnal activity and nocturnal rest. (Unpublished data gathered by M. Guignard, M. Lagoguey, and A. Reinberg.)

chronodesm whether or not the value in question is "normal." For a healthy adult with diurnal activity and nocturnal rest, a plasma cortisol level of zero is within the "normal range" if the blood sample is drawn at midnight (0000), while it is abnormal if obtained at 0800. On the contrary, a plasma cortisol of 20 μg/100 ml may well be considered evidence of pathology if obtained at 0000; it would definitively be considered normal if obtained at 0800 (Fig. 9).

The presentation of reference values as chronodesms constitutes a step forward in the appreciation and diagnosis of health and disease, specifically when dealing with a single datum. A single piece of data provided from the clinical laboratory through the use of sophisticated and precise instrumention has greater diagnostic value when related appropriately to the pertinent chronodesm made available by time series studies. In other words, a chronobiologic approach adds precision and avoids misinterpretation of clinical and laboratory data.

Summary

Various necessities of chronobiologic research have been presented. Subject standardization and synchronization as well as special considerations for data sampling, collection, and analysis using specific methodologies are indispensable for research of bioperiodic phenomena. Different types of investigative protocols are necessary depending on the nature of the research. The results of studies utilizing various kinds of chronobiologic protocols such as those used in detecting and quantifying rhythms in cell morphology (Chap. 3) and mitosis (Chap. 4), pathological processes and symptoms of human diseases (Chap. 5), and metabolism and effects of pharmaceutical agents (Chap. 6) and nutrients (Chap. 7) are presented later. Although the major focus of each of these chapters is the findings, appropriate detail about research procedures also is provided.

References

Apfelbaum, M, Reinberg, A, Nillus, P, and Halberg, F (1969) Rythmes circadiens de l'alternance veille-sommeil pendant l'isolement souterrain de sept jeunes femmes. Presse Médicale 77:879–882.

Aschoff, J (1960) Exogenous and endogenous components in circadian rhythms. Cold Spring Harbor Symp on Quant Biol 25:11–28.

Aschoff, J, Klotter, K, and Wever, R (1965) Circadian vocabulary. In: Aschoff, J, ed, *Circadian Clocks*. Amsterdam: North-Holland Publ. Co., pp. 10–19.

Aschoff, J, Fatranska, M, Giedke, H, Doerr, P, Stamm, D, and Wisser, H (1971) Human circadian rhythms in continuous darkness: entrainment by social cues. Science 171:213–215.

Aschoff, J (1981) Annual rhythms in man. In: Aschoff, J, ed, *Handbook of Behavioral Neurobiology*, Vol. 4. London: Plenum Press, pp. 475–487.

Barcal, R, Sova, J, Krizanovska, M, Levy, J, and Matousek, J (1968) Genetic background of circadian rhythms. Nature 220:1128–1131.

Batschelet, E, Hillman, D, Smolensky, M, and Halberg, F (1973) Angular-linear correlation coefficient for rhythmometry and circannually changing human birth rates at different geographic latitudes. Int J Chronobiol 1:183–202.

Bicakova–Rocher, A, Gorceix, A, and Reinberg, A (1981) Possible circadian rhythm alterations in certain healthy human adults (effects of a placebo). In: Reinberg, A, Vieux, N, and Andlauer, P, eds, *Night and Shiftwork: Biological and Social Aspects*. Oxford: Pergamon Press, pp. 297–310.

Boissin, J, and Assenmacher, I (1971) Entrainment of the adrenal cortical rhythm and of the locomotor activity rhythm by ahemeral photo-periods in the quail. J Interdiscipl Cycle Res 2:437–443.

Brody, AW, Vander, HJ, O'Halloran, PF, Connolly, JJ, and Schwertley, FW (1964) Correlation, normal standards, and interdependence in test of ventilatory strength and mechanics. Ann Rev Res Dis 89:214–235.

Brown, FA (1965) Propensity for lunar periodicity in hamsters and its significance for biological clocks theories. Proc Soc Exper Biol Med 120:792–797.

van Cauter, E (1974) Methods for the analysis of multifrequential biological time series. J Interdiscipl Cycle Res 5:131–148.

Cornelissen, G, Halberg, F, Stebbings, J, Halberg, E, Carandente, F, and Hsi, B (1980) Chronobiometry with pocket calculators and computer systems. La Ricerca in Clinica e in Laboratorio 10(2).

Czeisler, CA, Richardson, GS, Zimmerman, JC, Moore–Ede, MC, and Weitzman, ED (1981) Entrainment of human circadian rhythms by light–dark cycles: a reassessment. Photochem Photobiol 34:239–247.

Del Pozo, F, Jimenez, J, and De Feudis, F (1979) Method for the acquisition and analysis of chronopharmacological data. In: Reinberg, A, and Halberg F, eds, *Chronopharmacology*. Oxford: Pergamon Press, pp. 185–192.

De Prins, J (1975) Limitation des modeles mathèmatiques. Implications en ce qui concerne les transferts de méthodes. In: Delattre, P, ed, *Elaboration et justification des modèles. Applications en biologie*. Paris: Malone, pp. 243–253.

De Prins, J, Waetens, E, and Cornelissen, G (1976) Influence de la forme du signal sur la détermination de l'acrophase. Bulletin du Groupe d'Etudes des Rythmes Biologiques 8:123–129.

De Prins, J, Cornelissen, G, and Halberg, F (1977) Harmonic interpolation on equispaced series covering integral period of anticipated circadian rhythm in adriamycin tolerance. Chronobiologia 4:173 (abstract).

De Prins, J, Cornelissen, G, Hillman, D, Halberg, F, and Van Dijck. (in press) Harmonic interpolation yields paraphases and orthophases for biologic rhythms. Laboratoire des Etalons de Fréquence. Université Libre de Bruxelles Tervuren, Belgique pbl. No. 80, 1978, and Proc Int Conf Int Soc for Chronobiology, Pavia, 1978.

Descovich, GC, Montalbetti, N, Kuhl, JFW,

Himondos, S, and Halberg, F (1974) Age and catecholamine rhythms. Chronobiologia 1:163–171.

Dupont, W, Bourgeois, P, Reinberg, A, and Vaillant, R (1979) Circannual and circadian rhythms in the concentration of corticosterone in the plasma of the edible frog (*Rana esculenta l.*). J Endocrinol 80:117–125.

DuRuisseau, JP (1965) Seasonal variation of PBI in healthy Montrealers. J Clin Endocrinol Metab 25:1513–1515.

Gaultier, C, Reinberg, A, and Girard, F (1977) Circadian rhythms in lung resistance and dynamic lung compliance of healthy children. Effects of two bronchodilators. Respiration Physiology 31:169–182.

Gervais, P, and Reinberg, A (1976) The clinical significance of chronobiological methods for allergic asthma. In: McGovern, JP, Smolensky, M, and Reinberg, A, eds, *Chronobiology in Allergy and Immunology*. Springfield, Ill., Charles C Thomas, pp. 64–78.

Ghata, J, Reinberg, A, Lagoguey, M, and Touitou, Y (1977) Human circadian rhythms documented in May–June from three groups of young healthy males living respectively in Paris, Colombo and Sydney. Chronobiologia 4:181–190.

Guillemant, J, Eurin, J, Guillemant, S, and Reinberg, A (1979) Circadian and other rhythms in corticoadrenal cyclic nucleotides (cAMP–cGMP) of intact and hypophysectomized male, mature rats. Chronobiologia 6:101–105.

Gupta, BD, and Deka, AC (1975) Application of chronobiology to radio-therapy of tumor of oral cavity. Chronobiologia, 2 (Suppl. 1):25 (abstract).

Halberg, F (1973) Laboratory techniques and rhythmometry. In: Mills, JN, ed, *Biological Aspects of Circadian Rhythms*. London: Plenum, pp. 1–26.

Halberg, F, and Nelson, W (1978) Chronobiologic optimization of aging. In: Smith, HV, and Capobianco, S, eds, *Aging and Biological Rhythms*. London: Plenum, pp. 5–55.

Halberg, F, and Simpson, H (1967) Circadian acrophase of human 17-hydroxycorticosteroid excretion referred to midsleep rather than midnight. Human Biol 39:405–413.

Halberg, F, Halberg, E, Barnum, CP, and Bittner, JJ (1959) Physiologic 24-hour periodicity in human beings and mice, the lighting regimen and daily routine. In: Withrow, RB, ed, *Photoperiodism and Related Phenomena* in *Plants and Animals*. Washington, D.C.: A.A.A.S. 55:803–878.

Halberg, F, Engeli, M, Hamburger, C, and Hillman, D (1965) Spectral resolution of low-frequency, small amplitude rhythms in excreted ketosteroid; probable androgen-induced circaseptan desynchronization. Acta Endocrinol Suppl 103:5–54.

Halberg, F, Tong, YL, and Johnson EA (1967) Circadian system phase: an aspect of temporal morphology; procedure and illustrative examples. In: von Mayersbach, H, ed, *The Cellular Aspects of Biorhythms*. Berlin: Springer, pp. 20–48.

Halberg, F, Johnson, EA, Nelson, W, Runge, W, and Sothern, R (1972) Autorhythmometry. Procedures for physiologic self-measurements and their analysis. Physiol Teacher 1:1–11.

Halberg, F, Carandente, F, Cornelissen, G, and Katinas, GS (1977) Glossary of chronobiology. Chronobiologia, 4 (suppl. 1):1–189.

Halberg, F, Reinberg, A, and Lagoguey, M (1983) Circannual rhythms in man. Int J Chronobiol (in press).

Haus, E, and Halberg, F (1970) Circannual rhythm in level and timing of serum corticosterone in standardized inbred mature C-mice. Environ Res 3:81–106.

Klein, KE, and Wegmann, HM (1979) Circadian rhythms of human performance and resistance: operational aspects. In: AGARD lecture series no. 105, *Sleep, Wakefulness and Circadian Rhythm*. Neuilly S/Seine 92200 France: AGARD-NATO publications, pp. 2.10–2.12.

Marotte, H (1979) Etudes des rhythmes biologiques par analyse de variance: recherche expérimentale du rhythme circadien de la régulation thermique chez l'homme. Thèse Dr. ès-Sciences. Université Claude Bernard, Lyon France, Février, p. 348.

Martin, W (1981) Estimation of parameters of circadian rhythms, if measurements cannot be performed around the clock. The case of a band limited signal plus noise. In: Reinberg, A., Vieux, N., and Andlauer, P, eds, *Night and Shiftwork: Biological and Social Aspects*. Oxford: Pergamon Press, pp. 37–44.

von Mayersbach, H (1978) Die Zeitstruktur des Organismus. Arzneimittelforschung/Drug Research 28(11):1824–1836.

McGovern, MP, Smolensky, MH, and Reinberg, A (1977) Circadian and circamensual rhythmicity in cutaneous reactivity to histamine and allergenic extracts. In: McGovern, JP, Smolensky, MH, and Reinberg, A, eds, *Chronobiology in Allergy and Immunology*. Springfield, Ill.: Charles C Thomas, pp. 79–116.

Nelson, W, Tong, YK, Jueng–Kuen, L, and Halberg, F (1979) Methods for cosinor-rhythmometry. Chronobiologia 6:305-323.

Prevost, EJ, Smolensky, MH, Reinberg, A, and McGovern, JP (1980) Circadian rhythm of respiratory distress in asthmatic, bronchitic and emphysemic patients. In: Smolensky, MH, Reinberg, A, and McGovern, JP, eds, *Recent Advances in the Chronobiology of Allergy and Immunology*. Oxford: Pergamon Press, Ltd., pp. 237–250.

Procacci, P, Buzzelli, G, Passeri, I, Sassi, R, Viegelin, MR, and Zoppi, M (1972) Studies on the cutaneous pricking pain threshold in man, circadian and circatrigintan changes. Res Clin Stud Headache 3:260–276.

Reinberg, A (1971) Methodologic considerations for human chronobiology. J Interdiscpl Cycle Res 2:1–15.

Reinberg, A (1974) Aspects of circannual rhythms in man. In: Pengelley, ET, ed, *Circannual Clocks*. New York: Academic Press, pp. 423–505.

Reinberg, A, Vieux, N, Ghata, J, Chaumont, A-J, and Laporte, A (1979) Consideration of the circadian amplitude in relation to the ability to phase shift circadian rhythms of shift workers. Chronobiologia 6 (Suppl. 1):57–63.

Reinberg, A, Zagulla–Mally, Z, Ghata, J, and Halberg, F (1969) Circadian reactivity rhythms in human skin to house dust, penicillin and histamine. J Allergy 44:292–306.

Reinberg, A, Gervais, P, Halberg, Francine, and Halberg, Franz (1971) Trisentinel monitoring of air pollution by autorhythmometry of peak expiratory flow. *Proc 2nd Int Clean Air Cong*. New York: Academic Press, pp. 217–220.

Reinberg, A, Lagoguey, M, Chauffournier, JM, and Cesselin, F (1975) Circannual and circadian rhythms in plasma testosterone in five healthy young Parisian males. Acta Endocrinol 80:732–743.

Reinberg, A, Lagoguey, M, Cesselin, F, Touitou, Y, Legrand, JC, Delasalle, A, Antreassian, J, and Lagoguey, A (1978) Circadian and circannual rhythms in plasma hormones and other variables of five healthy young human males. Acta Endocrinol 88:417–427.

Reinberg, A, Vieux, N, Laporte, A, Andlauer, P, and Smolensky, M (1979) Chronobiological field studies of oil refinery shift workers. Chronobiologia 6 (Suppl 1):1–119.

Rutenfranz, J (1978) Schichtarbeit und biologische Rhythmik. Arzneimittel Forschung/Drug Research 28(11):1867–1872.

Scheving, LE, Sohal, GS, Enna, D, and Pauly, JE (1973) The persistence of a circadian rhythm in histamine response in guinea pigs maintained under continuous illumination. Anat Rec 175:1–7.

Simpson, HW, and Bohlen, JG (1973) Latitude and the human circadian system. In: Mills, JN, ed., *Biological Aspects of Circadian Rhythms*. London: Plenum Press, pp. 85–118.

Simpson, H, and Halberg, E (1974) Menstrual changes of the circadian temperature rhythm in women. In: Ferin, M, Halberg, F, Richart, RM, and Vande Wiele, RL, eds, *Biorhythms and Human Reproduction*. New York: John Wiley, pp. 549–556.

Smolensky, MH (1976) Chronobiologic aspects of cutaneous reactivity, an example of endogenous rhythmicity and implications upon the evaluation of environmental quality. In: Gervais, P, ed, *Asthme, Allergie Respiratoire et Environnement Socio-Ecologique*. Le Mont-Dore meeting, mai 1975. Imprimeca 19200 Ussel, pp. 41–60.

Smolensky, MH, Reinberg, A, Lee, RE, and McGovern, JP (1974) Secondary rhythms related to hormonal changes in the menstrual cycle. In: Ferin, M, Halberg, F, Richart, RM, and Vande Wiele, R, eds, *Biorhythms and Human Reproduction*. New York: John Wiley, pp. 287–306.

Smolensky, MH, Halberg, F, Harter, J, Hsi, B, and Nelson, W (1978) Higher corticosterone values at a fixed single timepoint in serum from mice 'trained' by prior handling. Chronobiologia 5:1–13.

Smolensky, MH, Halberg, F, Pitts, GC, and Nelson, W (1980a). The chronopharmacology of methylprednisolone: clinical implications of animal studies with special emphasis upon the moderation of growth inhibition by timing to circadian rhythms. In: Smolensky, MH, Reinberg, A, and McGovern, JP, eds, *Recent Advances in the Chronobiology of Allergy and Immunology*. Oxford: Pergamon Press, pp. 137–171.

Smolensky, MH, Reinberg, A, and McGovern, JP, eds. (1980b) *Recent Advances in the Chronobiology of Allergy and Immunology.* Oxford: Pergamon Press.

Sollberger, A (1970) Problems in the statistical analysis of short periodic time series. J Interdiscipl Cycle Res. 1:49–88.

Tammeling, GJ, De Vries, K, and Kruyt, EW (1977) The circadian pattern of the bronchial reactivity to histamine in healthy subjects and in patients with obstructive lung disease. In: McGovern, JP, Smolensky, MH, and Reinberg, A, eds, *Chronobiology in Allergy and Immunology.* Springfield: Charles C Thomas, pp. 139–149.

Weitzman, ED, Fukushima, D, Nogeire, C, Roffwarg, H, Gallager, TF, and Hellman, L (1971) Twenty-four hour pattern of the episodic secretion of cortisol in normal subjects. J Clin Endocrinol Metab 33:14–22.

Wever, RA (1965) A mathematical model for circadian rhythms. In: Aschoff, J, ed, *Circadian Clocks.* Amsterdam: North-Holland Pub. Co., pp. 47–63.

Wever, RA (1979) *The Circadian System of Man: Results of Experiments under Temporal Isolation.* New York: Springer-Verlag.

Winfree, AT (1980) The Geometry of Biological Time. *Biomathematics,* Vol. 8. New York: Springer-Verlag.

3

An Overview of the Chronobiology of Cellular Morphology

Heinz von Mayersbach

Temporal organization at the cellular level is evident for the eukaryote (Edmunds 1978; Ehret 1974; Goodwin 1963; Hastings and Keyman 1965; Hastings and Schweiger 1976; Schweiger et al. 1964; Vanden Driessche 1971, 1975), plant (Sweeney 1969), bird (Young 1978a,b), and human being (Ashkenazi et al. 1973, 1975). In this chapter, temporal patterns in cellular morphology are illustrated using the hepatic cell of the rodent. This example has been selected since the general properties and concepts of the temporal morphology of rodent cells are also common to other ones. Although cellular morphology rhythms are of interest in their own right, the materials of this chapter are especially relevant for understanding the other topics of this volume, i.e., chronopharmacology, chronochemotherapy, and chrononutrition.

Introduction

Over the past few decades, a great deal of research on 24-hr variation in cellular function has been conducted. It is almost impossible to compile the vast number of publications which have demonstrated statistically significant circadian variations in the chemical composition of organs, tissues, and blood. The prominence of these circadian oscillations is exemplified by the data of Fig. 1, a presentation of the amplitudes of various rhythms detected in normal, healthy laboratory rats fed *ad libitum*. During each 24-hr period every cellular component oscillates within a certain range. From the examples given in Fig. 1 and from many others, it is evident that the most stable component of tissue is water. For example, repeated investigations on the liver (Abicht 1976; Philippens and Abicht 1977) have shown that the water content varies only slightly over each 24-hr span without exhibiting significant circadian rhythmicity. This finding is in clear contrast to the observations on other biochemical constituents of the liver, which demonstrate striking circadian rhythmic changes.

Temporal variations in such biological components as hormones and enzymes, for example, are undoubtedly the expression of temporal alterations in metabolic processes. Since metabolic processes are based on cellular functions, the question arises: To what extent are structural manifestations during the circadian cycle visible

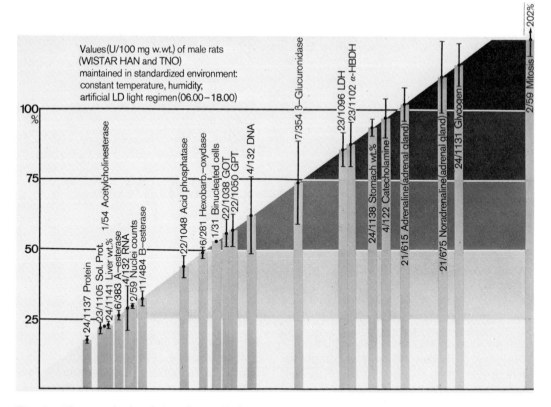

Fig. 1. The magnitude of circadian variations of organ components is given as percent deviation from the respective 24-hr mean. The values were derived from repeated investigations performed on standardized laboratory rats. (The lower number in the columns indicates how many experiments were conducted; the upper number represents the total animals studied; organs other than liver stated in columns.) Male rats (Wistar HAN and TNO) were maintained in a standardized environment of constant temperature, humidity, and an artificial LD regimen (L:0600–1800). (From von Mayersbach 1978.)

at the cellular level? Unfortunately, in contrast to the vast body of published analytic studies, the number of chronomorphologic investigations on mammalian tissues is quite small. However, based upon those cytological and histochemical studies reported thus far it is clear that:

1. Functional circadian variations coincide closely with profound, periodic reorganizations of the cell inventory, such as the nucleus, cell organelles, and other cytoplasmic constituents (Fig. 2).
2. As a result, the site and concentration of substrates, enzymes, and hormones, among other constituents of cells and tissues, appear quite different when traced by cytochemical and histochemical procedures depending on the time during the 24-hr span of study.
3. The temporal structure of cells essentially determines the time-dependent response to hormones, drugs, and poisons (see Chap. 6).

The intent of this chapter is to present an overview of the tremendous chronobiologic variation in cell morphology. It will become apparent that the configuration of cells and tissues in the normal, healthy organism periodically may even attain organizational states which are considered either

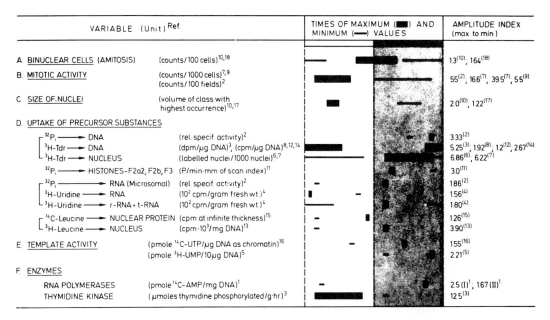

VARIABLE (Unit) Ref.	TIMES OF MAXIMUM (■) AND MINIMUM (—) VALUES	AMPLITUDE INDEX (max. to min.)
A. BINUCLEAR CELLS (AMITOSIS) (counts/100 cells)[10,18]		13[10]; 164[18]
B. MITOTIC ACTIVITY (counts/1000 cells)[7,9] (counts/100 fields)[2]		55[2]; 16.6[7]; 39.5[7]; 55[9]
C. SIZE OF NUCLEI (volume of class with highest occurrence)[10,17]		2.0[10]; 122[17]
D. UPTAKE OF PRECURSOR SUBSTANCES		
$^{32}P_i \longrightarrow$ DNA (rel. specif. activity)[2]		3.33[2]
^{3}H-Tdr $\longrightarrow$ DNA (dpm/μg DNA)[3], (cpm/μg DNA)[8,12,14]		5.25[3]; 192[8]; 12[12]; 267[14]
^{3}H-Tdr $\longrightarrow$ NUCLEUS (labelled nuclei/1000 nuclei)[6,7]		6.86[6]; 6.22[7]
$^{32}P_i \longrightarrow$ HISTONES-F2a2, F2b, F3 (P/min·mm of scan index)[11]		3.0[11]
$^{32}P_i \longrightarrow$ RNA (Microsomal) (rel. specif. activity)[2]		1.86[2]
^{3}H-Uridine $\longrightarrow$ RNA (10^2 cpm/gram fresh wt.)[4]		1.56[4]
^{3}H-Uridine $\longrightarrow$ r-RNA + t-RNA (10^2 cpm/gram fresh wt.)[4]		1.80[4]
^{14}C-Leucine $\longrightarrow$ NUCLEAR PROTEIN (cpm at infinite thickness)[15]		1.26[15]
^{3}H-Leucine $\longrightarrow$ NUCLEUS (cpm·10^3/mg DNA)[13]		3.90[13]
E. TEMPLATE ACTIVITY (pmole ^{14}C-UTP/μg DNA as chromatin)[16] (pmole ^{3}H-UMP/10μg DNA)[5]		1.55[16] 2.21[5]
F. ENZYMES		
RNA POLYMERASES (pmole ^{14}C-AMP/mg DNA)[1]		2.5(I)[1]; 1.67(II)[1]
THYMIDINE KINASE (μmoles thymidine phosphorylated/g·hr)[3]		12.5[3]

Fig. 2. Circadian variations of cell nuclei. The different nuclear activities are listed, and the occurrence of maximal and minimal values is demonstrated in relation to the light and dark periods of the different species investigated. References (as cited in the source for this figure) are Barbiroli et al. (1973),[1] Barnum et al. (1958),[2] Dallman et al. (1974),[3] Döring and Rensing (1973),[4] Earp (1974),[5] Echave Llanos et al. (1970),[6] Echave Llanos et al. (1971),[7] Eling (1967),[8] Jackson (1959),[9] Jerusalem et al. (1970),[10] Letnansky (1974),[11] Potter et al. (1966),[12] Rohde and Rensing (1973),[13] Ruby et al. (1973),[14] Sestan (1964),[15] Steinhart (1971),[16] Suppan (1966),[17] and Zhirnova (1969).[18] (From von Mayersbach 1981.)

"abnormal" or the consequence of experimental challenge. The findings from the field of modern cytology reviewed here were derived from research using histochemical tools. The predictable chronobiologic variability of cells and tissues, however, may essentially affect the manner in which the results of histotechniques, for example, are interpreted; unexpected findings may be viewed as the result of poor technique rather than expressions of circadian variability. Chronotechnical problems, although beyond the scope of this paper, have been considered; the interested reader is referred to another paper by the author (von Mayersbach 1981).

Circadian Rhythms in Cells

The main components of each living eukaryotic cell are the nucleus and the cytoplasm. The nucleus has two main functions,

each of which is linked with characteristic morphological features.

1. The nucleus contains the genetic material (genome) of the cell. During cell division the nucleus forms two identical daughter nuclei, each with a complete set of genes. Cell division is visualized by the appearance of a double set of chromosomes, representing a condensed, transportable form of the genes. The chromosomes undergo a series of spatial rearrangements known as mitotic figures.

2. The interphase is the span between two cell divisions. Among various types of tissues it ranges in duration from hours to weeks. In the interphase nucleus the chromosomes are not visible, but exhibit strongly basophilic chromatin (DNA-containing) granules and a clearly visible nuclear membrane (see Fig. 8). Further-

more, each interphase nucleus contains one or more RNA-producing nucleolus. During this stage, the nucleus serves as the regulatory center for all the metabolic processes involved in cell-specific functions.

Cell Division

One of the earliest chronobiologic discoveries was that the mitotic index (number of dividing cells) varies over 24 hr. Many studies have confirmed this observation. High-amplitude rhythms in mitotic activity have been found for various mammalian tissues as discussed in Chap. 4 and reviewed in detail by Scheving (1959), Scheving and Pauly (1960, 1967a,b, 1973), and Scheving et al. (1974b). A representative example is given in Fig. 3.

Pilgrim (1967) reported that the number of DNA-synthesizing cells varies significantly during each 24-hr period. Based on cytokinetic studies, Burns and Scheving (1975) reported circadian differences in the cell-cycle time; this finding was confirmed by Thorud et al. (1979). Several studies of the mitotic activity in liver tissue (Wilson and LeDuc 1948; Halberg 1957; Jackson 1959; Vonnahme 1974) have revealed circadian patterns similar in phasing to those of the cornea and skin. This latter observation suggests that the rhythm of cell proliferation is highly synchronized in different tissues of an organism.

Philippens (1979) analyzed the importance of various synchronizers on the circadian rhythm of mitotic activity using a very elaborate protocol of experimentally changed light–dark and feeding schedules. Clear evidence was obtained revealing that the circadian rhythm of mitosis in the rat cornea is specifically synchronized by the alternating light–dark cycle. In contrast, the substrate supply (food intake) was found to be the *Zeitgeber* (synchronizer) for the circadian rhythm of mitosis in the liver, which phase-shifted under the influence of altered feeding schedules. Since the periodic food intake of animals having unlimited access

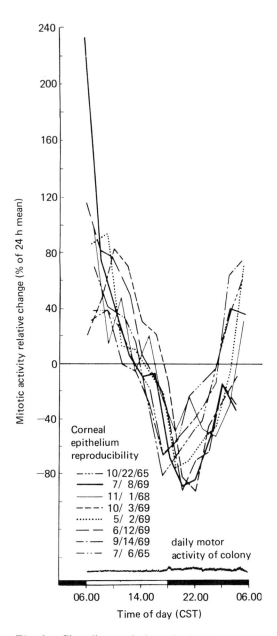

Fig. 3. Circadian variation of mitotic index in rat cornea. Investigations performed in different months of different years. (From Scheving et al. 1974b.)

to nutrients is governed by the light–dark schedule, it is apparent why the mitotic rhythms of the cornea and liver appear to be synchronized in rats housed under standardized conditions used for chronobiologic research.

The Interphase Nucleus

The size of the interphase nuclei is specific for each cell type. Likewise, the ratio of the nuclear volume to the cytoplasmic volume is also cell-type specific. An increase in the nuclear size is generally believed to be caused either by DNA duplication during the S phase preceding mitosis or by the expression of increased functional activity, appearing as a nuclear edema. Karyometric measurements of interphase nuclei, performed as early as 1934 by Caspersson and Holmgren, revealed pronounced "diurnal" variations in the nuclear size of liver cells. Since then, it has been demonstrated by many investigators that the nuclei of liver cells periodically undergo dynamic changes over each 24-hr span. Many of these changes, which have been enumerated by Philippens and Abicht (1977), are summarized in Fig. 2.

Circadian changes in the nucleolar components of the superior cervical ganglia (SCG) of rats have been reported as well (Pébusque and Seïte 1980, 1981a,b; Pébusque et al. 1981a,b). In their studies different but comparable subgroups of adult male rats, synchronized with L(0700–1900):D(1900–0700) and with food and water available *ad libitum,* were sacrificed at 2–3 hr intervals during a single 24-hr span. The SCG was removed and the mean volume of the nucleolar fibrillar centers and of the other nucleolar—fibrillar, granular, and vacuolar—components were determined by stereological analyses.

Temporal differences in the ultrastructure of the nucleolar components as a function of the circadian time are easily discernable in Fig. 4. The reticulated nucleolus in the sympathetic neurons of the SCG in rats sacrificed at 1500 contained only small-sized fibrillar centers with granular and vacuolar components dispersed throughout. The ultrastructure of the reticulated nucleolus of the sympathetic neurons of the SCG from rats sacrificed at 0100 appeared very different. Clearly apparent in Fig. 4 is a single voluminous fibrillar center (FC) along with many other smaller, dense fibrillar components located within a well-formed network as well as within the FC. Figure 5 presents a quantification of these changes in the nucleolar ultrastructure. The mean volume of the fibrillar centers, poorly visible in the SCG removed from animals during the light span (at 1500), increased in volume 13-fold on the average in animals sacrificed during the dark span (at 0100). The volume of the SCG nucleoli at 0100 also was elevated 1.7-fold over that at 1500.

The findings of Pébusque et al. are of interest for several reasons. Most pertinent to the contents of this chapter, however, is the implication that the ultrastructure of the nucleoli of even mitotically quiescent neurons undergoes systematic circadian rhythms in organization. Although an increase in nucleolar size is generally thought to reflect an increase in cellular activity, it is not known yet whether these rhythmic variations in the ultrastructure of the SCG nucleolus are correlated with an increased level of transcriptional activity. While it is well known that the cells of mature neuronal tissue are non-mitotic, it appears that processes within these types of cells display circadian rhythms. This is true not only for the nucleolus of the SCG, but for the shedding and degradation of the outer segment of the membranes of rods and cones, demonstrated by Young (1978a,b) for the chick retina.

Most somatic cells contain only one nucleus, but in several organs such as the liver a number of cells may contain two nuclei, thus being termed polyploidy. An increasing percentage of binucleated cells is generally regarded as a response to functional load. Philippens and Abicht (1977), Abicht (1976), and Röver and Philippens (1979) studied the relative number of binucleated cells in the liver of rats over the 24-hr span. They found, in animals maintained in LD 12 : 12 and fed *ad libitum,* a significant circadian rhythm with highest counts (28.54%) during the dark span and lowest counts (14.21%) during the light span (Fig. 6). This normally occurring temporal variation of

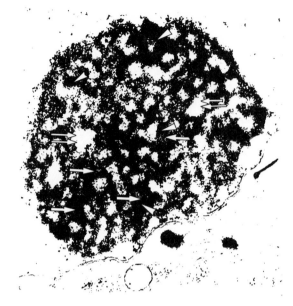

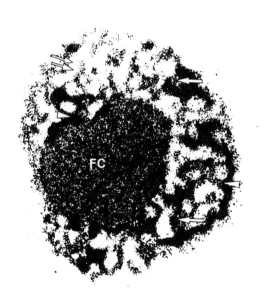

Fig. 4. **Upper portion** of figure shows section of reticulated nucleolus (×25 000) in sympathetic neurons of the SCG for a rat synchronized to L(0700–1900):D(1900–0700) and sacrificed at 1500. Small-sized fibrillar centers (*arrows*) are seen surrounded by a continuous layer of dense fibrillar (ribonuclearprotein) component which takes the form of a well-delimited network (*arrowhead*). The granular and the vacuolar components (*double arrows*) are easy to distinguish. **Lower portion** shows section of reticulated nucleolus in sympathetic neurons of the SCG of an identically synchronized rat sacrificed at 0100. One large voluminous fibrillar center (FC) and other small ones (*arrow*) can be seen. The dense fibrillar component is seen either near the FC or in the form of a well-delimited network (*arrowhead*). The double arrows point to the vacuoles. (From Pébusque and Seïte 1981b, reproduced with permission.)

polyploidy equals or even exceeds the relative increase in binucleated hepatocyte numbers found after the application of metabolic loads as detected in single-time-point (nonchronobiologically designed) investigations. The observed systematic circadian variation in binucleated cells is interpreted as the expression of amitotic divisions alternating with nuclear fusion processes. The cycles of structural rearrangements of the nuclear compartment basically reflect changing, although continuous, metabolic loads on the liver during each 24-hr duration.

Circadian changes in DNA concentration have been detected by several techniques. Barnum et al. (1958) first reported that ^{32}P-labeled precursors were incorporated at different rates in liver DNA, depending on the timing of their administra-

lysosomes, peroxisomes, Golgi apparatus, and centrosome (Fig. 8). In certain cells the organelles are characteristically located at certain cytoplasmic sites. For instance, in the cells of the proximal tubules of the kidney the mitochondria are located in the basal parts; in hepatocytes, the lysosomes are found mainly along the bile canaliculi. Organelles can be isolated by cell homogenization and recovered as organelle-specific fractions by differential centrifugation.

Mitochondria. Mitochondria are organized multienzyme systems possessing catabolizing oxidative processes. Under the electron microscope they reveal a double membrane. The inner one forms infoldings, the so-called *cristae mitochondriales* (cristae-type mitochondria, Fig. 8); the mitochondria of steroid-producing cells, such as the adrenal cortex, contain tubuli instead of cristae (tubuli-type). By use of the light microscope, mitochondria appear as fine rods or granules which can be visualized by histochemically tracing their enzymes, among

which SDH (succinate dehydrogenase) is preferentially used as a marker enzyme.

In quite a number of investigations organ- and species-dependent differences in the enzyme patterns of mitochondria have been identified, in addition to differences due to changing biological conditions such as aging (Iemhoff and Hülsmann 1971). Under experimental influences, mitochondria became very reactive (Aithal and Ramasarma 1971; Klima et al. 1971; Laguens and Gomez-Dumm 1967; Mäusle and Fröhlke 1971; Milner 1972; Rafael et al. 1970; Reith and Schüler 1971, 1972; Riede and Rohr 1970; Stenram 1969). Mitochondria exhibit remarkable heterogeneity within a single liver lobule as revealed by enzyme composition (Novikoff 1959). However, the question remains open as to the conclusiveness of many individual reports, which have failed to take into account the possible influence of circadian rhythmic changes as first demonstrated in the adrenals by Glick and his colleagues (1961b). Using liver preparations, we were able to demonstrate

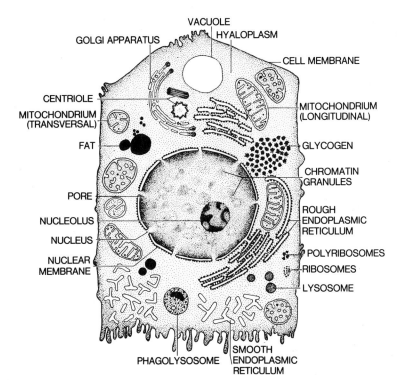

Fig. 8. Scheme of an interphase cell. (From von Mayersbach and Reale 1973.)

a strong circadian variation in SDH—activity, topographical distribution, and reaction–product appearance (von Mayersbach et al. 1964).

Philippens (1968; 1970; 1971) found that the circadian rhythm of SDH activity, irrespective of circadian stage, was strongest in the periportal region of the liver lobules. SDH circadian variations were apparent by differences in the extent of histochemical staining and by regional differences in strong reactions toward the central vein. Interestingly, despite the fact male and female rats basically displayed the same rhythmic variations in the topochemical distribution of liver SDH, the phasing was 180° (12 hr) apart; i.e., the SDH activity of the males was highest when that of females was lowest and vice versa (Fig. 9).

In other histochemical analyses, Philippens (1970; 1971; 1975) investigated *iso-lated mitochondria* of the same livers of rats utilizing quantitative biochemical methods. A significant circadian rhythm of SDH activity was detected as indicated by succinate-dependent oxygen consumption (succinate oxidase), cytochrome c reduction (succinate cytochrome c reductase), and by the nitro-BT reaction determined by a kinetic technique. Lowest reduction rates were manifested during the light span and highest ones during the dark span.

A highly interesting differential effect of the alteration of the light–dark synchronizer schedule on the in vivo activity of liver mitochondria was reported by Philippens (1973). The author subjected rats fed *ad libitum* for 6 weeks to an inverted light–dark schedule (LD 12:12, light 1800–0600) prior to investigation. The circadian rhythm of α-glycerophosphate dehydrogenase (mGPDH) determined in the isolated mito-

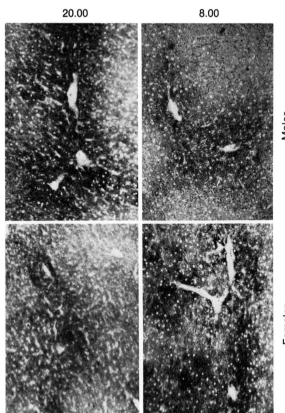

Fig. 9. SDH activity in rat liver mitochondria. The figure shows male and female rats at their respective lowest and highest SDH activity indicated by staining intensity and the extension of the strongly reacting area. (From Philippens 1971, reproduced with permission.)

chondrial fractions was phase-shifted in the same direction and amount as the shift of the synchronizing LD schedule, whereas the activity of the SDH continued to oscillate in the same manner as it did under the previous LD conditions (Fig. 10). Perhaps the resulting desynchronization due to phase shifting, eventhough occurring in only one subcellular compartment, contributes to the inhibition of weight gain in rats subjected to LD shifts (Philippens 1976).

Impressive and strong circadian variations of several mitochondrial enzymes (SDH, mGPDH, and NADH-tetrazolium reductase) in the parietal cells of the gastric mucosa of rats were demonstrated by Za-

viacic and Brozman (1978), with highest activities during the dark span (1800 and 2400) and lowest ones in the morning (0600). The times of highest activity observed in animals restricted from food intake for 24 hr before killing coincide with the span of food intake of control animals fed *ad libitum* and correlates well with the circadian differences in gastric HCL production.

The Ergastoplasm. Production of the cell's structural proteins, enzymes, and export proteins—such as secretory products, albumin, immunoglobulins, and enzymes—occurs in the ergastoplasm. Chemically, the ergastoplasm is composed of RNA and ba-

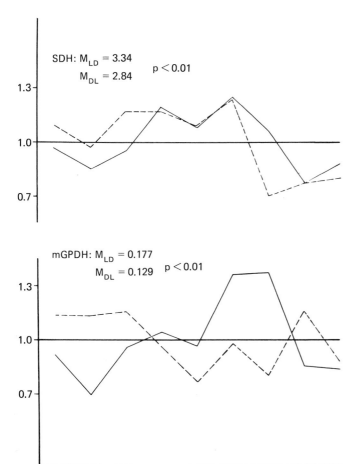

SDH: $M_{LD} = 3.34$
$M_{DL} = 2.84$ $p < 0.01$

mGPDH: $M_{LD} = 0.177$
$M_{DL} = 0.129$ $p < 0.01$

Influence of LD (———) and DL (--------) conditions on mitochondrial SDH and mGPDH circadian activities in (WS - TNO) rat livers: *relative values.*

Fig. 10. Influence of light shifts on mitochondrial enzymes. The activities of succinate dehydrogenase (SDH) and α-glycerophosphate dehydrogenase (mGPDH) were determined in isolated liver mitochondria. Groups of male Wistar rats (TNO) were subjected for 6 weeks to an inverted light–dark schedule (DL, L:1800–0600) and compared with those kept under the original 12:12 LD schedule (L:0600–1800). The rhythm of SDH activity is not influenced by this light shift, whereas mGPDH becomes synchronized to the new light schedule. All values scaled relative to the respective 24-hr mean M (set equal to 1), which are significantly lowered by inverting the light schedule. (From von Mayersbach, H, Philippens, K, and Scheving, LE (1977) Light—a synchronizer of circadian rhythms. In: *Proc. Intl. Soc. Chronobiol.* Milano: Il Ponte, pp. 503–510, reproduced with permission.)

sic proteins (histones). Electron microscopy reveals that the RNA appears in cell-specific, varying proportions either as free ribosomes and ribosome clusters (polysomes) or as ribosomes bound to membranes of the endoplasmic reticulum (ER). The ER itself is a membrane-delimited system of tubules, channels, and cisternae. If the membrane of the ER is studded with ribosomes, it is called rough-surfaced or granulated endoplasmic reticulum (RER) as depicted in Fig. 8. If the membrane is not associated with ribosomes, it is called smooth-surfaced or agranular endoplasmic reticulum (SER); the latter is mainly associated with lipid and steroid hormone synthesis.

Due to its RNA content, the ergastoplasm is negatively charged, which explains its strong binding capacities for (positively charged) basic dyes. Under light microscopic examination, the ergastoplasm is visible only in cells prominently involved in protein synthesis. Thus, in cells such as the liver, pancreas, and plasmocytes as well as in rapidly dividing cells such as blood stem and embryonic cells the ergastoplasm appears either as diffuse basophilia of the cytoplasm or as strong basophilic granules. Since these RNA-containing structures are involved in enzyme synthesis, their appearance after staining is correspondingly diffuse or granular when endoplasmic reticulum enzymes are demonstrated by histochemical methods. After cell centrifugation, free ribosomes, polysomes, and granules of ruptured RER form the microsome fraction; their enzymes are called microsomal enzymes.

The first systematic study of circadian changes in the microscopic appearance of RNA structures was presented by Müller (1971c) who showed that such variations exhibited a strict temporal relationship with rhythmic changes in the glycogen content of the same liver cells. The different circadian stages of RNA appearance can be summarized as follows: (1) At the time of maximal glycogen content (which in the nocturnally active rodent occurs during the morning hours), the RNA structure of the hepatocytes appears as heavily stained clots and granules. This description corresponds to the classic textbook picture of the basophilic bodies (also referred to as ergastoplasm and stalagmoid). (2) At the time of minimal glycogen content (in the evening), the RNA structure is weak and appears as diffuse basophilia of the cytoplasm. Between these extreme configurations, transitional stages are observable.

These qualitative and quantitative temporal variations in the basophilic structures of the hepatocytes are paralleled by the 24-hr differences in the concentration of several enzymes of the endoplasmic reticulum. Tracing the activities of the organophosphate-sensitive *B*-esterase (carboxylesterase, EC3.1.1.1) during the 24-hr span, this author (von Mayersbach et al. 1964; von Mayersbach 1967) observed different staining intensities representing different levels of enzyme activity and variable enzyme distributions not only within the liver lobuli but also within single cells where the enzyme reactions appeared either as rough granules or as diffuse or finely granulated stainings of the cytoplasm. A direct correlation between the circadian variations of the ergastoplasm in hepatocytes and the sites of glucose-6-phosphatase (G6P, EC.3.1.3.9) activity using both the light and electron microscope was reported by Müller (1971b). In his study, it was shown clearly that the cellular distribution of G6P previously regarded as "normal" is representative only of the circadian phase of high glycogen content; the coincidence of this state with the beginning of the usual hours of work by employees or scientists in research laboratories tends to explain the unanimity of the literature pertaining to the "normal" G6P distribution found in single-time-point studies.

Systematic rhythmic changes revealed by microscopy are coincident with statistically significant circadian variations as revealed by quantitative measurements of enzyme activities such as for carboxylesterase (von Mayersbach and Yap 1965), and G6P (Müller 1971b,c), as well as liver homogenate RNA.

Barnum et al. (1958) observed variations in the synthesis of microsomal RNA using ^{32}P incorporation. Using this same technique, Horvath (1963a, 1964), von Mayersbach (1967), and Eling (1967) reported large-amplitude circadian variations of the total liver RNA content. Döring and Rensing (1973) subsequently identified circadian variations of liver RNA resulting from 24-hr variation in the synthesis of individual RNA liver fractions. It is worthwhile to point out that quite a number of publications have dealt with the influence of protein synthesis inhibitors on the circadian pattern of various liver enzymes (inter alia, Hardeland 1973; Hardeland and Stephan 1974) thereby establishing, indirectly, the role of nucleic acids, especially RNA, in the regulation of cellular rhythms.

Lysosomes. The term "lysosome" originally was introduced by De Duve in 1969 to denote those cytoplasmic particles sedimenting with the fraction of light mitochondria; they are characterized by a remarkably high activity of several (about 36) hydrolases. Under the electron microscope, lysosomes appear as roundish dense bodies covered by a lipoprotein membrane. In light microscopic preparations, they are visible only by use of histochemical staining methods to trace their marker enzymes—acid phosphatase, β-glucuronidase, and arylesterase (an organophosphate-resistant A-esterase EC3.1.1.2). In biochemistry the same marker enzymes are used for lysosome studies. An absolute prerequisite for the histochemical demonstration of lysosomes is the use of appropriate methods for preparation to ensure preservation of both the membrane and enzyme activities of the lysosome.

The cytogenesis of lysosomes is not fully understood, but it is generally believed that lysosomes originate from the Golgi membrane, enveloping hydrolytic enzymes synthesized in the RER. Newly formed lysosomes are called primary lysosomes. The membranes of the lysosomes keep the highly concentrated hydrolytic enzymes separate from the surrounding cytoplasm, thus preventing hydrolytic self-destruction of the cell. The predominant functions of the lysosomes are:

1. Digestion of extraneous and worn-out cell constituents, such as the mitochondria. Extraneous materials which have entered the cell by phagocytosis and pinocytosis as well as worn-out cellular components are enwrapped by cytomembranes, thus forming phagosomes and autosomes, respectively. For the digestion of their contents the phagosomes and autosomes fuse with primary lysosomes to become larger-sized secondary lysosomes, which according to their content can be qualified as phagolysosomes or heterolysosomes and autophagosomes or autolysosomes (Fig. 11).
2. Transportation of enzymes destined for extracellular use across the cytoplasm. On the inner side of the cell surface, the lysosomal membrane fuses with the cell membrane and the enzymes are delivered by exocytosis to the extracellular space.

Autophagic processes play an important role in long-lived, stable parenchymal cells with minimal mitotic renewal, such as the parenchymal cells of the liver, kidney, and pancreas. In these cells the cytoplasmic components are partially renewed by replacement of several "out-of-use" structures and substances. A very interesting finding is that the autophagic breakdown of cellular waste material does not occur at random; it occurs instead in a temporally organized manner over each 24-hr span. Pfeifer (1977) demonstrated that the autophagic processes in hepatocytes, kidney tubular epithelium, and acinar cells of the exocrine pancreas predominantly occur during the environmental light span, i.e., during the resting phase of nocturnally active rats. A special form of autophagosomes are the glycogenosomes, mostly

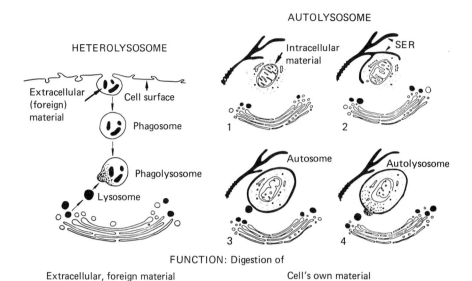

Fig. 11.　Development and functions of phagolysosomes. (From Dvorák, M (1974) Origin and development of lysosomes and peroxisomes. In: Dvorák M, ed. *Biogenesis of Cell Organelles*. Brno: JE Pukyne University Medical Faculty, pp. 59–86.)

β-glycogen-containing lysosomes. Initially, their appearance was mainly attributed to certain pathological conditions or associated with specific developmental stages such as in the liver of the newborn. However, Müller (1971c) observed glycogenosomes present also in the liver of normal adult rats. During the circadian stage of glycogen depletion, they are found predominately in the periportal sections of the liver lobules; while during the circadian stage of minimal glycogen content they are found predominately in the centrolobular region.

From the viewpoints of biological significance as well as histochemical (and biochemical) technology, the study of circadian rhythmicity in lysosomes has contributed to answering the following questions:

1. Are the lysosomes of the liver a heterogeneous population? This question emerged mainly from several nonrhythmic, that is single-time-point, studies. A question closely associated with this one is:
2. Can all lysosomes be traced by the use of a single marker enzyme if the lyso-

somes are heterogeneous? Despite the great volume of investigations, confusion still exists about the suitability of different marker enzyme techniques used to reveal lysosomes.
3. What is the significance of extralysosomal activities of lysosomal enzymes? In studies not using chronobiologic methods, such activities were found to a varying extent in both histochemical and biochemical preparations. The detection of a dual localization of lysosomal enzymes caused many controversies. The existence of extralysosomal enzymes was interpreted by some as an artifact resulting from inadequate techniques. Others ascribed this to enzyme displacement caused by escape from ruptured lysosomes, diffusion into the cytoplasm during fixation, or the use of unsuitable tissue preparations.

Using histochemical, electron microscopic, and biochemical tools in a series of studies, this author and his colleagues systematically investigated the activities of lysosomal marker enzymes most frequently used in histochemical and biochemical investigations: Acid phosphatase, β-glucuronidase, A-esterase, β-galactosidase, and arylsulphatase (Bhattacharya 1977; Bhattacharya and von Mayersbach 1976; von Mayersbach and Bhattacharya 1977; Groh and von Mayersbach, 1981a; Uchiyama et al. 1981).

Omitting the specific details of these investigations, the results can be summarized as follows:

1. Lysosomes exhibited marked circadian variations in number, size, configuration, and activity as well as in the position within the cell and predominant localization within the liver lobule.
2. The lysosomes revealed by different marker enzymes varied in their mean number and size. They appeared numerous and large when traced with the acid phosphatase and A-esterase reactions. In contrast they were much smaller and fewer in number with the β-glucuronidase reaction. They were lowest in number with the β-galactosidase reaction.
3. For each enzyme a dual localization was observed which gave rise to a circadian pattern in the staining background of the entire cytoplasm.
4. These circadian variations did not occur synchronously when the histochemical reactions were applied to sections of the same livers: each marker enzyme demon-

strated maximal and minimal lysosomal and extralysosomal activity at different clock hours.
5. Irrespective of the marker enzymes used, circadian variations were manifested in the form of three main types of lysosomal appearances as illustrated in Fig. 12. (1) Numerous, relatively small, and sharply configured granules outlined the bile canaliculi. (2) Fewer, but larger, strongly reacting granules were located near the bile canaliculi. (3) Very few weakly reacting bodies were seen; they were frequently ill-defined in shape or localization, thus giving the impression of being the result of a very poor technique.
6. Circannual influences drastically modified the rhythm of lysosomal enzymes in two respects. (1) The overall staining intensity as well as the extent of the circadian variation differed with season. This was confirmed by biochemical measurements on the same livers, likewise demonstrating significantly different mean circadian activities (mesors) and amplitudes between seasons. (2) The inter-circadian phases of high and low activity were found to systematically vary over the year (Table 1).

These results clearly indicate that the population of lysosomes is heterogeneous

Acid
Phosphatase   A-Esterase β-Glucuronidase

07.00

16.00

22.00

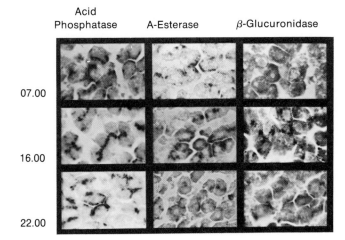

Fig. 12. Lysosomes revealed by three different marker enzymes. Note the asynchrony in the lysosomal appearance. (From von Mayersbach 1981.)

Table 1. *Biochemical Evaluations of Whole Liver Homogenates (Male Wistar Han Rats).*

	Exp. group	n	ANOVA p(F) ≦	r_c	24-hr Mean	SD	Δ ST–LD[a] p(t) ≦	Amplitude % 24-hr mean +	−	Total
Acid phosphatase										
January	ST	53	0.335	0.709	683.89	82.36	0.045	5.67	9.74	15.41
	LD	54	0.091		646.91	104.90		17.15	10.62	27.77
April	ST	54	0.0001	0.821	660.41	149.27	0.086	26.94	19.80	46.74
	LD	54	0.002		701.69	91.18		11.97	13.28	25.25
June	ST	54	0.0001	0.366	581.83	159.07	0.001	38.90	26.81	65.71
	LD	54	0.0001		694.39	190.41		49.85	31.03	80.88
September	ST	54	0.0001	0.197	565.55	142.30	0.161 n.s.	25.58	38.54	64.12
	LD	54	0.002		601.56	122.33		23.31	28.62	51.93
β-Glucuronidase										
January	ST	54	0.0001	0.986	42.89	18.42	0.649 n.s.	57.79	67.81	125.60
	LD	54	0.0001		41.37	16.17		41.82	59.29	101.11
April	ST	54	0.0001	0.584	37.90	7.49	0.84 n.s.	37.20	18.68	55.88
	LD	54	0.018		37.63	6.41		15.97	16.18	32.15
June	ST	54	0.0001	−0.365	32.05	5.85	0.23 n.s.	10.67	20.47	31.14
	LD	54	0.001		33.41	6.03		21.73	16.41	38.14
September	ST	54	0.0001	0.923	30.34	8.67	0.028	30.94	41.33	72.27
	LD	54	0.0001		34.03	8.51		31.53	38.14	69.67
Total esterase										
January	ST	54	0.0001	0.928	578.66	58.27	0.033	8.88	12.47	21.35
	LD	54	0.0001		607.03	77.09		12.56	14.77	27.33
April	ST	54	0.0001	0.787	422.50	97.54	0.063	46.17	25.76	71.93
	LD	54	0.0001		460.86	113.71		44.92	29.89	74.81
June	ST	54	0.0001	0.338	430.50	63.11	0.360 n.s.	17.07	15.76	32.83
	LD	54	0.0001		421.33	39.73		10.92	8.07	18.99
September	ST	54	0.001	0.597	561.67	68.81	0.008	13.35	9.77	23.12
	LD	54	0.0001		597.24	67.43		16.15	11.63	27.78

[a] n.s. = not significant.

Note: Group LD refers to animals kept under a conventional 12:12 hour LD system = control group (light 0600–1800); ST refers to experimental groups subjected to a staggered light system; n = number of animals investigated; p(F) = rhythm detection by analysis of variance = ANOVA; r_c = correlation coefficient group LD:ST (index of rhythm adjustment); ST-LD = difference of 24-hour mean values and statistical significance according to Student (t-) test; Amplitude = deviation in percent of 24-hr mean, + at peak time, − at trough time.

Source: von Mayersbach (1981).

at least with respect to the temporal pattern of enzyme activity. This heterogeneity is underlined by a distinct response of the different lysosomes to experimental challenges such as starvation and drug action. From a technical point of view, these observations indicate lysosomes cannot be revealed by tracing just a single marker enzyme. Consequently, it seems appropriate to specify lysosomes according to the marker enzymes used for their recognition:

phosphatasosomes, esterasosomes, glucuronidasosomes, etc.

Our studies (Groh and von Mayersbach 1981b) reveal that the periodic occurrence of extralysosomal activities during the 24-hr cycle is not due to technical artifact. At some circadian stages, even with improved methods such as membrane techniques generally considered capable of avoiding diffusion artifacts, the extralysosomal activities are more pronounced than those observable in classical tissue preparations in which enzyme activities are quenched by chemical fixation. Here, it should be stated that with respect to the concept of the cytogenesis of lysosomes, according to which the enzymes are synthesized in the ER, such extralysosomal activities are to be expected; the periodic appearance of marked RER-tubules (Uchiyama et al. 1981; see Fig. 13) found in our ultracytochemical study gives strong support for this concept.

Golgi Apparatus.   By applying special fixation and staining methods, the Golgi apparatus can be visualized in light microscopy preparations. The Golgi apparatus appears as a network of tubuli which is especially well developed in secretory cells. Electron microscopy has revealed that each cell possesses a Golgi apparatus composed of flat, discoidal cisternae and sacculi of smooth-surfaced membranes arranged in parallel, interconnecting with the ER.

The Golgi apparatus is involved in the production of secretions and in the cytogenesis of lysosomes. In both cases its function consists of packaging products synthesized in the ER. For secretion these products usually are modified by the addition of carbohydrates. In a glycoprotein-secreting cell, for example, the protein portion is synthesized in the RER and subsequently transported to the Golgi apparatus; there the carbohydrate is synthesized and added to the protein. The complete glycoprotein is then enveloped by a membrane, sequestered from the Golgi apparatus, and transported to the cell surface in the form of secretory granules.

Despite the many studies concerned with function-related changes, only recent ob-

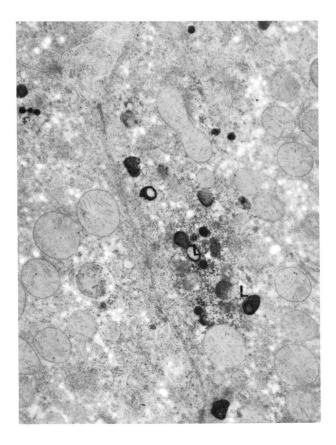

Fig. 13. Extralysosomal phosphatase activity as seen at the ultra-cytochemical level. Next to the lysosomes (L), reaction product is also localized in the ground plasm and attached to the ER. (From Uchiyama et al. 1981, reproduced with permission.)

servations indicate that the Golgi apparatus is subjected to circadian variations. This was shown in an ultracytochemical study on TPPase (thiamine pyrophosphatase) by Uchiyama et al. (1982). TPPase is regarded as an exquisite marker enzyme for the Golgi apparatus. Peaks of activity in rat hepatocytes occurred at both daily transitions from light to darkness and vice versa. At these times strong enzyme reactions were observed in almost all cisternae of *expanded* Golgi apparatus. During those time spans corresponding to middark and midlight, TPPase activity was generally lower and only a few, if any, of the lamellae of the *shrunken* and round-shaped Golgi complexes (Fig. 14) gave a positive reaction. In the rat liver, TPPase also was highly active in the walls of the bile canaliculi and, to a lesser extent, in the ER. At

these two sites, however, no clear circadian variation in activities was observed.

Cell Membrane. The cytoplasm is bordered by a membrane (cell membrane or plasma membrane, also known as the plasmalemma) which is visible only by electron microscope. The cell border visible in light microscopy preparations of several cell types actually is a rim of condensed cytoplasm, or exoplasm, underlying the cell membranes which is involved in transport processes. 5'-nucleotidase (5'adenosin-mono-phosphatase or AMP-A or EC 3.1.3.5) is regarded as an exquisite marker enzyme of plasma membranes, but confusion exists still about its reaction at other cellular sites. AMP-A activity found in the nuclei, nucleoli, and lysosomes has frequently been questioned. It is widely as-

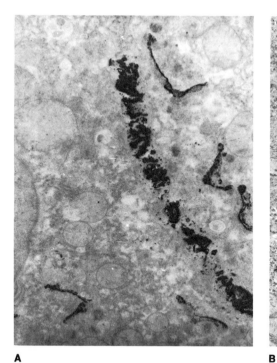

A

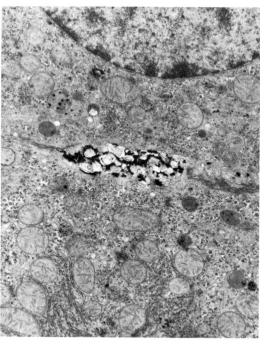

B

Fig. 14. TPPase reaction in Golgi apparatus. **A**: large and expanded Golgi apparatus showing strong TPPase activity at 2100. **B**: Golgi apparatus at 0500. Only a few spots of the reaction product are found in a small number of lamellae by which the Golgi apparatus is not clearly marked. (From Uchiyama et al. 1982.)

sumed that these sites of activity represent artifacts caused either by inadequate technique, nonspecific enzyme action, and/or nonspecific absorption of lead ions used as an indicator of the histochemical reaction for the detection of AMP-A. In a series of studies primarily concerned with the histochemical and biochemical technology of AMP-A estimation, prominent and systematic circadian variations were found (Klaushofer et al. 1979; Klaushofer and von Mayersbach 1979; von Mayersbach and Klaushofer 1979). Quantitative radiochemical analysis revealed that (1) the AMP-A activity of rat liver homogenates varies significantly during the 24-hr period, with a peak at 1300 and a nadir at 2200 for animals maintained on L(0600–1800):D(1800–0600); (2) AMP-A is consistently located in the membranes of the bile canaliculi and in the blood vessels exhibiting circadian variation in activities; and (3) additional activity is demonstrable in the nuclear membrane, nucleoli, and lysosomes during the dark span (Fig. 15).

Based on the tissue techniques applied in these studies, it can be concluded that the location of AMP-A activity at sites other than the cell membrane is caused neither by enzyme displacement nor by the nonspecific absorption of lead ions. Since in addition the possible action of nonspecific phosphatases on the substrate was excluded by proof of specificity using inhibitors, the different sites of AMP-A activity have to be considered as real and as an expression of the circadian turnover of hepatocytes.

Brush Border. Cells specialized for reabsorption, such as the enterocytes of the intestine, bear on their surface a brush border consisting of cylindrical cytoplasmic projections termed "microvilli," by which the surface area is greatly enlarged. The brush border zone is the site where a variety of enzymes involved in active transport are found. Lojda et al. (1976) investigated the intestinal enzymes of guinea pigs at different times over 24 hr using biochemical and histochemical means (Fig. 16). They dis-

covered statistically significant circadian variations in the activities of the brush border enzymes—alkaline phosphatase, amino peptidase, trehalase, and saccharase. These circadian variations were more pronounced in starved animals than in animals fed *ad libitum*. This observation is in accordance with the results obtained by Malis et al. (1977), who investigated the rhythmicity of several enzymes in the duodenum, jejunum, and pancreas of the guinea pig.

Paraplasm. The terms paraplasm or paraplasmic structures refer to various kinds of nonliving substances stored in the cytoplasm. These substances either serve as energy sources, in the case of glycogen and fat, or they play a role in other more specific biological functions as exemplified by melanin in the pigmented epithelium of the retina. The high-amplitude circadian rhythm in livers of animals fed *ad libitum*, first observed by Forsgren in 1928 using chemical determinations and by Holmgren in 1936 using histological stainings, can be regarded as the historical initiation of modern chronobiology. The circadian variations of liver glycogen will be discussed extensively in the subsequent section.

Functional Morphology

In the previous section of this chapter, the specific functions of the various cell components were outlined and evidence for circadian differences in their activities—as far as established—were reviewed. An economy of metabolic processes and the achievement of optimal cellular function can only be accomplished by a spatial arrangement of organelles and other components within the cell. Some intracellular organizations are regarded as typical for a number of organ-specific cells, e.g., the basal striation of the serous gland cell (parotid, pancreas), which is caused by the arrangement of its ergastoplasm. But it is also the experience of every histologist that the standard appearance of a certain cell type, as depicted in textbooks, cannot al-

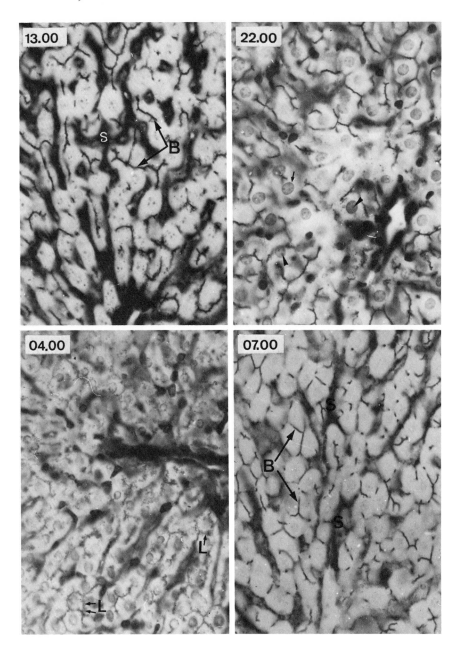

Fig. 15. Circadian variations of AMP-A activity in the rat liver. During the light period (0700 and 1300), AMP-A activity appears only in the bile canaliculi (B) and walls of sinusoids (S). During the dark span (2200 and 0400), additional activities are found in the nuclear membrane and nucleoli (*arrows*) and in the lysosomes (L) bordering the bile canaliculi. (From von Mayersbach and Klaushofer 1979.)

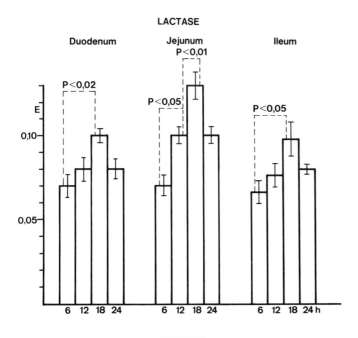

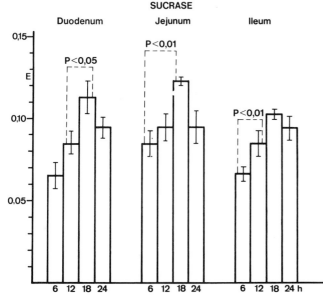

Fig. 16. Circadian variations of enzyme activities in guinea pig intestinal mucosa. The bars represent the histophotometric evaluation of histochemical reactions of the brush border zone. (Reproduced by courtesy of Prof. Lojda, Prague.)

ways be achieved. Pitfalls in attaining such are ascribed either to technical failures, postmortal changes, interindividual variances, or species-specific and sexual differences.

Since many incompatible biochemical processes are involved in cellular energy metabolism (Selkov 1979), it might be anticipated that not all of them can be executed within the cell at the same time and place. Therefore, it seems likely that alternating qualitative, quantitative, and spatial rearrangements of the organelles must take place in a fixed temporal sequence in order to cope with the necessary complex metabolic demands of life.

In fact, circadian rearrangements of the cellular inventory have been found and appear to be correlated with circadian variations in cellular functions, thus supporting and satisfying the aforementioned theoretical considerations and premises. Moreover, the extent of the observed cytological variations documented over 24 hr not only explains the discrepancies between findings sometimes reported in nonchronobiologic studies, but indicates that the "ideal" appearance of several cell types as given in textbooks represents only a characteristic state of a certain circadian phase—obviously that observed during the usual work hours of investigators in laboratories during which materials are harvested for investigation.

The consecutive phases of synthesis, storage, utilization, and depletion in the acinar cells of the submandibular gland of rats were demonstrated by Albegger et al. (1973) and Albegger and Müller (1973a,b). At the beginning of the rat's resting phase (about 0600), the acinar cells exhibit a well-developed RER representing the classical basal ergastoplasmic configuration (Fig. 17). The nuclei are large and contain a big nucleolus; the Golgi apparatus is expanded; there are only a few secretory granules in the cytoplasm. Shortly before the nocturnally active rats become active and commence feeding, around 1800, a radically different picture is exhibited. The ER is condensed to a small basal rim, the nuclei are small and almost pycnotic, the nucleoli are hardly visible, the Golgi apparatus are condensed, and the cytoplasm is stuffed with big secretory granules and large fusing secretory vacuoles.

Using morphometric methods, Müller et al. (1977) demonstrated circadian variations in the cell organelles of the exocrine pancreas. Differences in secretory states are well-known. Early histologists described phases of production and rest in secretory cells with which they correlated changes in the Golgi apparatus. Definitely new, how-

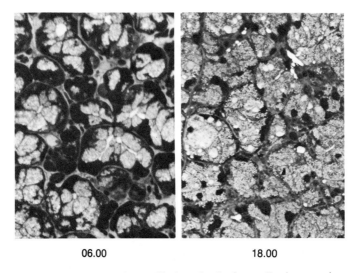

06.00   18.00

Fig. 17. Circadian variations in the submandibular gland of rats. In the morning, after the feeding span of the rats, this salivary gland exhibits the classic feature of serous gland acini exemplified by a strong ergastoplasm localized in the basal parts of the cell (**left**). Actually, these cells are exhausted by depletion of their secretory products utilized for fermentation of food stuffs. At the onset of the feeding span (evening, **right**), the cells are packed with secretory granules, some confluing to big secretory vacuoles. In this manner, the cells show similarities with mucous glands. The nuclei are condensed and pycnotic-like; the ER is reduced to a small rim at the base of the cells (semi-thin sections stained with toluidine blue in the original). (Reproduced by courtesy of Doz. Dr. K. Albegger, Salzburg.)

ever, is the knowledge that in the whole organ this turnover proceeds in a perfectly synchronized, circadian manner. Recently, it was shown that this type of functional temporal order is valid also for the endocrine pancreas. Thus, Polak et al. (1975) observed with immunohistochemical methods a statistically significant circadian rhythmicity of insulin and glucagon content, respectively, in the β- and α-cells of the islets of Langerhans.

Such successive on–off states of activity and rest in monofunctional cells seem quite feasible. Theoretically, it is conceivable that a structural reorganization of multifunctional cells is necessary to cope with different metabolic tasks. A state of functional activity for one particular process at one circadian stage coincides with a state of functional rest for another process at the same time and vice versa. This hypothesis is supported by the observed circadian fluctuations of glycogen and albumin metabolism in the liver, fluctuations which are correlated with ultramorphologic changes of enzymes involved in glycogen synthesis and degradation. In elaborate studies, Müller et al. (1966) and Müller (1970, 1971a–c) investigated the circadian changes of the electron microscopic structure and histochemistry of hepatocytes as well as the effects of experimental challenges such as starvation and phenobarbital intoxication over a 24-hr period. It was found that the hepatocytes of rats undergo successive changes between two extremes of cytological organization during each 24 hr. These are shown in Figs. 18 and 19. At the time of high glycogen content, which coincides in time with the interval between the end of the dark span until the first third of the light span for animals kept in L(0600–1800): D(1800–0600), the hepatocytes exhibit a structural organization stereotypically depicted as typical for the liver cell in all textbooks and electron microscopy atlases. That is, the rough endoplasmic reticulum (RER) forms stacks of tubules which are arranged in parallel and are rich in ribosomes, and which exhibit G6P activity. The

bile canaliculi appear narrow, and their ATPase activity is relatively low. This cellular arrangement is in great contrast with the cellular appearance exhibited at the time of the glycogen minimum which occurs at the end of the light and the beginning of the dark span. Only a very few glycogen granules of low molecular weight, mainly β-granules, can be seen. The stacks of the RER have almost disappeared, but single tubules of RER enwrap the mitochondria. The SER and the Golgi apparatus are very clearly visible at this time. The bile canaliculi are wide with short microvilli and exhibit high ATPase activity. Quantitative measurements of the albumin content by radial immunodiffusion (von Mayersbach 1978) demonstrate that the maximal albumin content coincides with the just defined morphologic state hitherto not described in the literature. Even during this stage some stacks of RER are present. The complete disappearance of the RER stacks occurs only when the circadian trough of the glycogen content rhythm is very low (0.8 mg/100 mg liver wet weight). Uchiyama and von Mayersbach (1981) reported that the ER stacks do not disappear completely unless the lowest glycogen content recorded during the 24-hour period is below an average minimum level of 2.2 mg/100 mg liver wet weight.

These ultramorphologic changes which are easily visible are not only accompanied by circadian changes in liver glycogen content; they also are paralleled by circadian variations in the activity of certain enzymes—glycogen synthetase and phosphorylase (Müller and Preuss 1976; Preuss 1977) as well as glucose-6-phosphatase (Müller 1971b). The histochemical analysis of these components reveals that the periphery of the liver lobules is the main site of glycogen turnover, whereas the central portions remain relatively stable.

Müller (1971c) observed that these typical morphologic changes continue even during prolonged (5-day) starvation. Under such experimental conditions, glycogen rhythmicity persists although at a very low

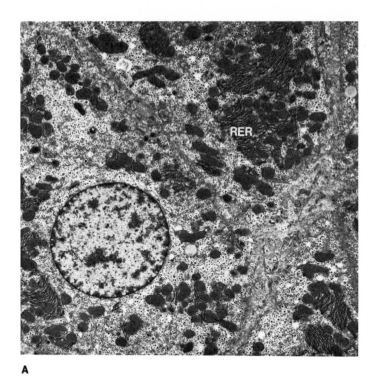

A

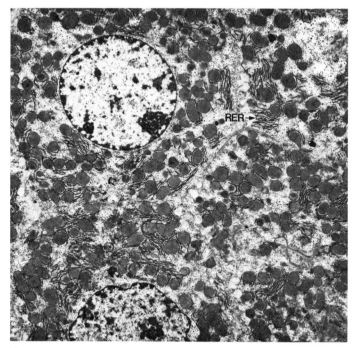

Fig. 18. Electron microscopic view of hepatocytes. **A**: At the time of high glycogen content (0700) typical stacks of RER tubules are seen arranged in parallel. **B**: At the time of the glycogen minimum (1900) the RER stacks have almost disappeared and each single mitochondrium is enwrapped by a RER tubule. (From Uchiyama and von Mayersbach 1981.)

B

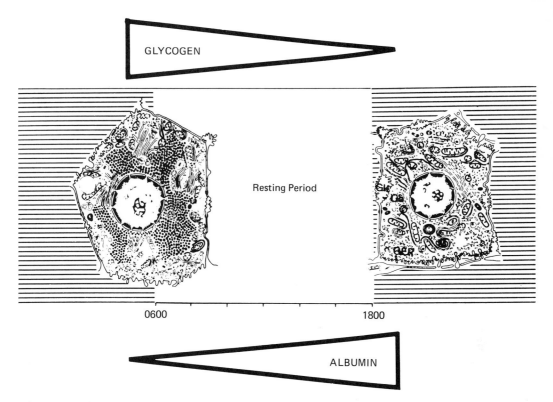

Fig. 19. Schematic illustration of the cytological reorganization and the accompanying functional changes in multifunctional cells in the liver of the rat. At the end of the activity period (onset of light), the liver cells contain their highest content of glycogen (*heavy dark dots*). The rough endoplasmic reticulum (RER) forms stacks of tubules arranged in parallel which are rich in ribosomes and exhibit strong G6P activity. Smooth endoplasmic reticulum (GER) is hardly visible. The bile canaliculi are narrow and their ATPase activity is relatively low. At the end of the resting period (onset of darkness) few glucogen granules are apparent. The stacks of RER have disappeared; their tubules now enwrap mitochondria. GER and Golgi apparatus (Go) become clearly visible. The bile canaliculi (Gk) are very wide and exhibit strong ATPase activity. At this time the albumin level in the liver is at its highest. These circadian features are not a direct consequence of food intake; they appear after deprivation of food for 4 days while also the glycogen circadian rhythm persists although with a reduced mesor. (Redrawn from electron microscopic investigations of Müller 1971c.)

level, as shown with chemical-quantitative methods (Holmgren 1938; Haus and Halberg 1966; Müller 1971c). Chiakulas and Scheving (1965) demonstrated persistence of the glycogen circadian rhythm in the liver of salamanders after 1 month of continuous food deprivation. This observation was confirmed by Sauerbier and von Mayersbach (1976) on the long-term "natural" starvation of hibernating dormice (*Glis glis*) restricted from food by their natural

continuous sleep for 3 months, during which the body temperature declined to between 3° and 6°C. The circadian activities of acid and alkaline phosphatase, nonspecific esterase, SDH, and cytochrome-c-oxidase in the epithelium of the duodenum varied almost in the same manner as that seen in non-hibernating dormice. Only mean (24-hr) level differences were found. The activity of the hydrolases was higher in nonhibernating animals, while that of the dehydrogenases was much higher in hibernating animals not having consumed food for three months.

Circadian rearrangement of the cellular inventory assures a sequence of cellular compartmentalizations so that incompatible processes involved with complex metabolic activities can occur within a single cell. In addition, the temporal organization of metabolic processes makes understandable the observation that an appropriate cellular response to an external stimulus can only be exerted during a defined span of the circadian system. This is underlined by experiments showing that circadian changes in responsiveness do not only occur in an entire organism, with its complex capacity for systemic regulation, but also in isolated organs. Rebolledo and Gagliardino (1971b) and Gagliardino and Rebolledo (1972) studied the response of isolated muscle of the diaphragm to an in vitro application of insulin by measuring the ^{14}C-leucine incorporation into the protein. The incorpo-

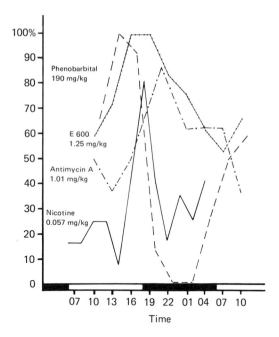

Fig. 20. Circadian variation of mortality rates of animal groups at different times following single treatments with certain poisons in fixed doses. (From von Mayersbach 1978.)

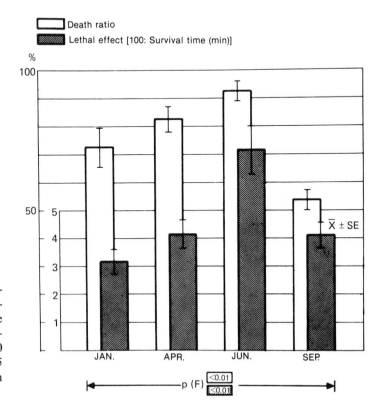

Fig. 21. Seasonal modification of the 24-hr mean mortality and of the lethal effect due to the intraperitoneal application of identical doses of E 600 (paraoxon) in a dosage of 1.25 mg/kg. (From von Mayersbach 1978.)

ration of protein is expected to be enhanced by insulin. Diaphragms were harvested from different groups of mice at 4-hr intervals during a 24-hr span and incubated both with and without the addition of insulin to the medium. Significant circadian fluctuations were found when the protein-specific activity values were plotted as a function of time. In studies without the addition of insulin, crests and troughs occurred at 0000 and 0800, respectively. The effectiveness of insulin on protein synthesis varied greatly. No effect was observed at 0000, while a large one was observed at 2000. Similar differences were found by Pessacq and Gagliardino (1975a) for the in vitro synthesis of glycogen after incubating rat diaphragms in a glucose-rich medium. In addition, the authors noticed quantitative differences between experiments conducted in September and December—spring and summer, respectively, in the Southern Hemisphere where the research was performed (La Plata, Argentina). The results of these in vitro studies are supported by in vivo studies on the metabolism of skeletal muscle of rats following insulin administration (Rebolledo and Gagliardino 1970, 1971a; Pessacq et al. 1971; Gagliardino and Pessacq 1974; Pessacq and Gagliardino 1975b).

From the findings presented in this chapter, it is evident that circadian and circannual changes of the ultrastructure are correlated with qualitative differences in cellular activities. These rhythmicities are so significant biologically, they greatly affect the manner in which toxic substances (Figs. 20 and 21) and medications are tolerated giving rise to both circadian and circannual chronotoxicities. Moreover, such rhythmic changes in cellular structure and function form the basis for understanding circadian and circannual rhythm-dependent differences in the metabolism and/or effects of medications and nutrients.

References

Abicht, J, and Philippens, KMH (1973) Circadian rhythmicity of liver DNA in rats. Int J Chronobiol 1:317.

Abicht, J (1976) *Die Circadianrhythmik des DNS-Gehaltes in der Rattenleber. Neue Untersuchungen unter Berücksichtigung der methodischen Fehlerquellen und der Circadianrhythmen anderer Leberwerte,* Dissertation (M.D.-Thesis). Hannover: Medizinische Hochschule (West Germany).

Aithal, HN, and Ramasarma, T (1971) Changes in the liver mitochondrial oxidation of succinate during cold-exposure. Biochem J 123:677–682.

Albegger, KW, and Müller, O (1973a) Der tagesrhythmische Sekretionszyklus der Glandula submandibularis der Ratte. Arch klin exp Ohren-Nasen-u. Kehlkopfheilkd 204:27–56.

Albegger, KW, and Müller, O (1973b) Zur Circadianstruktur der Glandula submandibularis. Arch klin exp Ohren-Nasen-u Kehlkopfheilkd 205:122–125.

Albegger, KW, Müller, O, and Albegger, C (1973) Quantitative microscopy of the circadian secretory cycle of the rat parotid gland. Int J Chronobiol 1:317–318.

Ashkenazi, YE, Ramot, B, Brok-Simoni, F, and Holtzman, F (1973) Blood leucocyte enzyme activities. I. Diurnal rhythm in normal individuals. J Interdiscipl Cycle Res 4:193–205.

Ashkenazi, YE, Goldman, B, and Dotan, A (1975) Rhythmic variation of sex chromatin and glucose-6-phosphate dehydrogenase activity in human oral mucosa during the menstrual cycle. Acta Cytologica 19:62–66.

Barbiroli B, Moruzzi, MS, Monti, MG, and Tadolini, B (1973) Diurnal rhythmicity of mammalian DNA-dependent RNA polymerase activities I and II: Dependence on food intake. Biochem Biophys Res Comm 54:62–68.

Barnum, CP, Jardetzky, CD, and Halberg, F (1958) Time relations among metabolic and morphologic 24 hours changes in mouse liver. Amer J Physiol 195:301–310.

Bhattacharya, R (1977) Circadian differences of lysosomes and their enzymes. Leopoldina Symposion Die Zeit und das Leben, Halle/Saale, März, 1975. Nova Acta Leopoldina 225:171–179.

Bhattacharya, R, and von Mayersbach, H (1976) Histochemistry of circadian changes of some lysosomal enzymes in rat liver. XVII Symposion Ges Histochemie, Bozen, 1974. Acta histochem Suppl 16:109–116.

Bollweg, L, and Maskos, S (1979) *Zirkadianrhythmik der DNS-Konzentration in Milz und*

Thymus von Ratten, Dissertation. Hannover: Medizinische Hochschule.

Burns, ER, and Scheving, LE (1975) Circadian influence on the wave form of the frequency of labeled mitoses in mouse corneal epithelium. Cell Tissue Kinet 8:61–66.

Caspersson, T, and Holmgren, H (1934) Variationen der Kerngrösse während der verschiedenen Phasen der Leberarbeit. Anat Anz 79:53–59.

Chiakulas, JJ, and Scheving, LE (1965) Periodicity in liver glycogen of urodele larvae. Comp Biochem Physiol 17:87–91.

Dallman, PR, Spirito, RA, and Siimes, MA (1974) Diurnal patterns of DNA synthesis in the rat: Modification by diet and feeding schedule. J Nutr 104:1234–1241.

Daoust, R (1958) The cell population of liver tissue and the cytological reference bases. Am Inst Biol Sci Pub 4:3–10.

De Duve, C (1969) The lysosome in retrospect. In: Dingle, JT, and Fell, HB, eds, *Lysosomes in Biology and Pathology,* Vol. I. Amsterdam: North Holland, pp. 3–40.

Döring, R, and Rensing, L (1973) Circadian rhythm of different RNA-fractions in rat liver and the effect of cyclohexamide. Comp Biochem Physiol B45:285–290.

Earp, HS III (1974) Glucocorticoid regulation of transcriptions. The role of physiologic concentrations of adrenal glucocorticoids in the diurnal variation of rat liver chromatin template availability. Biochim Biophys Acta 340:95–107.

Echave Llanos, JM, De Vaccaro, MEE, and Surur, JM (1970) 24-hour variations in DNA of the liver in young adult male mice. J Interdiscipl Cycle Res 1:161–171.

Echave Llanos, JM, Aloisso, MD, Souto, M, Balduzzi, R, and Surur, JM (1971) Circadian variations of DNA synthesis, mitotic activity and cell size of hepatocyte population in young immature male mouse growing liver. Virch Archiv (Cell Path.) 8:309–317.

Edmunds, LN (1978) Clocked cell cycle clocks. Implications toward chronopharmacology and aging. In: Samis, HV, and Capobianco, S, eds, *Aging and Biological Rhythms.* New York-London: Plenum Press, pp. 125–184.

Ehret CF (1974) The sense of time: evidence for its molecular basis in the eukaryotic gene-action system. Ad Biol Med Phy 15:47–77.

Eling, W (1967) The circadian rhythm of nucleic acids. In: von Mayersbach, H, ed, *The Cellu-lar Aspects of Biorhythms.* Berlin-Heidelberg-New York: Springer-Verlag, pp. 105–114.

Forsgren, E (1928) Mikroskopische Untersuchungen über die Gallenbildung in den Leberzellen. Z Zellforsch 6:647–688.

Gagliardino, JJ, and Pessacq, MT (1974) Diurnal variations in the action of insulin on muscle glycogen synthesis. J Endocrinol 61:171–177.

Gagliardino, JJ, and Rebolledo, OR (1972) Hormonal control of protein synthesis in muscle: an approach through the study of its circadian rhythm. Horm Metab Res 4:278–279.

Glick, D (1961a) *Quantitative Chemical Techniques in Histo- and Cytochemistry,* Vol. I. New York-London: Wiley, p. 58.

Glick, D, Ferguson, RB, Greenberg, LJ, and Halberg, F (1961b) Circadian studies on succinic dehydrogenase pantothenate and biotin of rodent adrenal. Amer J Physiol 200:811–814.

Goodwin, BC (1963) *Temporal Organization in Cells. A Dynamic Theory of Cellular Processes.* London: Academic Press.

Groh, V, and von Mayersbach, H (1981a) Histochemical tracing of lysosomal enzymes. Improved preparation technique for acid phosphatase, β-glucuronidase, acid-β-galactosidase and arylesterase in rat liver. Acta Histochem 69:1–11.

Groh, V, and von Mayersbach, H (1981b) Enzymatic and functional heterogeneity of lysosomes. Cell Tissue Res 214:613–621.

Halberg, F (1957) Young NH-mice for the study of mitosis in intact liver. Experientia 13:502–503.

Hardeland, R (1973) Diurnal variations in inducibility of hepatic tyrosine aminotransferase. Int J Biochem 4:357–364.

Hardeland, R, and Stephan, E (1974) Diurnal rhythms and post-transcriptional regulation of hepatic tyrosine aminotransferase and tryptophan oxygenase. J Interdiscipl Cycle Res 5:247–255.

Hastings, JW, and Keyman, A (1965) Molecular aspects of circadian systems. In: Aschoff, J, ed, *Circadian Clocks.* Amsterdam: North Holland Publ. Co., pp. 167–182.

Hastings, W, and Schweiger, HG (Eds) (1976) *The Molecular Basis of Circadian Rhythms* (Dahlem Konferenzen). D-1 Berlin (W. Germany): Abakon Verlag.

Haus, E, and Halberg, F (1966) Persisting circadian rhythm in hepatic glycogen of mice during inanition and dehydration. Experientia 22:113–114.

Holmgren, H (1936) *Studien über 24-stundenrhythmische Variationen des Darm-, Lungen- und Leberfettes,* Dissertation. Helsingfors.

Holmgren, H (1938) 24-Stundenvariationen des Gewichtes der Leber, Lunge und Milz der grossen weissen Ratte (*Mus norvegicus albinus*). Gegenbaurs Morphol Jahrb 81:653–668.

Horvath, G (1963a) Biorhythmische Veränderungen der Phosphorproteine und Nucleinsäuren. 8th Int. Congr. Biological Rhythms, Hamburg.

Horvath, G (1963b) Naturally occurring variations in rat liver DNA content. Nature 200:261.

Horvath, G (1964) Quantitativer und qualitativer Nucleinsäurebestand normaler Rattenorgane. II Int Kongr Histo-Cytochem, Frankfurt/Main, 1964. Berlin-Göttingen-Heidelberg: Springer-Verlag, p. 137.

Iemhoff, WGJ, and Hülsmann, WC (1971) Development of mitochondrial enzyme activities in rat small-intestinal epithelium. Eur J Biochem 23:429–434.

Jackson, B (1959) Time-associated variations of mitotic activity in livers of young rats. Anat Rec 134:365–377.

Jerusalem, Ch, Eling, W, and Yap, P (1970) Histochemische und elektronenmikroskopische Veränderungen der Leberzelle im Tagesrhythmus und unter experimentellen Bedingungen. Acta Histochem 36:168.

Klaushofer, K, and von Mayersbach, H (1979) Freeze substituted tissue in 5'-nucleotidase histochemistry. Comparative histochemical and biochemical investigations. J Histochem Cytochem 27:1582–1587.

Klaushofer, K, Mayer, D, Hummel, W, and von Mayersbach, H (1979) A double-labelling radioassay for the determination of 5'-nucleotidase activity. Enzyme 24:77–84.

Klima, J, Pfaller, W, Tiefenbrunner, F, and Plattner, H (1971) Respiratory activity and stereological organization of the chondriome of mouse liver: an attempt of correlation during growth. Cytobiól. 3:351–359.

Laguens, RP, and Gomez–Dumm, CLA (1967) Fine structure of myocardial mitochondria in rats after exercise for one-half to two hours. Cir Res 21:271–279.

Letnansky, K (1974) Zirkadiane Rhythmen bei der Phosphorylierung von Kernproteinen und ihre Bedeutung für die Zellproliferation. Wien Klin Wschr 86:250–252.

Lojda, Z, Malis, F, Havrankova, E, and Ruzickova, M (1976) Circadian rhythms of enzyme activities of rat and guinea pig enterocytes. Cs Gastroent Vyz 30:257.

Malis, F, Lojda, Z, Fric, P, and Slaby, J (1977) Zirkadianrhythmus einiger Verdauungsenzyme des Dünndarms und des Pankreas bei Meerschweinchen. III. Bilaterales Symp. CSSR-DDR. *Fortschritte der Gastroenterologie.* Karlovy Vary, pp. 182–183.

Mäusle, E, and Fröhlke, M (1971) Geschlechtsabhängige Grössenunterschiede der Mitochondrien in der Zona fasciculata der Nebennierenrinde der Ratte. Experientia 27:700–701.

von Mayersbach, H (1967) Seasonal influences on biological rhythms of standardized laboratory animals. In: von Mayersbach, H, ed, *The Cellular Aspects of Biorhythms.* Heidelberg: Springer-Verlag, pp. 87–99.

von Mayersbach, H (1978) Die Zeitstruktur des Organismus. Auswirkungen auf zelluläre Leistungsfähigkeit und Medikamentenempfindlichkeit. Arzneim-Forsch 28:1824–1836.

von Mayersbach, H (1981) Chronobiological aspects in histochemistry. In: Graumann, W, and Neumann, K, eds. *Handbuch der Histochemie,* Bd. 1, Teil 4. Stuttgart: G Fischer.

von Mayersbach, H, and Bhattacharya, R (1977) Circumannual variations of liver lysosomes of rats living under constant environmental conditions. Chronobiologia 4:131.

von Mayersbach, H, and Klaushofer, K (1979) Circadian variations of 5'-nucleotidase activity in rat liver. Cell Mol Biol 24:73–79.

von Mayersbach, H, and Reale, E (1973) *Grundriss der Histologie des Menschen, Bd. 1, Allgemeine Histologie.* Stuttgart: G Fischer Verlag.

von Mayersbach, H, and Yap, P (1965) Tagesrhythmische Schwankungen der Leberesterase. Histochemie 5:297–302.

von Mayersbach, H, Philippens, K, and Yap, P (1964) Die Einflüsse biologischer Tagesschwankungen auf fermenthistochemische Untersuchungen. II. Internat Congr Histochem Cytochem, 1964. Berlin-Göttingen-Heidelberg: Springer-Verlag, pp. 139–140.

Milner, AJ (1972) Corticotrophin-induced differentiation of mitochondria in rat adrenal cortical cells grown in primary tissue-culture—effects of ethidium bromide. J. Endocrinol 52:541–548.

Müller, O (1970) Die tageszeitliche Struktur der Leber und ihre Beziehung zur tagesrhythmischen Wirkung von Barbituraten. IX. Int Anatomen Kongreß, Leningrad.

Müller, O (1971a) Circadian rhythmicity in response to barbiturates. Naunyn Schmied Arch Pharmacol 270(Suppl.):R99.

Müller, O (1971b). Zur elektronenmikroskopischen Histochemie der Glucose-6-Phosphatase. Acta Histochem Suppl. 10:141–146.

Müller, O (1971c). *Die Circadianstruktur der Leber*. Hannover: Habilitationsschrift, Medizinische Hochschule.

Müller, O, and Preuss, D (1976) Circadiane Histochemie der Glykogen-Synthetase und -Phosphorylase in der Leber der Maus. XVII. Symp Ges Histochemie, Bozen, 1974. Acta Histochem Suppl. 16:145–147.

Müller, O, Jerusalem, C, and von Mayersbach, H (1966) Die Ultrastruktur der physiologischen Tagesschwankungen in Leberzellen von Ratten. Z Zellforsch 69:438–451.

Müller, O, Blatti, HR, and Gerber, B (1977) *Morphometrie des circadianen Sekretionscyclus der Acinuszellen im Rattenpankreas*. Aachen: 72. Vers. Anat. Ges.

Nicolau, GY, Apostol, G, and Milcu, S (1979) Effects of pinealectomy on the RNA, DNA, and protein circadian rhythms in the rat adrenal and testis. Chronobiologia 6:136.

Novikoff, AB (1959) Cell heterogeneity within the hepatic lobule of the rat. J Histochem Cytochem 7:240–244.

Pébusque, M-J, and Seïte, R (1980) Circadian change of fibrillar centers in nucleolus of sympathetic neurons: an ultrastructural and stereological analysis. Biol Cell 37:219–222.

Pébusque, M-J, and Seïte, R (1981a) Electron microscopic studies of silver-stained proteins in nucleolar organized regions: location in nucleoli of rat sympathetic neurons during light and dark periods. J Cell Sci 51:85–94.

Pébusque, M-J, and Seïte, R (1981b) Evidence of a circadian rhythm in nucleolar components of rat superior cervical ganglion neurons with particular reference to the fibrillar centers: an ultrastructural and stereological analysis. J Ultrastruct Res 77:83–92.

Pébusque, M-J, Dupuy-Coin, A-M, Cataldo, C, Seïte, R, Bouteile, M, and Moens, P (1981a) Three-dimensional electron microscopy of the nucleolar organizer regions (NORs) in sympathetic neurons. Biol Cell 41:59–62.

Pébusque, M-J, Robaglia, A, and Seïte, R (1981b) Diurnal rhythm of nucleolar volume in sympathetic neurons of the rat superior cervical ganglion. Eur J Cell Biol 24:128–130.

Pessacq, MT, and Gagliardino, JJ (1975a) Glycogen metabolism in muscle. The circadian influence on the in vitro model. Chronobiologia 2:205–209.

Pessacq, MT, and Gagliardino, JJ (1975b) Glycogen metabolism in muscle. Its circadian and seasonal variations. Metabolism 24:737–743.

Pessacq, MT, Rebolledo, OR, and Gagliardino, JJ (1971). Circadian variations of muscle metabolites. Experentia 27:1394–1395.

Pfeifer, U (1977) Tagesrhythmik der cellulären Autophagie. Leopoldina Symposion Die Zeit und das Leben, Halle/Saale, März 1975. Nova Acta Leopoldina 225:181–187.

Philippens, K (1968) Twenty-four hour periodicity of succinodehydrogenase in rat liver. III. Int Congr Histochem Cytochem New York, pp. 206–207.

Philippens, K (1970) Tagesrhythmische Schwankungen im Succino-dehydrogenasesystem. In: Hettler, LH, ed, *Abhdlg Dtsch Akad Wiss Berlin*. Berlin: Akademie Verlag, pp. 607–610.

Philippens, K (1971) Vergleichende Untersuchungen über biochemische Aktivitätsbestimmungen an Mitochondrien und histochemischem Reaktionsausfall. Acta Histochem Suppl 10:323–332.

Philippens, K (1973) Circadian activity patterns of two rat liver mitochondrial enzymes. Succinatedehydrogenase (SDH) and α-glycerophosphate dehydrogenase (mGPDH). Int J Chronobiol 1:350.

Philippens, K (1975) Manipulation of circadian rhythms. Naunyn Schmied Arch Pharmacol 287(Suppl.):R111.

Philippens, KMH (1976) The manipulation of circadian rhythms. Arch Toxicol 36:277–303.

Philippens, K (1980) Synchronization of rhythms to meal timing. In: *Principles and Applications of Chronobiology to Shifts in Schedules, with Emphasis on Man*. Alpen aan den Rijn, The Netherlands: Sijthoff and Noordhoff Int Pub, pp. 403–416.

Philippens, KMH, and Abicht, J (1977) Tagesrhythmik des Nukleinsäure-Stoffwechsels. Leopoldina Symposion Die Zeit und das

Leben, Halle/Saale, März 1975. Nova Acta Leopoldina 225:143–147.

Pilgrim, C (1967) Autoradiographic investigations with ³H-thymidine on the influence of the diurnal rhythm on cell proliferation kinetics. In: von Mayersbach, H, ed, *The Cellular Aspects of Biorhythms*. Berlin-Heidelberg-New York: Springer-Verlag, pp. 100–104.

Polak, JM, von Mayersbach, H, Van Mourik, M, and Pearse, AGE (1975) Circadian rhythms of the endocrine pancreas: A quantitative biochemical and immunocytochemical study. Acta Hepato-gastroenterol. 22:118–122.

Potter, VR, Gebert, RA, Pitot, HC, Peraino, C, Lamar, C Jr, Lesher, S, and Morris, HP (1966) Systematic oscillations in metabolic activity in rat liver and in hepatomas. I. Morris Hepatoma No. 7793. Cancer Res 26:1547–1560.

Preuss, D (1977) *Methodologische und biologische Aspekte für den histochemischen Phosphorylase- und Synthetase-Nachweis in der Leber,* Dissertation. Hannover: Medizinische Hochschule.

Rafael, J, Hüsch, M, Stratmann, D, and Hohorst, HJ (1970) Mitochondrien aus braunem und weißem Fettgewebe: Struktur, Enzymprofil und oxidative Phosphorylierung. Hoppe-Seylers Z physiol Chem 351:1513–1523.

Rebolledo, OR, and Gagliardino, JJ (1970) Circadian rhythm in the protein and RNA of mouse diaphragm. Acta Physiol Lat Amer 20:168–170.

Rebolledo, OR, and Gagliardino, JJ (1971a) Circadian variations of DNA in mouse diaphragm. Amer J Physiol 221:1481–1483.

Rebolledo, OR, and Gagliardino, JJ (1971b) Circadian variations of the protein metabolism in muscle. J Interdiscipl Cycle Res 2:101–108.

Reith, A, and Schüler, B (1971) The ultrastructure of mitochondria in relation to the lobular distribution of hepatocytes of the normal rat. J Ultrastruct Res 36:550.

Reith, A, and Schüler, B (1972) Heterogeneity of rat liver mitochondria as indicated by differential cytochrome-oxydase activities. J Ultrastruct Res 38:206.

Riede, UN, and Rohr, HP (1970) Atypische Lebermitochondrien adaptive Sonderformen? I. Ultrastrukturell-morphologische Untersuchung. Virch Arch Abt B Zellpath 8:350–356.

Rohde, B, and Rensing, L (1973) Circadian rhythm of 3H-leucine incorporation into isolated rat liver nuclei. J Interdiscipl Cycle Res 4:303–306.

Röver, S, and Philippens, KMH (1979) Circadian rhythm of binuclear rat liver cells. Response to phase-shifted light-dark cycle. Chronobiologia 6:149.

Ruby, JR, Scheving, LE, Gray, SB, and White, K (1973) Circadian rhythm of nuclear DNA in adult rat liver. Exp Cell Res 76:136–142.

Sauerbier, I, and von Mayersbach, H (1976) Circadianrhythmisch-histochemische Untersuchungen am Dünndarmepithel von Winterschläfern. XVII. Symposion Ges. Histochemie, Bozen, 1974. Acta Histochem, Suppl. 16:155–160.

Scheving, LE (1959) Mitotic activity in the human epidermis. Anat Rec 135:7–20.

Scheving, LE, and Pauly, JE (1960) Daily mitotic fluctuations in the epidermis of the rat and their relation to variations in spontaneous activity and rectal temperature. Acta Anat 43:337–345.

Scheving, LE, and Pauly, JE (1967a) Effect of adrenalectomy, adrenal medullectomy, and hypophysectomy on the daily mitotic rhythm in the corneal epithelium of the rat. In: von Mayersbach, H, ed, *The Cellular Aspects of Biorhythms*. Berlin-Heidelberg-New York: Springer-Verlag, pp. 167–174.

Scheving, LE, and Pauly, JE (1967b) Circadian phase relationships of thymidine-³H uptake, labeled nuclei, grain counts and cell division rate in rat corneal epithelium. J Cell Biol 32:677–683.

Scheving, LE, and Pauly, JE (1973) Cellular mechanisms involving biorhythms with emphasis on those rhythms associated with the S and M stages of the cell cycle. Int J Chronobiology 1:269–286.

Scheving, LE, von Mayersbach, H, and Pauly, JE (1974a) An overview of chronopharmacology. Eur J Toxicol 7:203–227.

Scheving, LE, Dunn, JD, von Mayersbach, H, and Pauly, JE (1974b) The effect of continuous light or darkness on the rhythm of the mitotic index in the corneal epithelium of the rat. Acta Anat 88:411–423.

Schweiger, E, Wallraff, HG, and Schweiger, HG (1964) Endogenous circadian rhythm in cytoplasm of acetabularia: Influence of the nucleus. Science 146:658–659.

Selkov, EE (1979) A unifying theory of the cell mechanism. Chronobiologia 6:155.

Sestan, N (1964) Diurnal variations of 14C-leucine incorporation into proteins of isolated rat liver nuclei. Naturwissenschaften 51:371.

Steinhart, WL (1971) Diurnal rhythmicity in template activity of mouse liver chromatin. Biochim Biophys Acta 228:301–305.

Stenram, U (1969) The ultrastructure of the liver in thyroid-fed rats. Z Zellforsch mikr Anat 100:402–410.

Suppan, PP (1966) Le cycle diurne hépatique. Acta Anat 65:584–593.

Sweeney, BM (1969) *Rhythmic Phenomena in Plants*. New York: Academic Press.

Thorud, E, Clausen, OPF, Aarnaes, E, and Bjerknes, R (1979) Circadian changes in cell cycle phase durations in murine epidermal basal cells. Chronobiologia 6:163.

Uchiyama, Y, and von Mayersbach, H (1981) Circadian variations of ultra-morphology and glycogen content in hepatocytes of light-manipulated rats. Gegenbaurs morphol Jahrb 127:452–463.

Uchiyama, Y, von Mayersbach, H, and Groh, V (1982) Circadian changes of thiamine pyrophosphatase activity in rat hepatocytes: A histochemical study at the electron microscopic level. Cell Mol Biol 28:245–254.

Uchiyama, Y, Groh, V, and von Mayersbach, H (1981) Different circadian variations as an indicator of heterogeneity of liver lysosomes. Histochemistry 73:321–337.

Vanden Driessche, T (1971) Les rythmes circadiens, mécanisme de régulation cellulaire. La Recherche 2:255–261.

Vanden Driessche, T (1975) Circadian rhythms and molecular biology. Biosystems 6:188–201.

Vonnahme, FJ (1974) Circadian variation in cell size and mitotic index in tissues having a relatively low proliferation rate in both normal and hypophysectomized rats. Int J Chronobiol 2:297–309.

Wilson, JW, and LeDuc, EH (1948) The occurrence and formation of binucleate and multinucleate cells and polyploid nuclei in the mouse liver. Am J Anat 82:353–391.

Young, RW (1978a) The daily rhythm of shedding and degradation of rod and cone outer segment membranes in the chick retina. Invest Ophthalm Visual Science 17:105–116.

Young, RW (1978b) Visual cells, daily rhythms and vision research. Vision Res 18:573–578.

Zaviacic, M, and Brozman, M (1978) Circadian rhythms of oxydoreductases in the rat gastric mucosa. Histochemical study. Acta Histochem 62:155–162.

Zhirnova, AA (1969) Relationships between diurnal rhythm in number of binuclear cells in rat liver and its glycogen-forming function. Byulleten "Eksperimental" noi Biologii i Meditsiny 68:98–100.

4

Chronobiology of Cell Proliferation
Implications for Cancer Chemotherapy

L. E. Scheving, J. E. Pauly, T. H. Tsai, and L. A. Scheving

Traditionally, cell proliferation within mammalian tissues has been assumed to be asynchronous or random. Numerous investigators who have studied this phenomenon have ignored the potential importance of temporal, particularly circadian, variation. Within the last 20 years, however, rhythmic change in cell proliferation has been incontrovertibly demonstrated in a variety of tissues and organs. In fetal and neonatal tissues, such variation appears to be primarily ultradian (Goodrum et al. 1974), whereas in adult tissues it also has a strong circadian component for both the S and the M phases of the cell cycle (Scheving and Pauly 1967). Furthermore, the proliferative response of cells to chemical, environmental, and hormonal stimuli also has been shown to be rhythmic, and this has important clinical implications. In spite of this evidence, some investigators continue to underestimate the importance of rhythmicity (Scheving 1981; Scheving and Pauly 1974). Circadian variation in cell proliferation in a number of tissues has been reviewed earlier (Scheving and Pauly 1973). The objective of this chapter is to consider more recent work and to demonstrate how an appreciation of such rhythms is advantageous in basic research on growth and treatment of growth-related disorders, including cancer chemotherapy.

Circadian Rhythms in Cell Proliferation and Analysis of Data for Rhythms in the Mitotic Index in Rodents

All normal tissues examined to date in adult mammals have been shown to undergo circadian variation when either the DNA synthesis (S) phase of the cell cycle or the mitotic index (M) is monitored along the 24-hr scale. Several examples of rhythms are exhibited in Figs. 1 and 2. Figure 1 illustrates chronograms of rhythms in the mitotic indices of the epithelia of the tongue and duo-

Professor Dr. Heinz von Mayersbach was a dear friend of all four of the authors. Many of the ideas expressed in this chapter were discussed often with him, especially while the senior author, as a 1973 Alexander von Humboldt awardee, was a guest in his laboratory for several months. The last author, as a fledgling scientist, also received much encouragement and advice from Professor von Mayersbach while researching epidermal growth factor, insulin, and glucagon, of which some of the results are discussed herein. This chapter is especially dedicated to Heinz von Mayersbach.

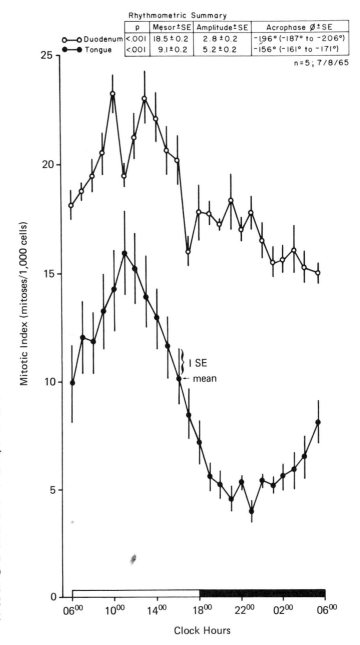

	p	Mesor±SE	Amplitude±SE	Acrophase ∅±SE
Duodenum	<.001	18.5±0.2	2.8±0.2	-196° (-187° to -206°)
Tongue	<.001	9.1±0.2	5.2±0.2	-156° (-161° to -171°)

Fig. 1. Chronograms illustrating the mitotic indices of the same animals in the duodenum (Scheving et al. 1972) and in the tongue (Gasser et al. 1972b) of the Sprague-Dawley rat. The rhythm in the tongue has a relatively high amplitude (A), whereas that of the duodenum is of lower A. The rhythmmometric summary presented in this and other figures is explained in the text. The abscissa shows the LD cycle to which the animals had been standardized for at least 2 weeks prior to the experiment with L(0600 to 1800).

denum. The mitotic index in the epithelium of the tongue has a high-amplitude rhythm, frequently dropping to a very low level at one circadian stage. On the other hand, the time-series mean (mesor) of the mitotic index in the duodenum stays rather high throughout the 24-hr span, but the amplitude of the rhythm remains rather low. Figure 2 presents the rhythmic pattern of the mitotic index in five different tissues for the same animals.

As stated in Chap. 2, when dealing with rhythmic time-series data, it is advantageous to quantify these objectively rather than simply "eye-ball" them from chronograms. A number of methods are available

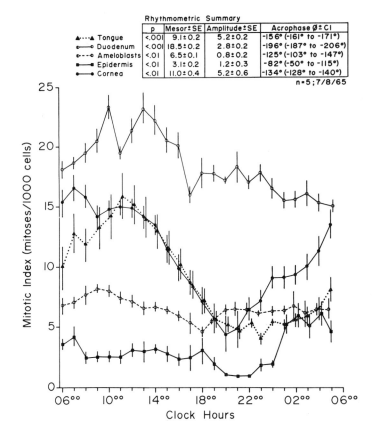

Rhythmometric Summary

	p	Mesor±SE	Amplitude±SE	Acrophase ∅±CI
▲····▲ Tongue	<.001	9.1±0.2	5.2±0.2	-156° (-161° to -171°)
∘——∘ Duodenum	<.001	18.5±0.2	2.8±0.2	-196° (-187° to -206°)
∘---∘ Ameloblasts	<.01	6.5±0.1	0.8±0.2	-125° (-103° to -147°)
■——■ Epidermis	<.01	3.1±0.2	1.2±0.3	-82° (-50° to -115°)
•——• Cornea	<.01	11.0±0.4	5.2±0.6	-134° (-128° to -140°)

n=5; 7/8/65

Fig. 2. A composite of chronograms illustrating the mitotic indices in five different tissues, all from the same animals. The duodenum and tongue data are reproduced from Fig. 1. Data for the cornea, epidermis, and the ameloblasts were previously published by Scheving and Pauly (1967), Scheving and Pauly (1977), and Gasser et al. (1972a), respectively. The trough levels in all tissues occur between 1800 and 2200, when lights were on from 0600 to 1800 and off from 1800 to 0600. It should be kept in mind that evaluations of the mitotic indices were made by five different technicians. The ameloblasts have the lowest amplitude rhythm, with rhythmicity statistically documented by Cosinor and variance analysis.

(Scheving 1980a). The one used most frequently in analyzing data considered in this paper is that described in Chap. 2, the so-called "Cosinor" (Halberg et al. 1972). Using the Cosinor, it is evident from Fig. 1 that with regard to the mitotic index of the rat the acrophase of the duodenum occurred about 2 hr 40 min later than that of the tongue, the mesor was about twice as high in the duodenum as in the tongue, and the amplitude was about two times greater for the tongue than for the duodenum.

Time-series data are often presented in several different ways. Figure 3 illustrates three different techniques of showing time-series data, all of which shall be used in this chapter. On the left are conventional chronograms illustrating the circadian variation found, on eight different dates, in the mitotic index of the corneal epithelium of the rat. The data are expressed as percent change from the 24-hr mean to facilitate

comparison. The number of animals (N) for each time point ranged from 7 to 14, with the majority of studies having an N of 8 per time point. Also shown just above the horizontal scale is the typical daily motor activity of the animals based on noises emanating from the colony. For a complete description of the method of animal standardization, determination of motor activity, and evaluation of the mitotic index, see Scheving and Pauly (1967). The chronogram on the right represents the summary of all eight studies expressed as absolute values (±SE). Note the mitotic index drops to zero or almost zero at certain circadian stages. The rhythmometric summary is shown above. The polar plot on the bottom is another way of displaying the data obtained by a fit of eight sets of time series to a 24-hr cosine curve. A 24-hr duration is simply equated to a 360° circle. The amplitude, shown as a directed line from the cen-

RHYTHMOMETRIC SUMMARY

CONDITION OF EXPERIMENT $L_{06-18}D_{18-06}$	N OF RATS	P	SE/C	MESOR ± SE	AMPLITUDE ± SE	ACROPHASE Ø ± SE
07-06-65	10	.001	.09	14.9 ± .6	9.81 ± .09	-138 (-128 то -149)
09-14-65	14	.001	.10	12.4 ± .6	7.72 ± .10	-119 (-108 то -131)
10-22-65	8	.001	.15	11.6 ± .6	5.64 ± .15	-179 (-161 то -197)
11-01-68	7	.010	.25	7.5 ± .7	3.79 ± .25	-140 (-111 то -168)
05-02-69	8	.001	.12	7.4 ± .5	5.58 ± .12	-125 (-110 то -140)
06-12-69	8	.001	.13	9.1 ± .8	7.61 ± .13	-135 (-119 то -151)
07-08-69	8	.020	.27	8.5 ± 1.6	7.96 ± .27	-120 (- 89 то -151)
10-03-69	8	.001	.09	10.4 ± .5	7.57 ± .09	-155 (-146 то -166)

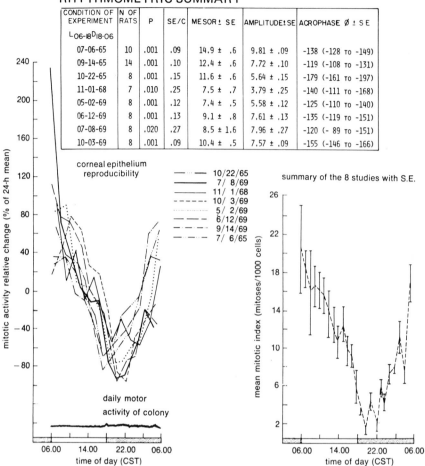

corneal epithelium reproducibility

- 10/22/65
- 7/ 8/69
- 11/ 1/68
- 10/ 3/69
- 5/ 2/69
- 6/12/69
- 9/14/69
- 7/ 6/65

summary of the 8 studies with S.E.

daily motor activity of colony

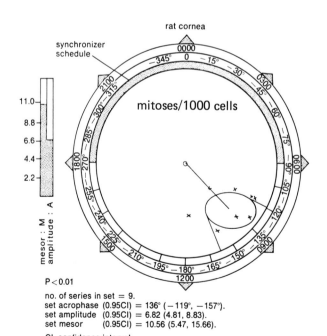

rat cornea

synchronizer schedule

mitoses/1000 cells

mesor : M
amplitude : A

P < 0.01

no. of series in set = 9.
set acrophase (0.95CI) = 136° (−119°, −157°).
set amplitude (0.95CI) = 6.82 (4.81, 8.83).
set mesor   (0.95CI) = 10.56 (5.47, 15.66).

CI, confidence interval.

ter to the point on the periphery representing the time from midnight to the computed time of the acrophase (in this case $-136°$ or 0904 CST), is 6.8 with confidence limits from 4.8 to 8.8 mitoses per 1000 cells counted. The mesor and confidence limits (CI) are 10.5 (CI = 5.4–15.6) mitoses per 1000 cells counted. The fit was highly statistically significant with $P < 0.01$. The 95% confidence ellipse constructed by a computer is centered on the end of the vector. If the ellipse were to cover the center of the circle (usually called the pole), the fit would not be considered significant for a given level of statistical confidence. Note that the synchronizer schedule indicates the dark span occurred between 1800 and 0600, CST. Whenever mention is made of a mesor or acrophase, it implies the analysis was done by Cosinor. For a complete description of this method refer to Chap. 2 and/or Halberg et al. (1972).

Rhythms in DNA Synthesis in Animals: Variation in Mesor, Amplitude, Phase, and Waveform

The mesors and amplitudes of the cell proliferation rhythms in the intact animal vary regionally, i.e., between organs; between tissues of a single organ; and finally, because of mitotic nesting (Scheving 1959; Burns et al. 1973) and stem cells, between the cells of a given tissue. We have studied extensively the DNA synthesis rhythms in many different organs, including the digestive tract. Circadian rhythms in several different regions of the digestive tract are illustrated in Fig. 4 (Scheving et al. 1978).

Our results in general indicate that the means and amplitudes of rhythms for different tissues show considerable variation.

It is readily apparent that large variation exists in the mesor and amplitudes of mitotic rhythms between tissues of various organs and/or sites within the same organ. For example, in one study using adult male mice, the data for DNA synthesis in the digestive tract were analyzed by the Cosinor method. The mesor was lowest in the tongue, 1.3 times greater in the esophagus, 2.8 times greater in the nonglandular stomach and rectum, 3.7 times greater in the proximal colon, 4.0 times greater in the duodenum and ileum, 4.5 times greater in the glandular stomach and jejunum, and 5.3 times greater in the caecum. Although variation may be found from one study to another, we believe, based on the data from a number of studies, that the comparative figures given above for the different regions of the gut are indicative of a typical pattern in mice standardized to 12 hr of light alternating with 12 hr of darkness.

Our results reveal that the DNA synthesis rhythm in the duodenum has the lowest amplitude in the gut, but still it is clearly rhythmic. Figure 5 summarizes six different studies done by us; the range of change along the 24-hr scale for the duodenum, from one study to another, usually falls between 30 and 50%. Recognition that this tissue has a low-amplitude rhythm is important since many studies on basic cell kinetics have used this rather atypical region of the digestive tract (Scheving et al. 1977a,b).

Proximal and distal to the duodenum the amplitude of DNA synthesis rhythms in

---

Fig. 3.   In the middle on the left is a conventional chronogram showing the circadian variation in the mitotic index of the epithelium of the rat cornea on eight different dates. Also shown is the daily motor activity of the colony based on noises emanating from it. The chronogram to the right represents the summary of all 8 studies expressed as absolute values ±S.E. The dates of study and the number of animals used are given in the first two columns of the rhythmometric summary displayed above the chronograms. The data are expressed as percent change from the 24-hr mean to facilitate comparison. The polar plot (*bottom*) is a display of the data obtained by a fit of the 8 sets of time-series data (shown in the tabular rhythmometric summary) to a 24-hr cosine curve; the technique is described in Chap. 2.

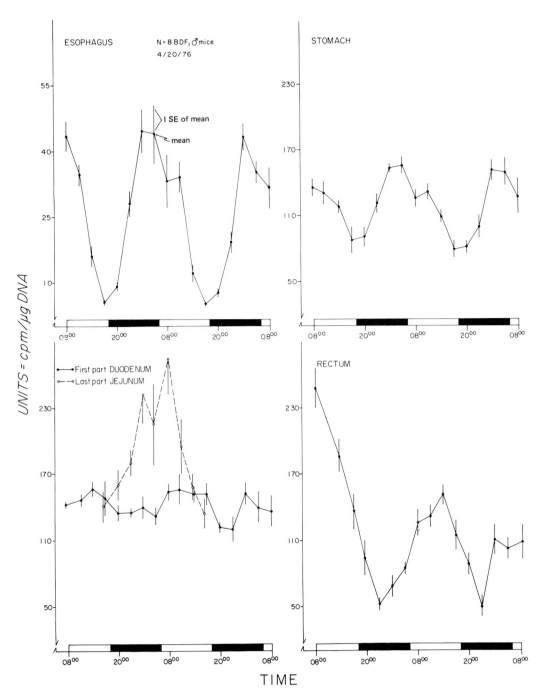

Fig. 4. Chronograms illustrating the rhythmic patterns of ^{3}H-thymidine, [^{3}H]TdR, incorporation into DNA over a 48-hr span in 5 different regions of the alimentary canal of male $CD2F_1$ mice. The abscissa represents the LD cycle to which the mice were standardized: L(0600-1800). The lowest amplitude rhythm was found in the duodenum. (Reproduced from Scheving et al. 1978.)

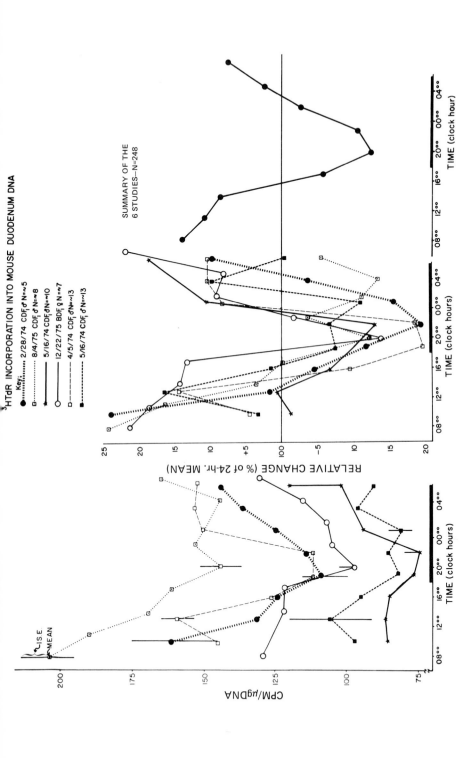

Fig. 5. A composite of chronograms for DNA synthesis in the duodenum of mice based on [³H]TdR incorporation into DNA. Tissues were obtained from control animals used in a variety of different experiments in our laboratory on different dates. Although the study was not designed to test for this, there clearly was a high degree of reproducibility in the phasing of the different rhythms. The mesors varied greatly as did the amplitude (A), and these can be explained. The point to emphasize is that although the A may be small, there is a clear-cut rhythm in DNA synthesis in the duodenum. For the sake of clarity, standard errors are shown only for the high and low points for each chronogram. In general, from one study to another, the trough is the most fixed phase of a rhythm; this is clearly evident in this series of data. (Reproduced from Scheving et al. 1977a.)

the digestive tract gradually increases, being greatest in the oral and anal ends where the mesor of DNA synthesis is the lowest. This variation in amplitude could reflect either regional difference in mucosal extent and cell composition or circadian variation in the distribution of positive or negative growth-controlling signals.

The tissues having the greatest amplitude DNA synthesis rhythms in the digestive tract, namely the tongue, esophagus, stomach, colon, and rectum—not necessarily tissues having the highest levels of DNA synthesis—are also the ones most prone to cancer. The significance of this observation has not yet been determined. Interestingly, these tissues also exhibit the greatest and most consistent growth response to epidermal growth factor (EGF), a polypeptide isolated from the submandibular salivary gland, which we believe plays an important positive role in the control of growth in the digestive tract (Scheving, L. A., et al. 1979, 1980). The role EGF may play in cell proliferation is further discussed below.

Variation in amplitude also occurs in nondigestive-tract tissues. The corneal epithelium and the ovary (Fig. 6) exhibit high- and low-amplitude rhythms, respectively, in cell proliferation (Scheving 1981). As mentioned above, evidence of DNA synthesis and mitotic figures in the corneal epithelium may be virtually absent at certain times of the day (at certain circadian stages), but then may increase as much as 20-fold over a 24-hr span. In the ovary, the amplitude of the DNA synthesis rhythm is low as is the mesor.

The mitotic index in the uterine epithelium of the rat was reported to be devoid of circadian rhythmicity by Bertalanffy and Lau (1963). Krueger et al. (1975), however, demonstrated clearly that the mitotic index in this same tissue was characterized by a very high-amplitude rhythm; the variation between the lowest and highest recorded means along the 24-hr scale represented a 1100% change. Reasons why Bertalanffy and associates frequently reported the absence of rhythms in many normal tissues,

including the cornea (Bertalanffy and Lau 1962a) and the digestive tract (Bertalanffy 1960), have been discussed by us (Scheving et al. 1972). The point to be made is that these investigators are still being widely cited without mention of the evidence to the contrary that certain tissues are devoid of rhythms. Moreover, in standardized, randomly selected rodents one would expect the mesor and perhaps even the amplitude of the DNA synthesis rhythm in the ovary and uterine epithelium to vary as a function of the estrous cycle since weekly, monthly, and annual cycles can modulate circadian rhythms (see Chap. 6).

In addition to variation in the mesor and amplitude of circadian cell rhythms, variation in the phasing of DNA synthesis

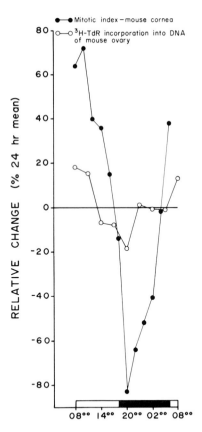

Fig. 6. Chronograms illustrating mitotic-index rhythms in corneal epithelium of mice and in the incorporation of [³H]TdR into DNA in the ovary of the same mice. (Reproduced from Scheving 1981.)

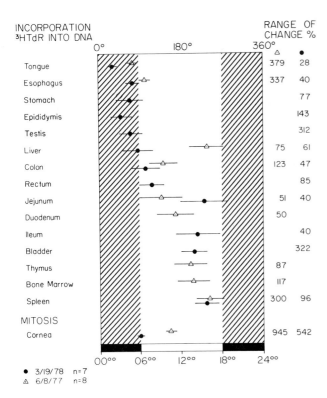

INCORPORATION
³HTdR INTO DNA

RANGE OF
CHANGE %

Fig. 7. An acrophase map, approximating the peak of the circadian cycle in either the incorporation of [³H]TdR into DNA or in the mitotic index of the corneal epithelium of mice. The acrophase (ϕ) is represented by a dot or triangle, and the bars extending out from the dots or triangles represent the 95% confidence limits. The shaded portion represents the 12-hr D phase of the environmental LD cycle. The range of change reflects the difference between the lowest and highest time-point means, with the lowest mean equal to 100%; values were rounded to the nearest integer. (Reproduced from Scheving 1981.)

rhythms also is known. The acrophase map illustrated in Fig. 7 (Scheving 1981) shows the phasing for 10 different tissues studied in one investigation (6/8/77) and for 13 tissues from a later investigation (3/19/78). Unfortunately not all tissues could be compared for reproducibility; however, it should be pointed out that neither study was designed initially to test for reproducibility. Perhaps the differences observed between studies on the same tissue reflect weekly, monthly, or seasonal changes (von Mayersbach 1967) or even the age of the mice. It is of interest that all sets of data shown in Fig. 7 demonstrate a statistically significant fit to a 24-hr cosine curve.

The study of rhythms in cells also reveals variation in the waveform of rhythms. In the digestive tract, the DNA synthesis rhythm tends, from one study to another, to be strongly monophasic in the oral, esophageal, stomach, and anal regions. Yet it occasionally is irregularly monophasic or even multiphasic in the re-

gions between the stomach and anus. This suggests that the cells dividing in the tongue, esophagus, stomach, and rectum progress through the cell cycle with a greater degree of synchrony than do those in the small intestine, caecum and colon. The technique of whole-organ analysis of DNA synthesis, however, may not give the best resolution of the inherent rhythmicity in cell proliferation within an organ, because it fails to discriminate between the rhythmic tendencies of regionally or functionally different subpopulations of cells. In other words, a multiphasic rhythm may represent monophasic rhythms of several different subpopulations of cells combined.

Synchronization of Circadian Rhythms in Cell Proliferation

Both the light–dark (LD) cycle and meal timing have been shown to influence, and even to synchronize, circadian rhythms in cell proliferation. However, the effect of either potential synchronizer on different organs and tissues varies. We shall first consider the synchronizing effect of the LD cycle with emphasis on the mitotic index of the corneal epithelium of the rodent.

Effect of the LD Regime on Cell-Proliferation Rhythms

In female rats standardized to a LD 12:12 cycle, with food available *ad libitum,* the trough of the mitotic index rhythm in the corneal epithelium occurs shortly after the time of transition from L to D, while the

peak occurs at or shortly after the transition from D to L (Fig. 8). The strong sychronizing effect of the LD cycle on this rhythm becomes evident when the LD cycle is inverted 180° (12 hr). The rhythm of the mitotic index becomes completely phase-shifted within a week and remains so (at least until the 12th day). The profile of the rhythm in plasma corticosterone measured in the same rats is also shown on the bottom in Fig. 8; it also becomes inverted completely within the 7-day span (Scheving and Pauly 1974). It should be realized that not all rhythmic variables phase shift this rap-

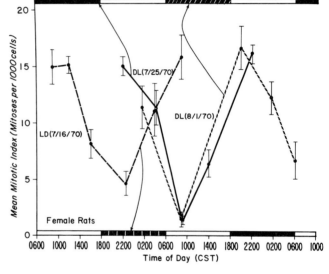

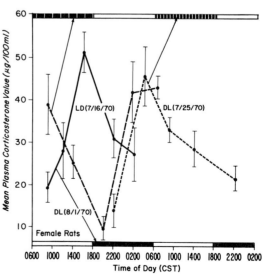

Fig. 8. In each of these two groups of chronograms, the curves identified as LD (7/16/70) illustrate the typical rhythmic pattern for the mitotic index (*upper chronogram, dashed line*) and for serum corticosterone (*lower chronogram, solid line*) in the rat. Note the inverse relationship between the two variables. The curves identified as DL (7/25/70) represent the pattern seen for both variables 7 days after reversal of the LD cycle. Note the complete shift in phasing for both variables and again the same inverse relationship between the two variables. The curves labeled DL (8/1/70) represent the 12th day after the reversal of the LD cycle, indicating that the reversed rhythm for both variables is "locked in" to the LD cycle. In all cases N = 5. (Reproduced from Scheving and Pauly 1973 and Scheving et al. 1974b.)

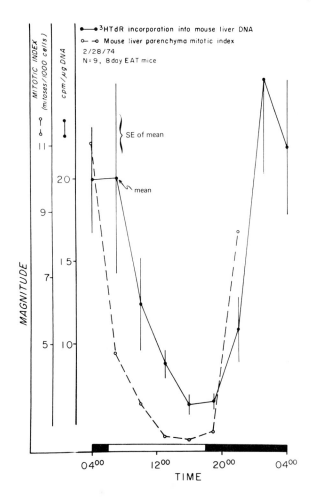

Fig. 9. Comparison of the phasing of the rhythm in mitotic index of mouse liver parenchyma with that in DNA synthesis based on the labeling index of the parenchymal cells subsequent to incorporation of [³H]TdR into DNA. Cell proliferation had been stimulated by the presence of an 8-day-old Ehrlich ascites tumor in the abdominal cavity. The liver itself was not yet invaded by the tumor cells. The curves, which represent M and S phases of the cell cycle, are not separated by 12 hr as has been previously reported. (Reproduced from Scheving et al. 1977b.)

idly; some have been shown to require at least three weeks. The incorporation of tritiated thymidine, [³H]TdR, into DNA in the spleen is one good example of a rhythm that does not completely invert within 7 days when mice are subjected to a change in the LD cycle; three weeks seems to be a sufficient span.

It has been reported, based primarily on data extrapolated from in vitro studies, that the duration of DNA synthesis in the epithelial cells of the cornea is about 10 hr, and that the peak of synthesis occurs about 10 hr prior to the peak of the mitotic index rhythm. However, data obtained by us as well as others simply do not support this view. The phasings of the DNA synthesis rhythm (S) and the mitotic index rhythm (M) are separated by a few hours, at most. Both rhythms usually peak, in animals

standardized to LD 12 : 12, during the latter part of the D phase or even at the very beginning of the L phase (Scheving and Pauly 1967). This observation has significance because in the intact animal there are spans of time when the troughs of both the S and M stages of the cell cycle are occurring and other spans when the peaks (or even other phases of their rhythms) can be predicted. This pattern of phasing also has been found for the corneal epithelium (Chumak 1963), duodenum (Sigdestad et al. 1969; Scheving et al. 1972), intact adult liver (Scheving et al. 1977b), and the epidermis of mice (Tvermyr 1969). Using the flow microfluorometric technique, Rubin (1981) has also shown a similar phenomenon in the epithelium of the mouse tongue. Figure 9 compares the phasing of the rhythm in DNA synthesis with that in the mitotic index of the liver in

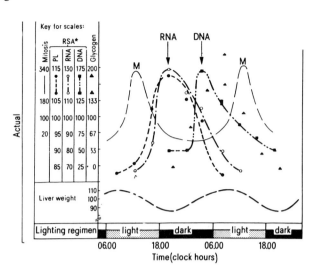

Fig. 10. From these data it appears that there is a considerable interval of time between the synthesis of RNA and DNA and mitosis in the regenerating liver of mice (Barnum et al. 1957). Of course in our liver model (Fig. 9), cells were stimulated to proliferate by a different method. *RSA = relative specific activity. (For further details see above reference and Halberg 1959.)

mice bearing a tumor. Those results might seem to differ from those first reported by Barnum et al. (1957) for the immature mouse liver for which the peaks in DNA synthesis and the mitotic index were separated by many hours, as shown in Fig. 10 (Halberg 1959; Nash and Echave Llanos 1971); it should be emphasized that the systems studied were different.

A possible explanation for the smaller than might be expected difference in phasing between the mitotic index and the DNA synthesis rhythms is that these represent two different populations of cells. The wave of synthesis for today may reflect the wave of mitoses on the following day. It also is possible that G_2 may be of very short duration, thus permitting rapid conversion from S to M (Burns and Scheving 1975; Scheving and Burns 1977). [For further consideration of the phasing and duration of the synthesis and mitosis stages of the cell cycle, see studies by Scheving and Pauly (1967, 1973).]

We have studied the cell-proliferation rhythms in various tissues and organs under several conditions, including short photoperiods (LD 8 : 16), long photoperiods (LD 16 : 8), continuous darkness (DD), continuous light (LL), and blindness. The major effect of altering the photoperiod is an alteration in the waveform of the rhythm.

Circadian Rhythms in Cell Proliferation in the Absence of the LD Cycle

When rodents are placed in either DD or LL, they no longer are subjected to the normal synchronizing effect that the LD cycle has on cell-proliferation rhythms. In the corneas of animals subjected to DD or to blindness, the colony rhythm in the mitotic index persists, but a change in phasing is evident (Fig. 11). Continuous light (LL) in contrast has a more drastic effect on the colony rhythm in this organ, evident by a reduction or flattening of the amplitude of the rhythm (Fig. 12).

It is not known why LL has such an effect (Scheving et al. 1974d; Scheving 1976; Scheving and Pauly 1977). On the one hand, the apparent loss of a rhythm may reflect depression of the sympathetic nervous system by L and resulting cessation of circadian variation in various mitogens, such as EGF, by glands involved in the control of circadian temporal structure. Chemical sympathectomy has been shown to suppress the colony circadian variation of DNA synthesis in the small intestine (Klein 1979). The circadian rhythm of the content of EGF in the submandibular salivary gland appears to be dependent on the activation of the sympathetic nervous sys-

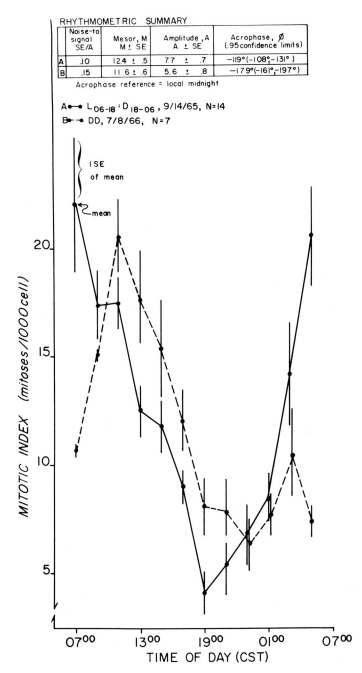

RHYTHMOMETRIC SUMMARY

	Noise-to signal SE/A	Mesor, M M ± SE	Amplitude, A A ± SE	Acrophase, ∅ (.95 confidence limits)
A	.10	12.4 ± .5	7.7 ± .7	−119°(−108°−131°)
B	.15	11.6 ± .6	5.6 ± .8	−179°(−161°,−197°)

Acrophase reference = local midnight

A •—• L$_{06-18}$: D$_{18-06}$, 9/14/65, N=14

B •—• DD, 7/8/66, N=7

Fig. 11. Comparison of rhythm seen in the mitotic index of the corneal epithelium of rats maintained in artificially controlled, LD 12:12 and DD schedules. Note the phase shift of the colony rhythm in animals in DD (the acrophase in DD occurred at 1100 rather than at 0800 as in LD). Note also that in the rhythmometric summary the *noise-to-signal ratio, SE/A,* represents an earlier method of estimating the significance of the data using the Cosinor technique. If a ratio is 0.33 or less, the data are considered to show a statistically significant fit to a cosine curve. (Reproduced from Scheving et al. 1974.)

tem, since it is abolished by superior cervical ganglionectomy (Krieger et al. 1976). Alternatively, the lack of rhythmicity in LL may only reflect the breakdown of colony rhythms. However, it has been shown through longitudinal studies on individual mice in LL that circadian rhythms of motor activity, temperature, and histamine responsiveness persist (Scheving et al. 1973), but the phasing of these rhythms differs between individual rodents. Thus, a comparison of the average values obtained for a group of mice at different time points over a 24-hr span may belie the extent of rhythmic

RHYTHMOMETRIC   SUMMARY

	Noise-to signal SE/A	Mesor, M M ± SE	Amplitude, A A ± SE	Acrophase, Ø (.95 confidence limits)
A	.10	12.4 ± .5	7.7 ± .7	−119° (−108°, −131°)
B	.39	12.3 ± .3	1.2 ± .4	−80°
C	.38	12.9 ± .5	2.1 ± .8	−54°

Acrophase   reference = local midnight

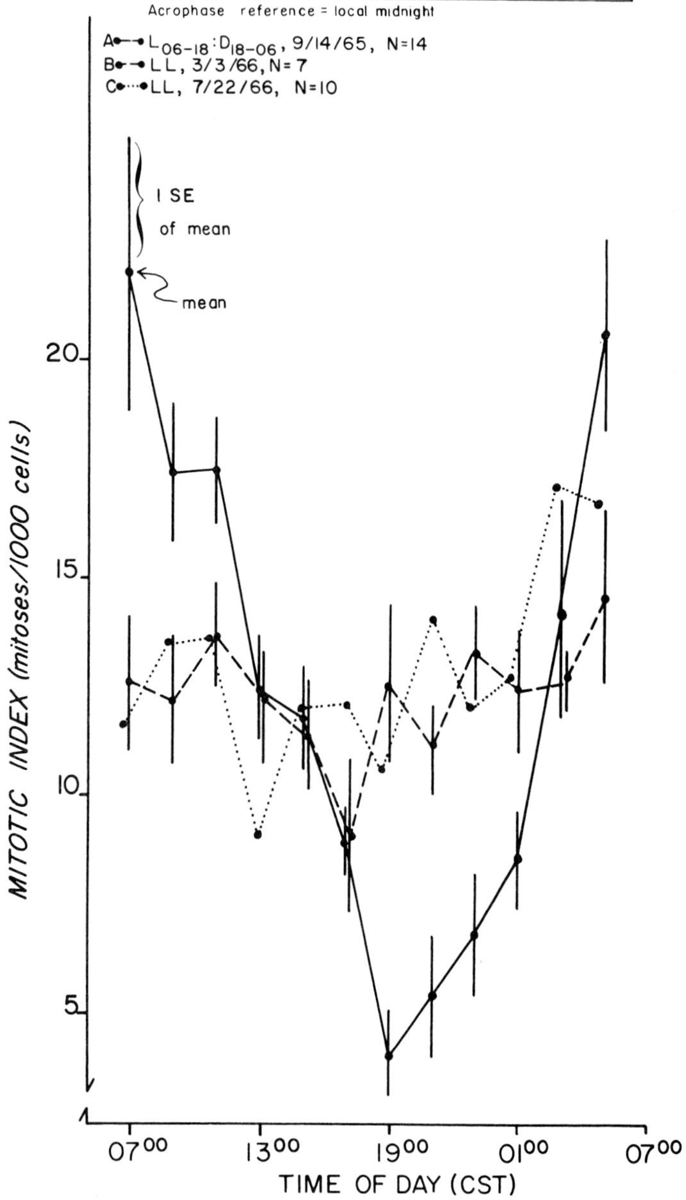

A●—●L$_{06-18}$:D$_{18-06}$, 9/14/65, N=14
B●—●LL, 3/3/66, N=7
C●····●LL, 7/22/66, N=10

Fig. 12. A comparison of rhythms in the mitotic indices of the corneal epithelium of rats maintained in an artificially controlled LD 12:12 (lights on from 0600 to 1800 and off from 1800 to 0600) with those in rats maintained in LL at 600 lux (two studies). Note a flattening of the curves and reduction of the amplitude in LL conditions. (Reproduced from Scheving et al. 1974c.)

variation in individual mice. The problem of carrying out longitudinal sampling in individual mice makes it difficult to evaluate this hypothesis for mitosis. The senior author, however, has seen some unpublished data (which seem to be no longer available) of the late Gordon Rosene which demonstrated, by longitudinal sampling (repeated biopsy) on individual mice subjected to LL, the persistence of the mitotic index rhythm in the pinna epidermis.

The effect of LL on DNA synthesis

rhythms in different tissues of the adult mouse illustrates once again the need for caution in extrapolating from data obtained on one tissue to a different tissue. For example, if one examines data for the effect that LL has on only the tissues with the most prominent rhythms, it might be concluded that LL suppressed only the amplitude of the rhythm in DNA synthesis. Our results, however, indicate that this is not the case. For example, LL results in a reduction in the mesors of the DNA synthesis rhythms in the tongue, esophagus, stomach, duodenum, caecum, colon, rectum, liver, testes, and epididymis, as well as a reduction in the amplitudes of all of the above tissues except for the duodenum, caecum, and epididymis. In mice standardized to a LD 12:12 synchronizer schedule, most of these tissues were not only the most rhythmic, but also the most responsive to the mitogenic effects of EGF (Scheving, L. A., et al. 1979, 1980). Also, such tissues tend to exhibit peak DNA synthesis under normal conditions late in the D phase or very early in the L phase. In contrast, LL results in an increase in both the mesors and amplitudes of the rhythms in the spleen, thymus, bone marrow, and bladder and in the amplitudes of the rhythms in the duodenum, jejunum, ileum, and caecum. Such tissues are the ones which generally are the least responsive to EGF; in fact, EGF at times inhibits DNA synthesis in some tissues. Also, DNA synthesis in these tissues of mice standardized to normal conditions tends to peak later in the L phase than in the other tissues.

Effect of Meal Timing on Cell-Proliferation Rhythms

When feeding is restricted to a single 4-hr interval within the 24-hr LD cycle, the rhythms in DNA synthesis and the mitotic index in the corneal epithelium are relatively resistant to change (Fig. 13). Therefore, for this tissue the lighting schedule appears to dominate meal timing in the sychronization of cell proliferation (Schev-

ing et al. 1974c; Philippens et al. 1977). Although the LD schedule acts to synchronize the corneal epithelium rhythm, it does not generate it as evidenced by the persistence of the rhythm in mice that are either blinded or raised in DD (Fig. 11). The transition from L to D may cause changes in the corneal epithelium, itself, or in the local concentration of a mitogen that leads to increased DNA synthesis and the ultimate division of the target cells. In other organs, such as those involved in hemopoiesis or digestion, the restricted feeding schedule appears to be able, eventually, to dominate or at least to compete with the LD schedule in the synchronization of DNA synthesis. This is illustrated in Fig. 14 for eosinophil levels in the blood of mice (Pauly et al. 1975).

Normally, feeding behavior, motor activity, and DNA synthesis increase at about the time of the L-to-D transition in animals fed *ad libitum* and synchronized to LD 12:12. When feeding is restricted to a single 4-hr period some time during the LD 12:12 span, the peak in DNA synthesis in organs, such as the duodenum, esophagus, tongue, spleen, and bone marrow, shifts in time to coincide with the time that food is presented. This shift is not immediate; it takes from several days to more than a week, depending upon the interval when the feeding time occurs in relation to the LD 12:12 cycle. Thus, the effect of meal timing, itself, can be said to be circadian-stage dependent, at least in certain organs or tissues. For example, in comparison to both *ad libitum* feeding and other restricted feeding schedules, a 4-hr feeding span during the latter part of the L span dramatically increases the amplitude of the circadian rhythm in DNA synthesis in the duodenum, spleen, and bone marrow (Figs. 15–17) (Scheving et al. 1976). In some organs, such as the esophagus, the shift of the rhythm is complete following a week of restricted feeding, regardless of the feeding span. In other organs, such as the tongue, the extent of shift in the original monophasic rhythm depends on the time of the feeding period in

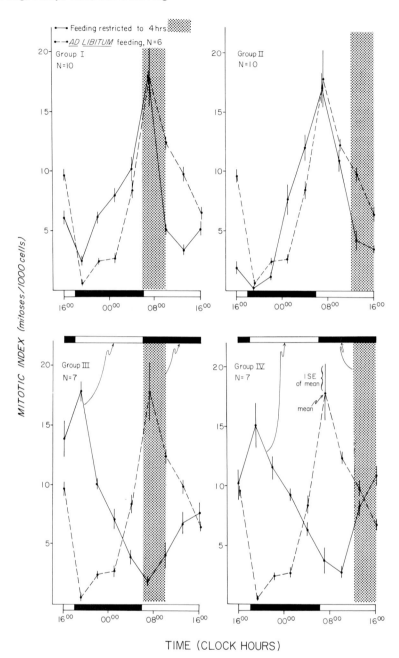

Fig. 13. Effect of 4 hr feeding schedules (shaded areas) on the mitotic-index rhythm in the mouse corneal epithelium. The LD cycle to which the animals were subjected is depicted on the horizontal axis of each chronogram. Within each group of mice (CD2F₁), controls were fed *ad libitum* and experimental mice were restricted in their access to food each day to 12 hr during the first week, 8 hr the second week, 6 hr the third week, and 4 hr during the fourth and fifth weeks (*shaded areas*). The mitotic-index rhythms remained remarkably synchronized to the LD cycle. In all instances, time was local clock hour (CST). (For details of this study, and for the data in Figs. 14–18, see Scheving et al. 1974b.)

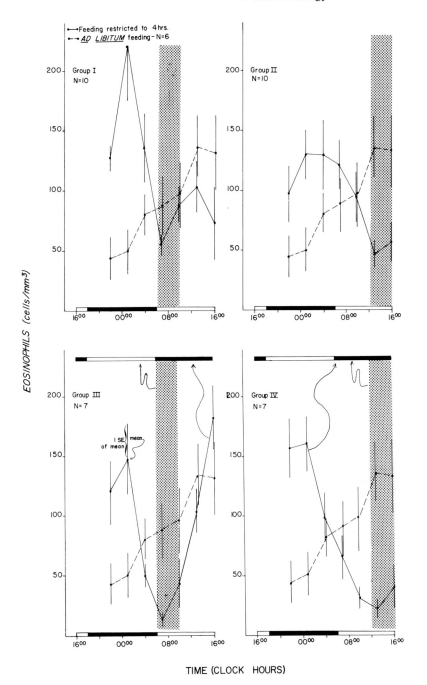

Fig. 14. The effect of restricted feeding schedules on eosinophil levels in mice in the same animals described in Fig. 13 (the data were published earlier by Pauly et al. 1975). Unlike the mitotic index of the cornea, the feeding schedule strongly synchronized the eosinophil rhythm.

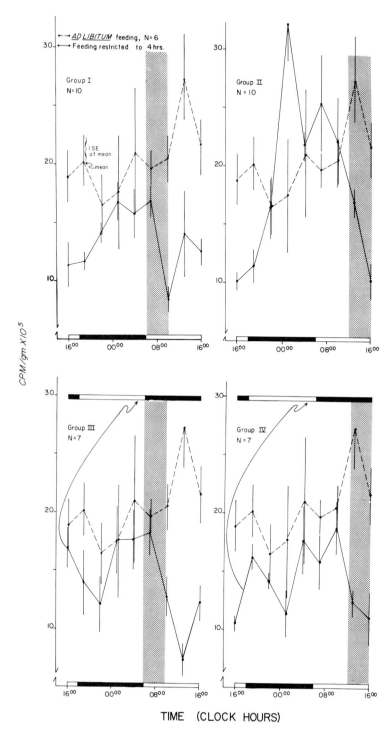

Fig. 15. The effect of restricted feeding schedules on the rhythm in [³H]TdR incorporation into the DNA of the duodenum in the same mice described in Fig. 13. Feeding synchronizes the rhythm in that the trough of the rhythm always occurs at or just after feeding.

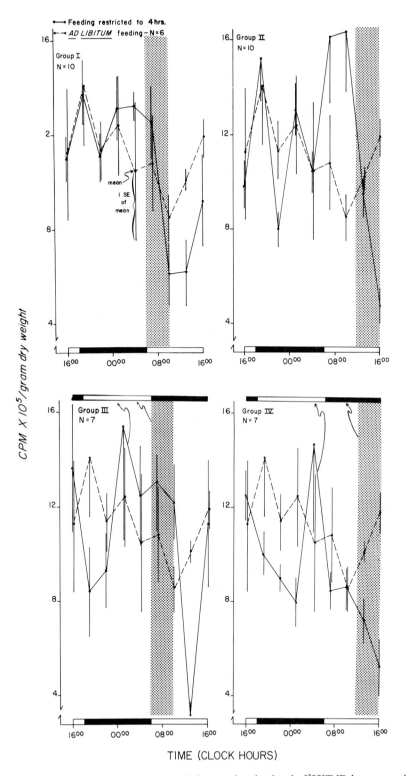

Fig. 16. The effect of restricted feeding schedules on the rhythm in [³H]TdR incorporation into the DNA of the spleen in the same mice described in Fig. 13. Feeding synchronizes the rhythm.

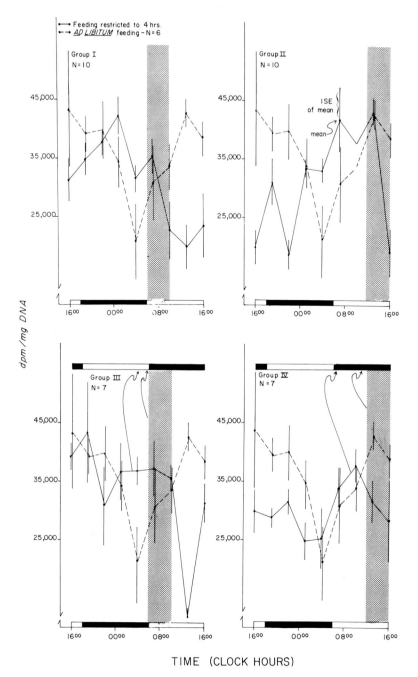

Fig. 17. The effect of restricted feeding schedules on the rhythm in [³H]TdR incorporation into DNA in the bone marrow of the same mice described in Fig. 13. The data shown in Figs. 15–17 have been published in part (Scheving et al. 1976). We have hypothesized previously that since the restriction of food could largely override the effect of the LD cycle for the duodenum, spleen, and bone marrow, meal-timing might be used advantageously in man for optimizing the effects of radiotherapy or chemotherapy. This hypothesis still remains to be tested in man; we wish to reemphasize the importance of attempting this.

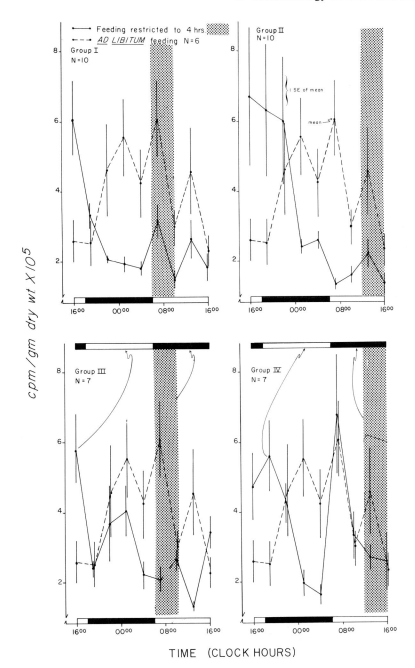

Fig. 18. The effect or restricted feeding schedules on the rhythm in [³H]TdR incorporation into the DNA of the tongue in the same mice described in Fig. 13. These data have not been published previously.

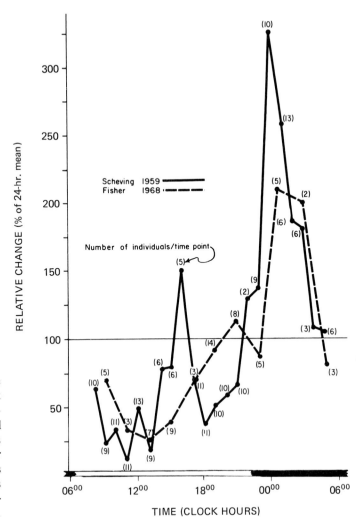

Fig. 19. Reproducibility of the mitotic-index rhythm in the adult human epidermis. Standard errors have been omitted to avoid a cluttered graph. (For details see Scheving 1959 and Fisher 1968.) The reproducibility was further documented 20 years later with two time-point samplings (Zagula-Mally et al. 1979).

relation to the LD cycle. For example, in the tongue of mice fed late in the D span (Fig. 18), but not in the esophagus (data not shown), the DNA synthesis rhythm becomes biphasic: one phase appears to be cued by food presentation and the other by the onset of darkness. One *cannot generalize* about the effect of meal timing as a synchronizer of rhythms based on studies done on one or two variables. Extensive data obtained on the cornea of rats and on other variables in the rat by Philippens et al. (1977) further support this conclusion.

The ability to phase shift some rhythms both within and among organs, thereby increasing the synchronization of cell-prolif-

eration rhythms in the intact animal simply by altering meal timing or the LD cycle, could provide a useful strategy for predictably shifting normal cells to a phase of the cell cycle more resistant to radiotherapy or chemotherapy (Scheving et al. 1976a). Furthermore, the combination of environmental and hormonal challenges involving the administration of a combination of mitogens, such as EGF, insulin, glucagon, and fibroblast growth factor (FGF), could be a powerful tool to accomplish this end. Indeed, it has been reported that immunocytoma-bearing rats survived longer following adriamycin treatment when meal timing was restricted to the early part of the L span (Nelson et al. 1974; Halberg et al. 1977; Halberg et al. 1979a). Further work is required to determine how environmental, hormonal, and perhaps social factors can be used to manipulate cell-proliferation rhythms in the mouse and in man in order to shield normal cells from the toxic effects of radiotherapy or chemotherapy (Scheving et al. 1977a, 1980).

With regard to man, only two tissues (in addition to circulating blood cells), the epidermis and the bone marrow, have been analyzed for rhythmic variation in mitotic index. Cell proliferation in both tissues (Figs. 19 and 20) has been shown not only to display a circadian rhythm, but also to peak around midnight, when man is normally beginning rest or sleep. The available data indicate, as has been shown for the circadian rhythms of serum prolactin and melatonin, that the cell-proliferation rhythms in pre-

dominately diurnally active man are not necessarily 180° (12 hr) out of phase with those in the nocturnal mouse. To see this one has only to compare the mitotic index rhythm in the epidermis of the rat (Fig. 2) with the same rhythm in the epidermis of man (Fig. 19). Thus, species-specific differences occur with respect to the time of peak cell proliferation in a tissue or organ. We emphasize, however, that the phasing of many rhythms when measured in the nocturnally active rodent and diurnally active man are 180° (12 hr) out of phase, e.g., steroids (Fig. 21).

The Sleep–Wake Cycle and Rhythms in Cell Proliferation

It has been asserted frequently that the highest levels of cell proliferation are asso-

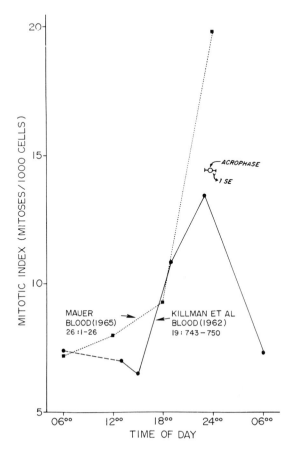

Fig. 20. The mitotic-index rhythm in the bone marrow of a group of young men (*dotted line*) and the mitotic rhythm in bone marrow obtained from a single individual (*solid line*) along the 24-hr domain. (For details see references shown in the figure.)

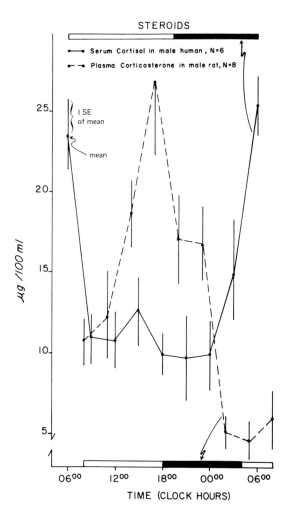

Fig. 21. Corticosterone level in rats standardized to a LD 12 : 12 cycle and fed *ad libitum*, and cortisol levels in presumably healthy young males (meal times: 0640, 1245, and 1645; rest or sleep from 2100 to 0600). We stress that the phasing of all rhythmic variables in the diurnally active man is not necessarily the inverse of that in the nocturnally active rodent as seen here. Consequently, one must not generalize when data are available from one and not the other. (Reproduced from Scheving and Pauly 1974.)

ciated with sleep, and data obtained on animals are given to support this claim. However, our results indicate that a relationship between sleep and cell proliferation does not exist for all tissues. In many organs, particularly in the digestive tract of adult mice standardized to LD 12 : 12, DNA synthesis and mitosis increase shortly after the animal begins eating and when there is an increase in motor activity, both of which are associated with the onset of darkness. In these tissues, peak levels of DNA synthesis are reached in the D span, when the animals are still active, or early in the L span. In other tissues, such as the bone marrow, spleen, and occasionally in the je-

junum and ileum, the peak in DNA synthesis occurs during the latter half of the L span, when the animals are resting (Fig. 7). Thus, caution is indicated when extrapolating from data obtained on one tissue to another or, in the case of the intestinal tract, from one region to another. Some data on man, described above, might seem to support the hypothesis that cell proliferation is associated with sleep because the two tissues thus far analyzed, epidermis and bone marrow, do show the majority of mitotic activity occurring at night. It must be kept in mind, however, that the data are limited and more extensive animal data do not fully support such a hypothesis.

Mechanisms of Circadian Rhythms in Cell Proliferation

Effect of Light–Dark Cycles and Meal Timing

Do the L-to-D transition and meal presentation have a direct synchronizing effect on target cells, perhaps by an alteration of cellular response to growth-control signals, or is the effect an indirect one, mediated through the synchronizer-induced release of growth-controlling signals? There are several possibilities. First the nutritional and abrasive effect of meals may play a direct role in the proliferation rhythm of the digestive tract. The nutritional effect would be analogous to the requirement of quiescent cells in vitro for certain low-molecular-weight components, such as glucose and amino acids, prior to entry into the S phase of the cell cycle. Second, the effects of certain components of the meal may play a direct role in evoking the secretion of mitogens, just as glucose stimulates pancreatic beta cells to secrete insulin. Third, the L-to-D transition and meal presentation acting neurally or hormonally on certain hypothalamic nuclei, for example, the suprachiasmatic and ventral medial nuclei, could induce local or systemic discharge of positive growth-controlling signals, such as EGF and insulin, possibly through the action of the sympathetic nervous system. The second and third possibilities would provide cells with the polypeptide hormones found in serum, saliva, and amniotic fluids, and possibly in other fluids, such as tears, that are required for cells in vitro to enter the S phase. Fourth, mesenchymal changes could affect the epithelial response to growth-promoting factors. Finally, these environmental stimuli might either directly or indirectly affect the rhythms in the number of the biochemical properties of the cell-surface receptors for positive growth factors, including membrane-associated biochemical events such as the phosphorylation of proteins or phospholipase activity.

Effect of Epidermal Growth Factor on DNA Synthesis In Vivo

We recently have been studying the effect of various peptides, including EGF, insulin, glucagon, and ACTH, on the DNA synthesis rhythms in the intact animal model. We have studied and reported on the effects of EGF on DNA synthesis in 20 different tissues (Scheving, L. A., et al. 1979, 1980; Yeh et al. 1981). Figures 22 and 23 show examples of DNA synthesis stimulation in the esophagus and rectum of mice 4, 8, and 12 hr after injection of EGF. Several conclusions relative to EGF have been reached. First, our results suggest EGF plays an important role in positive growth control of many tissues, particularly the cornea and the digestive tract. Second, different tissues exhibit considerable variation in their responsiveness to EGF 4, 8, and 12 hr after injection (EGF was injected into different groups of mice at five different clock hours to determine the circadian-stage dependency of EGF). For example, the cornea, tongue, and esophagus, which were the most rhythmic tissues studied, consistently responded to EGF with increased DNA synthesis 4, 8, and 12 hr after injection. On the other hand, the glandular and non-glandular stomach, colon, and rectum responded only after 8 and 12 hr. The lung and aorta responded only after 8 hr, and the liver and testes after 12 hr. Third, there are certain circadian stages when the stimulatory effect of EGF appears to be maximally potentiated. For example, injection of EGF at 1500 into mice standardized to L(0600–1800) : D(1800–0600) resulted in a striking, generalized increase in DNA synthesis 4 hr later, at 1900, particularly in the parotid, thymus, and small intestine, which at other times failed to respond to EGF. Interestingly, the serum concentrations of various hormones such as insulin, gastrin, and hydrocortisone peak during this period of time when the rate of feeding increases (Scheving, L. A. et al. 1980). Fourth, our results indicate that EGF can

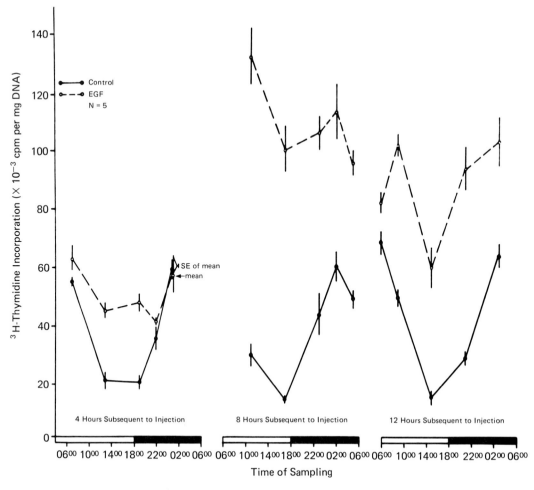

Fig. 22. Effect of EGF on [³H]TdR incorporation into the esophagus is plotted versus time of sacrifice for the different injection times. Mice were killed at either 4, 8, or 12 hr after each timed injection. (Modified from Scheving, L. A., et al. 1979.)

inhibit DNA synthesis at certain times in several tissues, including the small intestine, thymus, bone marrow, and spleen. Although the relationship between rhythmicity, response to exogenous EGF, and the potential to undergo transformation remains to be elucidated, the EGF cell-surface effector system has been implicated in the in vitro chemical and viral transformation of certain cell types. This is evidenced by the fact that transformed cells, in contrast to their normal counterparts, exhibit a decreased requirement for exogenous EGF to undergo cell proliferation (Cherington et

al. 1979). In such cells a tumor growth factor seems to be substituted for EGF.

EGF, itself, has been shown to be co-carcinogenic in the induction of certain skin tumors (Roberts et al. 1976). Recently, it has been shown in rats that the removal of the submandibular gland, the major source of EGF, results in a reduction in the number of dimethylbenzanthracene-induced tumors of the colon (Li et al. 1980). Furthermore, the induction of submandibular gland sarcomas with this same chemical has been shown to be circadian-stage dependent (Halberg 1964). This same chemical in adult

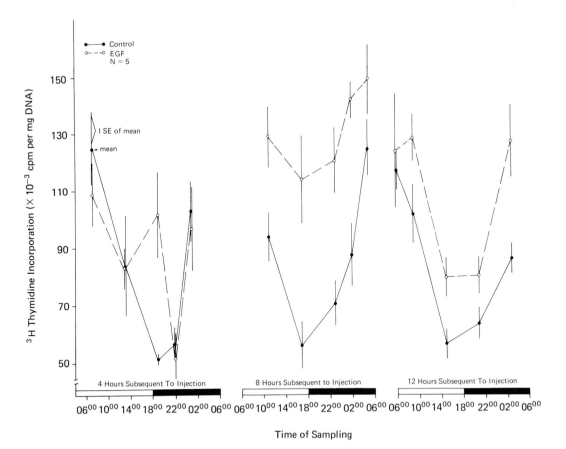

Fig. 23. Effect of EGF on [³H]TdR incorporation into the rectum is plotted versus time of sacrifice for the different injection times. Mice were killed at either 4, 8, or 12 hr after each timed injection. (Modified from data of Scheving, L. A., et al. 1980.)

male rodents appears to be most carcinogenic at a time when the glandular content of EGF is expected to be highest (Krieger et al. 1976). Recent evidence in addition suggests that EGF may also affect gastrointestinal motility. We frequently observe stomach engorgement in the absence of increased feeding in mice injected intraperitoneally 4 hrs earlier with EGF (20 µg/mouse) (Fig. 24) or with α-adrenergic saliva, which contains high concentrations of EGF (Murphy et al. 1980). Others have reported that EGF structurally affects rat parietal cells (Gonzalez et al. 1981), inhibits spontaneous movements of the guinea pig intestinal tract in vitro (Takayanagi 1980), and transiently inhibits sheep appetite

(Panaretto et al. 1982). Mahotra (1967) showed that when human saliva, which contains EGF, is premixed with food, gastric emptying is delayed. Furthermore, the secretion of EGF into the saliva of mice standardized to 12 hr of light alternating with 12 hr of dark appears to be greatest when mice begin to feed and become active, namely late in the light span and early in the dark span (Krieger et al. 1976).

The above results suggest that oral and intestinal mechanisms involving EGF secretion may play a role in the hormonal regulation of stomach emptying and appetite. The presence of EGF in cerebrospinal fluid (CSF) suggests that central mechanisms may be involved as well (Hirata et al. 1982).

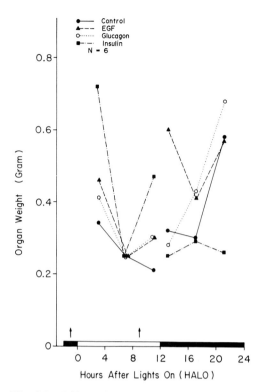

Fig. 24. Effect of EGF, insulin, and glucagon on stomach weight at various times after administration. The peptides were administered at two different circadian stages (see *arrows*). Sampling was at 4, 8, and 12 hours after injection. See text for more complete explanation.

In this regard, two interesting observations seem to implicate the effect of EGF. First, the demonstrated ability of transformed cells to secrete immunologically distinct molecules that can interact with the EGF cell-surface receptor implies that anorexia observed in some cancers may be related to the presence of ectopic EGF-like molecules (Todaro et al. 1982). Second, the delayed gastric emptying reported in pregnant women (Ryan and Pellecchia 1982) may be related to elevated EGF serum concentrations.

We have recently demonstrated for the first time that both insulin and glucagon affect the incorporation of [³H]TdR into DNA of the esophagus, stomach, duodenum, jejunum, ileum, colon, rectum, and spleen of the adult female mouse. They do so in dif-

ferent ways and at different circadian stages. The effects of these hormones were complex, but several generalizations emerged. (1) Insulin tended to increase the incorporation of [³H]TdR into DNA in the examined organs, whereas glucagon tended to decrease it. (2) Insulin was more effective in stimulating the incorporation of [³H]TdR into DNA when injected either at the end of the dark span or the beginning of the light span, as opposed to the end of the light span or the beginning of the dark span. (3) Insulin had its greatest effect on [³H]TdR incorporation into DNA in the glandular stomach and rectum, whereas glucagon had its greatest effect on the colon and spleen. (4) The effects of both insulin and glucagon were different from those of epidermal growth factor, as revealed in the earlier studies mentioned above. Our results suggest that insulin, glucagon, and epidermal growth factor play important roles in the control of various endodermally derived organs (Scheving, L. A. et al. 1982).

Are In Vivo Cell-Kinetic Studies that Ignore Rhythmicity Compromised?

Cell-kinetic studies that ignore rhythmicity are compromised. An obvious illustration of this is seen in the estimation of cell-generation time.

Examinations of cell generation time in many tissues have been made using the once-popular FLM (frequency of labeled mitosis) method originally defined by Quastler and Sherman (1959). In fact, the gut epithelium, which we have demonstrated to be extremely rhythmic, was used as the tissue of choice by Quastler and Sherman because they believed that it divided randomly. Reasons for this erroneous view have been discussed (Burns and Scheving 1975; Scheving and Burns 1977c). Obviously this method can no longer be considered reliable for the in vivo system, yet despite this it still was used by some at the time this paper was first drafted (Laurence et al. 1979; Klein 1979; and others).

We have shown that if one injects [³H]-TdR when the mitotic index is lowest in the corneal epithelium, about 2100, and analyzes the cell proliferation in this tissue in a conventional manner, then $G_{2+1/2M} = 8$ hr, and $T_S = 5.4$ hr. If [³H]TdR is injected at the time of highest mitotic activity, at 0900, then $G_{2+1/2M} = 4$ hr and $T_S = 12.2$ hr (Burns and Scheving 1975) (Fig. 25). Cell-kinetic studies which ignore circadian variation may be very misleading, and all published generation times obtained using this method need to be reevaluated with techniques that take into consideration the basic rhythmicity. Current studies using the flow microfluorometry technique appear promising for resolving cell-proliferation rhythms (Rubin 1981; Laerum and Aardal 1981). Rubin et al. (1983) have carried out extensive studies comparing the method of [³H]TdR incorporation into DNA with the flow cytometry method (FCM). The two methods were very similar for demonstrating rhythms in certain tissues, thus validating the method we use. The FCM method

has a distinct advantage over the older method in that it is rapid. However, it has the disadvantage of not being suitable for tissues where it is difficult or impossible to obtain a homogenous cell suspension, which is the case in many parts of the intestinal tract (Rubin et al. 1983).

Circadian Rhythms in Division of Cells Growing In Vitro

Twenty-six years ago, Hupe and Gropp (1957) reported that a 24-hr rhythm occurred in the rate of cell proliferation in chick embryonic cells growing in vitro; this represented a study with sampling only over a single 24-hr span and with no reported attempt to reproduce the results. In the Sixties, we carried out a rather large series of studies in an attempt to confirm this earlier work using other cell lines; we did not, however, attempt to repeat their work precisely. Unfortunately we did not publish the findings at that time because we believed the results were not definitive.

In the Seventies, Langer and Rensing

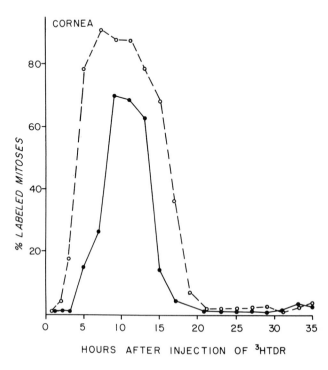

Fig. 25. The frequency of labeled mitosis method (FLM) was used to determine the duration of the S phase of the cell cycle in the epithelium of the mouse cornea. The *dashed line* represents the data obtained from mice that were injected with [³H]TdR at 0900 and killed at frequent intervals thereafter. The *solid line* represents data obtained from mice that were injected with [³H]TdR at 2100 and killed at frequent intervals thereafter. (For complete details see Burns and Scheving 1975.)

(1972), Hardeland (1973), Goedeke and Rensing (1974), and Rensing and Goedeke (1976) claimed to have demonstrated circadian rhythms in primary liver cells growing in vitro for (1) nuclear size, (2) oxygen consumption, (3) activity of thyrosine aminotransferase, (4) protein synthesis, and (5) DNA content in both normal liver cells and in the rat hepatoma cell. For each variable studied, their data covered only a single 24-hr span. Moreover, the authors claimed that the DNA rhythm in vitro was similar to that in normal liver cells in vivo; the impression conveyed to us is that these authors believed such rhythms may be synchronized to the LD cycle.

In view of the above work, our earlier findings now seem more relevant, even though we do not consider them to be definitive. We summarize them here for the first time.

Our approach was to establish initial cultures in milk dilution bottles. After about one week or 10 days, or when the cells had formed a confluent sheet, the cultures were trypsinized and the contents of several milk bottles pooled. Identical aliquots were taken from the pooled source of suspended cells and placed in 48 Leighton tubes containing cover slips and 1 ml of medium. The cells were then cultivated in an atmosphere of 5% CO_2 for a period of one week or 10 days, with two or three changes of medium during this span. Cells were sacrificed by beginning at a particular hour of an experimental day and fixing the contents of either two Leighton tubes hourly, or 4 tubes every 2 hr over a 24-hr span. Cover slips, on which the cells had grown in monolayers, were periodically removed from the Leighton tubes, washed with 70% alcohol, stained with Harris hematoxylin, and mounted on slides. A minimum of 2000 cells were counted on each slide, except in the case of HeLa cells, where 3000 cells were counted. As a precautionary measure, many of the mitotic counts were repeated by a second observer who had no knowledge of the previous results. When the data of the two counters were compared, the

major difference was a small discrepancy in the mean values of mitotic indices. Moreover, the timing of the peak and low values of the mitotic indices over the 24-hr spans was very similar for the two observers, thus giving us confidence that the fluctuations observed were not due to an artifact of counting. We used either primary or permanent lines of cells. All cultures were subjected to 12 hr of light (0600 to 1800) alternating with 12 hr of darkness (1800 to 0600); it should be noted that we also carried out studies on cells in continuous light (LL) and in continuous darkness (DD), but they are not reported herein because the results were not much different from those obtained from cells grown in LD cycles.

An analysis of the mitotic rate in a primary strain of human epidermal cells originally obtained from a 40-year-old man (LES) is shown in Fig. 26A. The overall 24-hr mean mitotic index was 3.5. There was a rather dramatic fluctuation around this mean with the peak in mitosis during the D phase. This was one of our first studies and at the time it was interesting, especially since the rhythm had a phasing similar to that reported for the rhythm known to characterize the in vivo human epidermal cells as evident from comparison of the plots in Figs. 19 and 26A (Scheving and Gatz 1955; Scheving 1959). In another early study on a primary cell line obtained from tonsil tissue removed from an adult patient, there was dramatic fluctuation around the 24-hr mean; however, the peak was very sharp (Fig. 26B).

Such studies were rather encouraging to us and seemed to confirm, although on different cell lines, the early finding of Hupe and Gropp (1957); they were deficient, however, just as were the original studies of Hupe and Gropp, because they represented only a single 24-hr span of sampling. We, therefore, decided to sample from the same culture line over several 24-hr spans. The infant prepuce was selected for this investigation simply because it was growing in our laboratory and had been obtained from the foreskin of a newborn infant; thus, we were

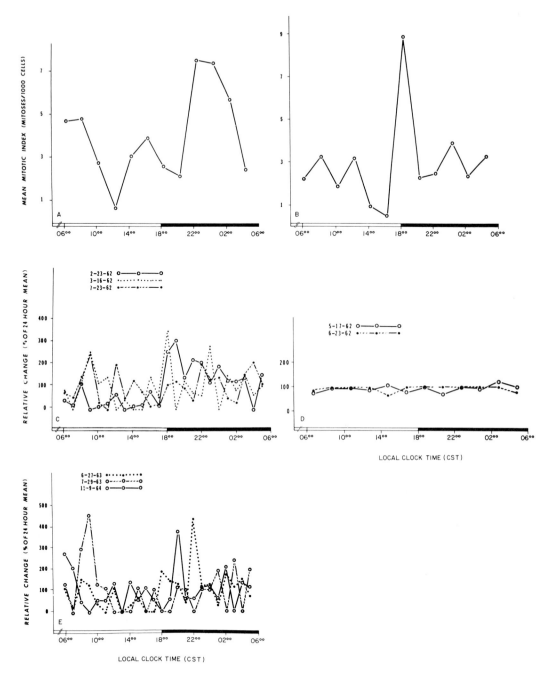

Fig. 26. **A** Fluctuation in the mitotic index of cells growing as a monolayer, in vitro; the source of the cells was a piece of human skin obtained from the forearm of a 40-year-old subject. Each point represents the mean of four such cultures; samples were obtained at bihourly intervals. The cells growing in the incubation chamber were subjected to 12 hr of light alternating with 12 hr of darkness as illustrated on the abscissa. Peak mitotic activity was recorded between 2230 and 0230. **B** Mitotic-index rhythm in cells from human tonsil. **C** Three different studies on tissues obtained from new-born infant prepuce. Samples were obtained at hourly intervals. **D** HeLa cells behaved differently in that they did not fluctuate as much as the other cells. **E** Mitotic-index rhythm in rat cornea cells growing in vitro. (None of these data were previously published.)

dealing with a primary culture. The data obtained from the mitotic counts on cultures of these cells (Fig. 26C) were plotted as relative changes of the hourly mean mitotic indices from the overall mean mitotic index. This was done simply to facilitate comparison of the different studies, since the 24-hr means varied. The data recorded on 2/23/62 revealed that the highest rate of mitotic activity in the culture occurred at 1900. The mitotic index at that time was 300% above the overall daily mean index. In general, these data also were encouraging in that they suggested that most of the cell division had taken place during the dark span. A second analysis, less than a month later, demonstrated a far more variable pattern (Fig. 26C); and a third study, done about four months later, showed a highly irregular pattern of cell division. The daily 24-hr mean mitotic index was 2.4 on 2/23/62; it was 1.3 on 3/16/62; and it was 3.3 on 7/23/62. There was no consistent finding among the three studies (Fig. 26C), unless one would attach significance to the fact there was a relatively low incidence of cell division between 1200 and 1800 in all three.

About this same time, we were using HeLa cells in our laboratory for other purposes and decided to do a similar analysis of their mitotic behavior using investigative methods identical to those used for the infant prepuce. The data in Figure 26D, plotted as relative changes of the bihourly mean from the 24-hr mean, point up the fact that the highly fluctuating cell-division rate seen in cultures of infant foreskin and other systems studied was absent in HeLa cell cultures (Fig. 26D). Two other 24-hr studies were carried out in addition to the two just discussed, and comparable results were obtained. The overall mean mitotic indices of HeLa cells were considerably higher than those of any other cells tested; an overall mean index of 18.8 was recorded on 5/17/62 and one of 21.4 was recorded on 6/23/62. In some cultures (not reported here), the daily mean cell-division rate in HeLa cultures ranged from as high as 45 dividing cells per 1000 cells counted to as low as 8/1000 cells.

In all cultures, however, fluctuations about the daily mean were not of sufficient magnitude to indicate any rhythmicity of mitotic rate. In this respect, the HeLa cells behaved quite differently from any of the nonmalignant cell lines we studied.

Earlier in vivo studies by us (unpublished) indicated that the infant prepuce was not characterized by a circadian rhythm. In fact, the pattern of fluctuation in vivo was more ultradian than circadian. These results were confusing to us because they were in conflict with earlier work, frequently cited (even to this day), claiming a circadian rhythm for the human infant prepuce (Cooper and Schiff 1938). Before accepting the finding of the earlier work as dogma, one should evaluate it carefully. Cooper and Schiff used only 13 specimens throughout the entire 24-hr span. We used a great many more specimens. In our opinion, the question of whether the newborn prepuce displays circadian rhythms needs to be reevaluated. Based on our own experience, we believe the waveform of the in vivo mitotic index rhythm in the human infant prepuce to be ultradian. Due to an unfortunate accident of flooding, our data were lost before they could be published. It is hoped that someone will repeat these studies.

It was with this background on the prepuce of the above-mentioned in vivo studies that we decided to do another in vitro study using a source of cells different from human prepuce since perhaps we had not selected in the above-mentioned study the most appropriate tissue. Rat corneal cells that had been growing in our laboratory for 3 years (76th subculture) were selected. In this respect, the corneal cells differed from the infant prepuce, human skin, and tonsillar cells which were primary cell cultures, none of which survived culture for more than a year because of some gradual nonspecific degeneration. The cells of the cornea cultures were heteroploid as determined by chromosome numbers.

The data obtained from mitotic counts on the rat corneal cells are plotted in Fig.

26E as the relative change of the individual hourly mean indices from the overall 24-hr mean. It is clear that the fluctuating nature of the cell-proliferation rate, which was characteristic of the infant prepuce, adult skin, and tonsillar tissue cultures, could also be seen in the corneal cell cultures. Curiously, on each sampling day, only one acute major peak in mitotic rate was observed. The peaks of the rhythms in the various studies were not in phase—that is, they did not occur at the same clock hour. All samples, however, demonstrated peak values of about the same magnitude, with the values being about 400% above the overall mean mitotic rate. Therefore, it might appear that the mitotic rate of rat corneal cells in culture was rhythmic over the 24-hr span, but the temporal occurrence of peak values was shifting in time. Was this an expression of "free running" within the culture of cells?

We conclude that there was no evidence from our own work that cell proliferation in vitro is synchronized to the LD cycle; nor can this be concluded with confidence from any of the work reported in the literature to date. To solve the problem of whether we are dealing with a free-running circadian rhythm or a type of ultradian fluctuation needs much more investigation using a system in which the cultures being monitored are carefully controlled and in which continuous samples can be obtained easily over several consecutive days at frequent intervals. Until this is done, identification of any specific frequency is unlikely. Fortunately, facilities today are much better than those available to us over 20 years ago.

It should, however, be of great interest or even concern to those engaged in cell-culture work to know that from hour to hour the metabolic behavior of their cultures may vary dramatically, as has been demonstrated for cell proliferation. Although we do not know the reasons for this fluctuation, we feel confident that we can rule out environmental temperature changes, since in our system temperature was carefully controlled. It was also of in-terest to note the rather unusual difference in the oscillatory behavior between HeLa cells and all other nonmalignant types. We have no explanation of this except to speculate that malignant cells have lost this ability to oscillate in a manner similar to normal cells.

Cell-Proliferation Rhythms in Tumors

A number of workers have reported evidence for and against circadian variation in the mitotic index of several different tumor types when studied at different times along the 24-hr domain in both animals and human beings. Among the first such studies was that of Dublin et al. (1940), who studied the mitotic activity of a human carcinoma of the large intestine. They simply removed specimens once during the day (1000–1200) and once during the night (2000–2400) and, finding little difference, concluded that no circadian variation was present.

Animal Models

Among the first adequately designed studies for rhythm exploration in animals were those of Blumenfeld (1943) who demonstrated the occurrence of mitotic rhythms in various healthy tissues of rabbits and mice. He then compared the mitotic activity of the presumably normal epidermis with that of a carcinoma induced in the same animals by the topical application of 3-methylcholanthrene. Unlike the normal epidermis, the induced epidermal carcinoma did not show a 24-hr synchronized circadian rhythm (Fig. 27F). The interpretation of this finding was that the malignancy represented an "escape" of the tumor from physiologic control of cell proliferation. A series of studies by Bertalanffy and Lau (1962b), Bertalanffy (1963a,b), and Bertalanffy and McAskill (1964) failed to detect any circadian variation in several tumor models, among them being spontaneous mammary gland adenocarcinoma in C3H/HeJ mice. As mentioned

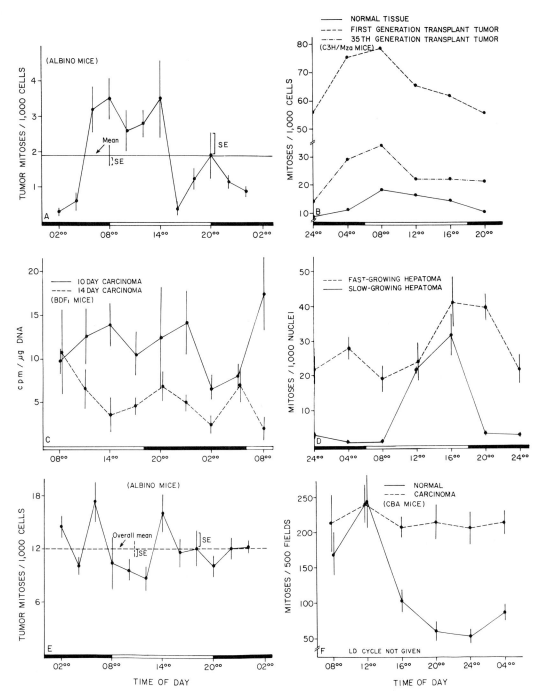

Fig. 27. **A** Circadian mitotic-index rhythm in spontaneous mammary tumors in mice; 96 "A"-strain mice were used (from Rosene and Halberg 1970). **B** Mitotic rhythm in normal mammary epithelium in mice in the first generation of a transplanted mammary carcinoma and in the 35th transplant generation of the same tumor (from Badran and Echave Llanos 1965). **C** The pattern of variation along the 24-hr scale in 10- and 14-day-old Lewis lung carcinoma in BD2F$_1$ mice. Although there is little evidence of a circadian rhythm, there is as much as 320% variation (from Burns et al. 1979). **D** Daily fluctuation in the mitotic activity of a fast-growing (SSIK) and a slow-growing (SSIH)

earlier, these workers have often failed to detect any circadian variation *even* in normal tissues. Nash and Echave Llanos (1971) reported a circadian rhythm in DNA synthesis of a slow-growing hepatoma (SS1H), but the variation was not as prominent as in a fast-growing hepatoma (SS1K) (Fig. 27D). Moreover, Badran and Echave Llanos (1965) reported the persistence of circadian rhythmicity in the mitotic activity of mammary carcinoma of C3H/Mza female mice and found that this tumor persisted over 35 transplant generations carried out over a 3-year period (Fig. 27B). Rosene and Halberg (1970) demonstrated the presence of a high-amplitude change along the 24-hr scale in mammary carcinoma in "A" mice (Fig. 27A). We believe that this well-designed study is especially relevant because the tumors studied were spontaneous in origin.

Burns et al. (1979) reported statistically significant differences in the uptake of [^{3}H]TdR into DNA in 10-day and 14-day transplanted Lewis lung carcinoma (Fig. 27C). The differences observed along the 24-hr scale were as great as 320%. There was, however, no evidence from their limited data of any circadian pattern. We also have carried out repeated studies on three other experimental mouse tumor models; they include: (1) the transplanted L1210 leukemia, (2) the Ehrlich ascites tumor, and (3) the mammary adenocarcinoma. An impression from studying the data of our collected studies is that when the tumor cells of different models are transplanted while still in the exponential growth phase, they are very likely to exhibit more of an ultradian (high-frequency) than a circadian variation. We have found that occasionally, when the data of a particular study are plotted over a single 24-hr span, a typical circadian pattern may emerge. But our impression is that this is not likely to be predictable from one study to another, especially in the transplanted tumor model. Evidence to support such a view comes from Rosene and Halberg (1970) who reported the absence of a circadian rhythm in transplanted Ehrlich ascites carcinoma in adult "A" mice (Fig. 27E), while Rubin et al. (1983) found rhythms in the G_1, S, and G_2 phases of the cell cycle in male Swiss mice using the FCM technique.

Human Models

Voutilainen (1953) carried out a series of studies on 21 patients with malignant tumors. Repeated biopsies were taken from the tumors of these patients along the 24-hr scale (longitudinal sampling). The patients were then irradiated (each one at a different interval of time after the first sampling), and another series of biopsies were carried out on all the patients at 2-hr intervals over a single 24-hr span, just subsequent to radiation. Thus, Voutilainen was able to compare the pattern of mitotic activity in subjects who had been sampled sufficiently far in advance of the radiation with the pattern in the same subjects immediately after irradiation (Fig. 28A).

hepatoma. Significantly higher mean values of mitotic activity are observed during light (L) than during darkness. The fast-growing hepatoma presents higher values than the slow-growing hepatoma during darkness, but the values for the 2 hepatomas are not different from one another during part of the L span. The circadian amplitude is higher in the slow-growing hepatoma and approached that found in the normal immature liver (from Echave Llanos and Nash 1970). **E** Variation along the 24-hr scale in an Ehrlich ascites tumor transplanted into "A" mice; no circadian variation is evident (Rosene and Halberg 1970). **F** Mitotic activity in an epidermal carcinoma compared with that in the normal epidermis of the rat (sampling at 4-hr intervals for a period of 24 hr). Note that there is no circadian variation in the tumor, whereas there is a characteristic circadian variation in the normal epidermis. The author failed to give the LD cycle to which the animals were standardized. (Reproduced with permission from Blumenfeld 1943.)

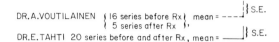

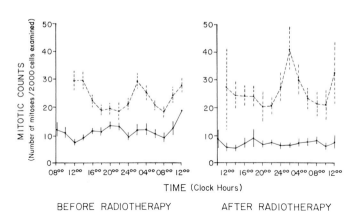

Fig. 28. Mean mitotic counts on serial biopsies from human malignancies, before (*left*) and after (*right*) radiotherapy. In the Tähti (1956) series of data (10 patients, *solid lines*) a biopsy was taken from each tumor at 2-hr intervals during the 24-hr span preceding exposure to X-rays and for 24 hr immediately after radiotherapy. Thus, 24 samples were obtained from each patient during a 48-hr span. Voutilainen's (1953) data (*dashed line*) were obtained from 21 patients with malignant tumors. The studies were similar, except that Voutilainen did not sample from the same tumor immediately before irradiation as did Tähti. These were tumors of several types (squamous cell, basal cell, and mammary carcinomas). When Garcia-Sainz and Halberg (1966) further analyzed these same data using the Cosinor, a clear-cut rhythm could be detected for the data on the mammary carcinoma but not for the squamous or basal cell carcinomas.

Following this, another herculean study was carried out by Tähti (1956) on 20 patients with exophytic ulcerated malignant tumors (Fig. 28B). A biopsy was taken from each tumor at 2-hr intervals during a 24-hr span immediately preceding exposure of the patients to X rays and again during another 24-hr span immediately after radiotherapy. In all, 24 samples were obtained from the tumor of each patient during a single 48-hr span. The major difference between the two studies was that Voutilainen did not sample the tumors immediately before irradiation as did Tähti. The conclusion of both authors, based upon examination of the data which are displayed in Fig. 28, was that prior to irradiation they were dealing with a bimodal rhythm.

Garcia-Sainz and Halberg (1966), using a Cosinor program for analyzing time series data, reevaluated the data from both the above studies. Although originally the three kinds of tumors were considered all together, in the re-analyses, the different tumors were separated into (1) squamous, (2) basal cell, and (3) mammary carcinoma types and tested separately for the presence of circadian variation. The conclusion from the special statistical evaluation of Garcia-Sainz and Halberg was that a statistically significant circadian rhythm could be demonstrated only for the mammary carcinoma data.

It is of interest to us that in both of the above studies, but especially in that of Voutilainen, maximum mitotic activity took place around midnight, which is the time when we and others had reported the occurrence of highest mitotic activity in the normal human epidermis as shown in Fig. 19 (Scheving and Gatz 1955; Scheving 1957; Fisher 1968; Zagula-Mally et al. 1979). This also was the time when Killman et al. (1962) and Mauer (1965), while evaluating human bone marrow for circadian variation, found the highest mitotic index (Fig. 20). It is our opinion that this similarity of phasing is not likely to be a coincidence, but of course this has not been proven.

Chemotherapy and Radiotherapy

At least two approaches can be taken when exploring the effect that the underlying rhythmicity in cell proliferation may have on the response to chemotherapy or radiotherapy. One way would be to concentrate on the rhythms (or lack of rhythms) found in the tumors themselves. Another is to concentrate on administering the treatment so as to minimize damage to normal cells that are vulnerable to either or both modes of treatment. We leaned toward the latter approach, that is, to protect in time the normal tissues such as the bone marrow and intestinal tract against the potent toxic effects of treatment—a "shielding in time" of the normal tissues—while still attacking the tumor (Scheving et al. 1974b, 1977a). This has been done experimentally by first determining host toxicity rhythms for certain agents and then applying the information gained to devise optimum schedules for the administration of particular chemotherapeutic agents in tumor-bearing animals.

Host Toxicity Rhythms

The host resistance to 1-β-D-arabinofuranosylcytosine (ara-C) (Fig. 29) illustrates what is meant by circadian variation in host toxicity. In our laboratory, a single fixed dose of ara-C administered once daily for 6 days to different subgroups of mice at different time points may kill as many as 78% of the animals, if injected at one time point, and as few as 15% of those injected at another time (Cardoso et al. 1970; Scheving et al. 1974a).

Subsequent work by Haus et al. (1972) applied this finding to the treatment of leukemic mice. In an initial study, a potentially lethal dose of 240 mg/kg ara-C was administered intraperitoneally to mice that had been inoculated with either 1×10^6 or 1×10^7 leukemia cells. Treatment was initiated 2 days (44 hr) after tumor-cell inoculation and was repeated on days 6, 10, and 14. On each treatment day, the total dosage of the drug was divided into 8 doses which were given at 3-hr intervals over a 24-hr span. The doses given at the various injection times, however, varied in amount according to a sinusoidal pattern. The amounts ranged from 7.4 mg/kg given at the time of the animals' lowest resistance to the drug (as predicted from earlier studies) to 67.5 mg/kg given at the predicted time of highest resistance. Even the smallest dose, given when the host was most susceptible, exerted some therapeutic antitumor activity (Halberg et al. 1973).

Such experimental chronotherapy succeeded in approximately doubling the survival time of leukemic mice compared to the controls that were treated without chronobiological consideration. The daily course of treatment using the nonchronobiological approach consisted of administering eight equal doses at 3-hr intervals over the 24-hr span. This treatment schedule had been described by Skipper et al. (1967) as the current (at the time these studies were initiated) best treatment for the mouse L1210 leukemia model.

Although the advantage of treating leukemic mice according to a sinusoidal schedule was clear-cut from the work reported by Haus et al. (1972), it seemed of interest to use a larger sample limited to tolerance per se in order to attempt an unequivocal demonstration of rhythmic variation in host susceptibility to ara-C. Studies were done us-

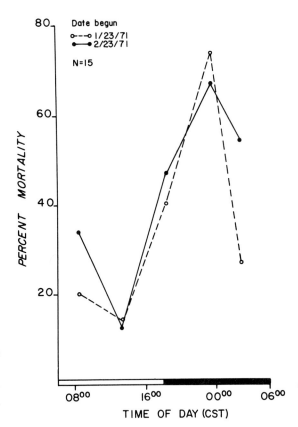

Fig. 29. Circadian susceptibility rhythm of BD2F₁ mice to arabinosylcytosine (ara-C) given on five consecutive days at single, defined, circadian-system phases. (Reproduced from Scheving et al. 1974a.)

ing the same experimental design and on the same day at both Little Rock, Arkansas, and Minneapolis, Minnesota. In each laboratory, 9 groups of 20 normal mice each received 4 courses of ara-C treatment beginning 2/7/73. In each course, a total dose of 240 mg/kg ara-C was divided among 8 separate injections given at 3-hr intervals. One group of mice received equal doses of ara-C at each time point (the reference schedule). The 8 other groups received the same total dose per course, but on one of several different sinusoidal schedules as illustrated in Fig. 30. As predicted from the earlier work, survival time after treatment with ara-C on different sinusoidal schedules differed significantly. Moreover, the sinusoidal schedules which yielded the longest or shortest survival times were remarkably similar in the two laboratories (Scheving et al. 1976b).

Chronotherapy of L1210 Leukemia Using the Single Drug Ara-C

Thus far we have considered reports dealing with variation only in mortality and survival time from acute drug toxicity in both normal and leukemic mice. It was of interest to determine whether an increase in cure rate could be obtained. Skipper et al. (1967) had reported that when mice bearing an inoculum of 1×10^5 L1210 tumor cells were treated with 120 mg/kg ara-C (15 mg/kg every 3 hr for 24 hr) on days 2, 6, 10, and 14 after tumor inoculation, generally most animals were cured. They also reported, using only 8 animals, that 62% of mice bearing 1×10^6 leukemic cells were cured using the above treatment protocol. In a comparable study using 10 mice, they reported that 50% were cured; however, in 2 subsequent studies (using 10 animals in each), no cures were obtained at this disease stage. These studies are mentioned because the claim was made (Rose et al. 1978), while commenting on the merits of a chronobiological approach to chemotherapy, that Skipper and his co-workers could, without a chronobiological approach, cure 62% of animals bearing the above-mentioned tumor load. None of our studies (using the same animal strain) or those of our collaborators, using hundreds of mice bearing this tumor load, have resulted in such high cure rates

as were *sometimes* found by Skipper and his coworkers when treatment was ara-C. We caution that the claim of a 62% cure rate mentioned above should be evaluated in light of all the data available from the laboratory in question.

To date, the best cure rate that we or our collaborators can achieve consistently with such an advanced disease stage (an inoculum of 1×10^6 leukemia cells) and using the single drug, ara-C (120 mg/kg per course and 4 courses of treatment given on days 2,

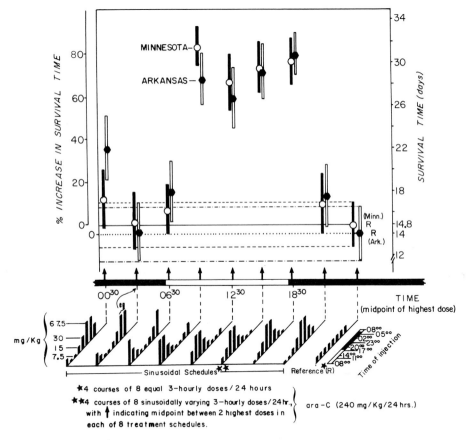

Fig. 30.   Survival times of CD2F$_1$ mice on different drug-administration schedules (*top*) and timing of doses of ara-C (*bottom*) in sinusoidal and reference (*R*) schedules. All treatment schedules comprise 4 courses, each consisting of a total of 240 mg/kg/24 hr. When the same total dose of ara-C is given, certain sinusoidal drug-administration schedules are definitely better tolerated by mice than are other sinusoids or than was a conventional (at the time the study was done) reference treatment schedule of 8 equal doses over a 24-hr span. Also, note unequivocal reproducibility of chronotoxicity of ara-C in experiments done on the same days in different laboratories in different geographic locations. (Reproduced from Scheving et al. 1976.)

6, 10, and 14), is between 20% and 28%. Increasing or decreasing the dosage does not improve this. If the dosage is increased, overwhelming toxicity prevails; if it is decreased, the leukemia prevails. We believe that the above is the most realistic cure rate to be expected for this stage of the disease, using $CD2F_1$ or $BD2F_1$ mice. Let us point out this cure rate could be consistently obtained *only* by using the *chronobiological* approach. When using a *homeostatic* approach, the cure rate in our studies was usually lower, being about one-half or even less than that achieved by the chronobiological approach. For example, in one study using 282 leukemic mice (141 on each treatment schedule) the cure rate (60-day survivors) was 23% for those treated on a chronobiological schedule but only 11% for those treated on a nonchronobiological schedule (Kühl et al. 1974). Such findings have been consistent, being detected both in Arkansas and Minnesota. Rose et al. (1978), in an attempt to confirm the findings of Haus et al. (1972), carried out studies in which they reported variation in host toxicity, thus confirming what has been reported earlier. Rose and his co-workers also reported that they did not find the therapeutic advantage claimed by Haus et al. (1972) using chronobiologically designed treatment schedules. It is important to recognize that they did not utilize the same experimental design. Rose and his colleagues administered only 1 or 2 courses of treatment, whereas Haus and others administered 4 courses. The fewer courses of treatment represent a significant alteration in protocol and were not very likely to manifest the full advantage of chemotherapy. [For further comments relative to the studies of Rose et al. (1978), see Halberg et al. (1979b,c), Burns and Scheving (1980), and Scheving et al. (1974).]

The Principle of Equal Toxicity

A comment should be made regarding the argument that one cannot compare two treatment schedules for a given drug—even though the total dosage given is the same— if the resulting acute drug toxicity in the host turns out to be unequal. In light of chronobiological variation, the classic concept of equal toxicity has to be questioned. A pertinent situation may be the case of an extremely toxic dose of a drug which one might elect not to use in a nonchronobiological treatment schedule, whereas its use in the timed treatment approach would be feasible. With such a drug, it may well be that the dose in a conventional regimen found to be equitoxic to the dose in a chemotherapeutically optimized regimen would be so low that it would be ineffective. A comparison of equitoxicity which disregards time may have little meaning (Haus et al. 1979).

Chronotherapy of L1210 Leukemia Using a Two-Drug Combination of Ara-C and Cyclophosphamide (CTX)

To obtain consistently better than a 28% cure rate using ara-C in any manner against 1×10^6 L1210 leukemia cells with treatment initiated on the second day, it was obvious a second drug was required in combination with ara-C. The second drug chosen was CTX and the results are illustrated in Fig. 31. In this study, mice were inoculated with 1.2×10^6 leukemia cells and treatment was initiated 44 hr later. Four courses (at intervals of 4 days) of ara-C were given (120 mg/kg per course) to all mice, and it was administered in one of the "best sinusoidal" schedules previously described. Each group of 20 mice also received 15 mg/kg CTX once per course, but each group of 6 received it at a different circadian stage. Only 2 mice out of 140 died from what might have been attributed to acute toxicity; all others that died did so from leukemia. As is evident, the cure rate ranged from 44%–94% along the circadian domain. When comparable animals bearing an identical tumor burden were treated with the same drugs and dosage given without chronobiological consideration, 30% died from acute drug toxicity. Those that sur-

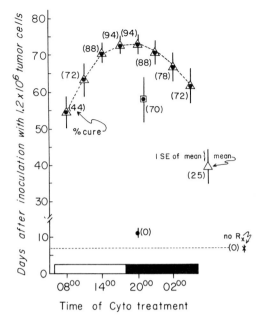

Fig. 31. Survival time and percentage of cures in L1210 leukemic mice treated with ara-C plus cyclophosphamide (CTX). The △ implies the best sinusoidal ara-C treatment schedule. The □ implies the reference treatment schedule. The ● implies that CTX was administered, in combination with ara-C, once per course to each mouse; however, different groups received it at different circadian stages ▲. The percentage of cures (percentage alive 75 days after tumor inoculation) is shown in parentheses. Time of the CTX administration is indicated on the horizontal scale. The groups that did not receive CTX are shown just right of the time scale. N = 20 for each group. (Reproduced from Scheving et al. 1977c.)

age of either drug as little as 10%, as might be necessary in order to treat according to the conventional (nonchronobiologic) approach, the leukemia would prevail.

Chronotherapy of L1210 Leukemia Using More than Two Drugs

Subsequent studies using more than two drugs against a larger tumor load than that described above have shown similarly that the chronobiological approach for treating L1210 leukemia is superior to the homeostatic one (Burns et al. 1979; Scheving et al. 1980). For example, we found that when 5×10^6 L1210 leukemia cells were injected and when treatment with a combination of five drugs commonly used in the clinic was initiated 44 hr later using the chronobiological approach, it was possible to attain a cure rate of 88% (range from 44 to 88%) as shown in Fig. 32. There were no deaths due to drug toxicity; all animals dying did so from leukemia (Fig. 33). This cure rate was not possible using the same five drugs with the homeostatic approach, from which 54% and 64% died due to acute toxicity (Figs. 32 and 33). Mean weight loss from 4 courses of treatment at the best circadian time (time of highest cure rate) was 2.5 g, whereas in the homeostatically treated animals it was 6.8 g. Thus, there is evidence that the "quality of life" for the treated mouse was improved by chronotherapy as well.

Circadian Variation in Sequencing of Two Drugs Used in Combination

In still more recent studies using two drugs and only one course of treatment consisting of 100 mg/kg CTX and 5 mg/kg adriamycin (ADR), after administration of 1×10^5 L1210 leukemia cells 4 days prior to treatment, it was shown that a dramatic circadian variation in response could be obtained. The variation in cure rate (mice alive and apparently free of disease 75 days after tumor inoculation) as a function of treatment time ranged from 8% to 68% in male ani-

vived the acute drug toxicity, however, were cured for this particular tumor load (Scheving et al. 1977c). The point to be made is that by giving agents in a chronobiological manner we have been able to eliminate the drug-induced death due to toxicity while still using an effective dose. There seemed to be little merit in attempting to treat by the conventional approach after adjusting the dosage so that toxicity would be equal to that of the chronobiologic approach. Previous studies had led us to conclude that if we were to reduce the dos-

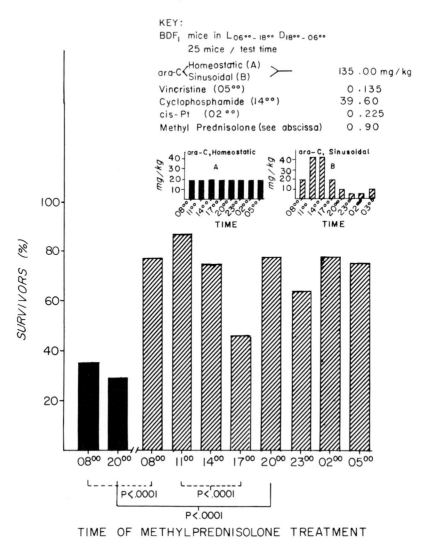

Fig. 32. Between 1130 and 1230, all (CD2F₁) mice were weighed and injected intraperitoneally with 5.0 × 10⁶ L1210 leukemia cells; the control group which received no treatment was injected with leukemia cells last. Treatment was initiated 45 hr later, beginning at 0800. Eight groups of animals received 135 mg/kg of ara-C over the 24-hr span administered on the sinusoidal schedule as follows: 15.88 mg/kg at 0800, then at 3-hr intervals, 38.25, 38.25, 15.88, 8.44, 4.22, 4.22, and 8.44 mg/kg. All of these mice also received 39.6 mg/kg of C (*Cyclophosphamide*) at 1400, 0.135 mg/kg of V (*Vincristine*) at 0500 and 0.225 mg/kg of CP (*cis-Pt*) at 0200. Each of these 8 groups was given 0.9 mg/kg of P (*Methylprednisolone*) once during the 24-hr span, one group receiving it at 0800, the second group at 1100, and so on at 3-hr intervals. The 9th and 10th groups (*black bars*) recived ara-C on a homeostatic (equal dose) treatment schedule of 16.88 mg/kg/3 hr, with 39.6 mg/kg of C at 1400, 0.135 mg/kg of V at 0500, and CP at 0200. One of the groups (8) received 0.9 mg/kg of P at 0800 and the other (9) at 2000. Four courses of treatment were administered to all groups with a 3-day interval between courses; all animals were weighed at the beginning (0800) of each course. The percentage of cured (tumor-free) animals in each group was determined on the 75th day after tumor inoculation. We do not know of any other report where such a large tumor load was cured with no deaths due to acute drug toxicity which was the case for the chronobiologically treated group. (Reproduced from Scheving et al. 1980.)

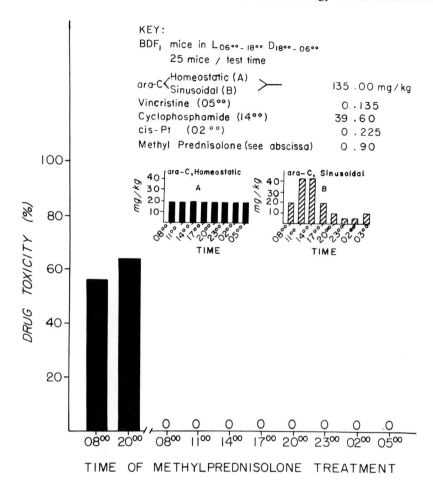

Fig. 33. Percentage of deaths from acute drug toxicity in the same study described in Fig. 32. An important finding was that none of the chronobiologically treated animals died from acute drug toxicity, whereas 54 and 64% of those treated on the homeostatic schedule died. (Reproduced from Scheving et al. 1980.)

mals standardized to LD 12:12 (Fig. 34). Similarly, in females standardized to LD 8:16, the cure rate ranged from 0 to 56% depending upon the stage of the mouse circadian system when treatment was given (Fig. 34). No cures were obtained with either drug alone. The maximum cure rate was recorded when the two drugs were administered during the early part of the D portion of the LD cycle (whether LD 12:12 or LD 8:16), whereas maximum mortality occurred following treatment early in the L span. Such variation also was seen in the length of survival of those mice that died; thus, both survival time and cure rate are

circadian-stage dependent (Scheving et al. 1980E).

In this same study, the data also showed that the maximum therapeutic advantage was obtained when the two drugs were separated by 2- or 3-hr intervals and that this effect of drug sequencing was strongly circadian-stage dependent (Fig. 35).

Additional Data from Toxicity Studies Relative to Chemotherapy

It has been questioned whether one should expect a large variation in host resistance when using a long-acting drug such as

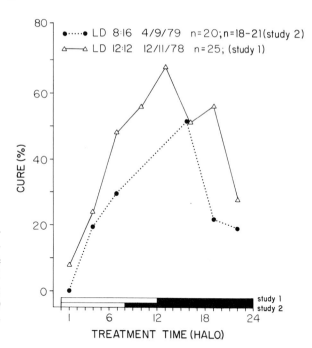

Fig. 34. Variation in cure rate of leuke-mic mice depending on the timing of com-bined treatment with cyclophosphamide (CTX) and adriamycin (ADR). Study 1 (*solid line*) on male mice in LD 12:12; study 2 (*dotted line*) on female mice in LD 8:16. *HALO* = hr after lights on. (Repro-duced from Scheving et al. 1980.)

ADR. To answer this, Kühl et al. (1973) gave a potentially lethal dose of ADR to both inbred Bragg albino mice and Fischer rats. They injected different subgroups from each species with 17.9 mg/kg at either 0800 or 2000 and found that 10% of those mice receiving ADR at 0800 died, whereas 55% of the mice receiving it at 2000 died. This finding was further investigated in greater detail in the same laboratory

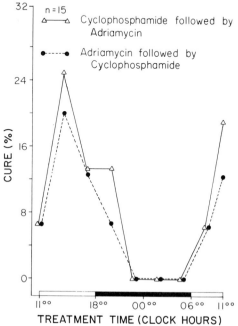

Fig. 35. Effect of drug sequence and interval (prob-ably confounded by circadian variation) in response of leukemic mice to cyclophosphamide and adriamy-cin. First drug given at 1100 (approximately midlight) and second drug given either concomitantly or 3, 6, 9, 12, 15, 18, 21, or 24 hr later. We conclude from these data that the best way of administering these two drugs in combination is to separate them by 2 or 3 hr. One might argue that this may hold true if the first drug is given near midlight (as was the case in this study), but may not be the case if the first drug is administered at another circadian stage (for example, during middark). Admittedly, the outcome might be completely different; however, it seems clear that circadian variation in response should be considered in any study of sequencing of drugs (Scheving et al. 1980).

(Sothern et al. 1977) in 5 different toxicity studies using a total of 858 inbred male mice with frequent intervals of sampling along the 24-hr domain. The results of these studies demonstrated unequivocally that the maximum mortality to ADR occurred around mid-D and that the host was more resistant to the drug around mid-L. It was further found that this rhythm in susceptibility could be modified by restricting the intake of food to the first 4 hr of the daily L span.

Nelson et al. (1974) conducted experimental chronotherapy studies and reported the advantage of treating immunocytoma-bearing LOU rats with ADR at certain stages of the circadian system. In animals fed *ad libitum*, the longest survival time occurred in those animals treated at the beginning of the D span; the shortest survival times were associated with those animals treated during the L span.

Philippens and Scheving (1979) calculated the difference in survival rate between NMRI mice bearing untreated Ehrlich ascites tumors and those treated at specific clock hours daily for 10 days, and reported

that it varied dramatically depending upon the stage of the mouse circadian cycle when treatment with ADR was given. For example, in a group of mice treated daily with a dosage of 1.75 mg/kg/day of adriamycin for 10 days at 1900 (1 hr into the D span), the mean survival time (calculated as the time when 50% of the animals had died) was 48 days longer than the mean survival time for the untreated mice. However, those mice treated at 0700 [1 hr into the L phase of the daily LD cycle (LD 12:12)] died even before the untreated control animals.

High-amplitude host toxicity rhythms also have been documented for daunomycin and vincristine (Halberg 1980). Simpson and Stoney (1977) found melphalan (L-Pam) when given to different subgroups of mice at different circadian stages produced a rhythm in the number of nucleated femur marrow cells evident 4 days after treatment. This finding, demonstrating that damage to the normal bone-marrow cells is circadian-stage dependent (Fig. 36), is important since lethality to the host is due in part to bone marrow depression.

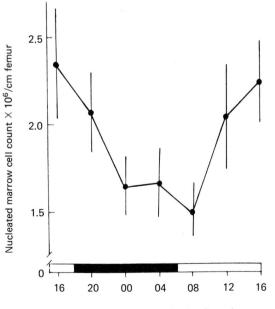

Fig. 36. Melphalan was injected intraperitoneally into 7 different subgroups of CFLP albino mice, and cell counts were made 96 hr after the injection. It is clear that bone-marrow depression is greatest in those groups which received the drug close to the end of the D span and around the transition from D to L. (Reproduced from Simpson and Stoney 1977.)

Conclusions

Clearly the response to both long-acting and short-acting drugs is circadian-stage dependent. This variation in response to different drugs may be interpreted as reflecting the rhythmic variation in the biochemistry of a large number of variables within the organism over the 24-hr period (Scheving 1980a–d). The circadian variation of susceptibility in the principal target organs of these drugs, such as the bone marrow and gut, plays a prominent part in generating the temporal variation in susceptibility seen in the host. At the present time, the mass of experimental data leads to the obvious conclusion that attempts must be made to bring such concepts into the clinic.

On the preventive side, there may be an advantage in monitoring and comparing a rhythmic variable, such as breast temperature, at the site of a tumor to that in normal tissue—the rationale being that the tumor site will manifest a higher metabolic rate and even an altered tumor rhythm (Simpson 1976; Halberg et al. 1979a). This may enable one to detect a tumor by monitoring the temperature over it even before it becomes palpable. A great deal of interest has arisen in this concept of prevention; it has led to the development of the "chronobra" which is so constructed that continuous temperature recordings can be made simultaneously from many different sites on a mammary gland (Simpson and Mutch 1981; Halberg et al. 1979a).

With respect to treatment, it is unfortunate that it took almost 50 years between the time of the first observation of circadian variations in cell proliferation to the application of these findings on an experimental basis to cancer chemotherapy or prevention. We have only just reached the stage when most scientists accept without question the existence of and the potential importance of such rhythms, even though they may still ignore them in experimental design. Based on the facts, we must abandon the erroneous concept that somehow sampling at the "same time of day" takes

care of the "rhythm problem" (Scheving 1976).

We are confident that there will not be a similar span of 50 years before the importance of rhythmicity to cancer biology and treatment in the clinics is adequately explored. One pioneering study recently reported has shown in the clinic that both the pharmacokinetics and the kidney toxicity of *cis*-platinum can be dramatically reduced in patients with advanced cancer by timing this drug relative to biological rhythms (Hrushesky et al. 1980, 1982; Lévi et al. 1980). Halberg (1977), in collaboration with Gupta of India (Gupta and Deka 1975), has reported that the timing of radiotherapy in relation to a marker rhythm (tumor temperature) determines the *rate* of regression of perioral tumors. Moreover, it has been reported that human bone marrow toxicity from adriamycin is statistically significantly reduced by its circadian timing (Hrushesky et al. 1981, 1982). Even more important, Hrushesky recently reported a response rate of 100% in a preliminary study of 12 patients with advanced—stages 3 and 4—ovarian carcinoma, who were treated with a chronobiologically designed two-drug chronotherapy regime. Over 80% of these responses were complete (total disappearance of all measurable disease). This 100% response rate compared favorably with a 42% response rate for 19 comparable control ovarian cancer patients who received the same two agents in the same doses but at random circadian stages. The duration of response was also highly statistically significantly different between the two groups ($P < 0.0001$) (Hrushesky et al. 1981) in favor of those 12 cancer patients who received chronotherapy.

Circadian cytokinetics, pharmacokinetics, endocrinology, immunology, and toxicology can no longer be ignored but must be used to treat human cancer more effectively and eventually to prevent some varieties of malignancies. The major shortcoming of classical noncircadian cytokinetics has been the inability to directly translate in vitro advances from the petri dish to the cancer patient. It has been thought that this has been because of the recognition that the in vitro synchronized cell population behaves differently than the in vivo populations which have classically been assumed to be nonrhythmic with regard to cytokinetic parameters. The realization that there is relative synchrony along the circadian time scale within all in vivo cell populations is the only solution for cytokinetics as a practical, clinically relevant tool for the treatment of cancer patients. If the basic rhythmicity inherent in the organism is not ignored, we believe this will greatly benefit cancer patients.

Some of the work reported herein was supported by grant CA-14388 from the National Cancer Institute and grant OH-00952 from the National Institute of Occupational Safety and Health.

References

Badran, AF, and Echave Llanos, JM (1965) Persistence of mitotic circadian rhythm of a transplantable mammary carcinoma after 35 generations: Its bearing on the success of treatment with endoxan. J Natl Cancer Inst 35:285–290.

Barnum, CP, Jardetzky, CD, and Halberg, F (1957) Nucleic acid synthesis in regenerating liver. Tex Rep Biol Med 15:134–147.

Bertalanffy, FD (1960) Mitotic rates and renewal times of the digestive tract epithelia in the rat. Acta Anat 40:130–148.

Bertalanffy, FD (1963a) Mitotic rate of methylcholanthrene induced subcutaneous fibrosarcoma. Naturwissenschaften 50:648–659.

Bertalanffy, FD (1963b) Mitotic rate of spontaneous mammary gland adenocarcinoma in C3H/HeJ mice. Nature 198:496–497.

Bertalanffy, FD, and Lau, C (1962a) Mitotic rate and renewal time of the corneal epithelium of the rat. Arch Ophthalmol 68:546–550.

Bertalanffy, FD, and Lau, C (1962b) Rates of cell division of transplantable malignant rat tumors. Cancer Res 22:627–631.

Bertalanffy, FD, and Lau, C (1963) Mitotic rates, renewal times and cytodynamics of the female genital tract epithelia in the rat. Acta Anat 54:39–81.

Bertalanffy, FD, and McAskill, C (1964). Rate of cell division of malignant mouse melanoma. J Natl Cancer Inst 32:535–545.

Blumenfeld, CM (1943) Studies of normal and abnormal mitotic activity. II. The rate and periodicity of the mitotic activity of experimental epidermoid carcinoma in mice. Arch Pathol Lab Med 35:667–673.

Burns, ER, and Scheving, LE (1975) Circadian influence on the waveform of the frequency of labeled mitoses and mouse corneal epithelium. Cell Tissue Kinet 8:61–66.

Burns, ER, and Scheving, LE (1980) Circadian optimization of the treatment of L1210 leukemia with 1-beta-D-arabinosyl cytosine, cyclophosphamide, vincristine and methylprednisolone. Chronobiologia 7:41–51.

Burns, ER, Uyeda, CK, and Scheving, LE (1973) Mitotic nests in human vaginal smears and cultures of amphibian cells. Oncology 27:92–96.

Burns, ER, Scheving, LE, and Tsai, TH (1979) Circadian rhythms in DNA synthesis and mitosis in normal mice and in mice bearing a Lewis Lung Carcinoma. Eur J Cancer 15:233–242.

Cardoso, SS, Scheving, LE, and Halberg, F (1970). Mortality of mice as influenced by the hour of day of drug (ARA-C) administration. Pharmacologist 12:302 (abstract).

Cherington, PV, Smith, BL, and Pardee, AG (1979) Loss of epidermal growth factor requirement and malignant transformation. Proc Natl Acad Sci 70:3937 (abstract).

Chumak, MG (1963) Mitotic cycle of epithelium cells of cornea in mice. Studied by means of thymidine tagged with tritium. Dokl Akad Nauk SSSR 149:960–962.

Cooper, ZK, and Schiff, A (1938) Mitotic rhythms in human epidermis. Proc Soc Exp Biol Med 39:323–324.

Dublin, WB, Gregg, RO, and Broders, AC (1940) Mitosis in specimens removed during the day and night from carcinoma of large intestine. Arch Path 30:893–395.

Echave Llanos, JM, and Nash, RE (1970) Mitotic circadian rhythm in a fast growing and a slow growing hepatoma. Mitotic rhythm in hepatomas. J Natl Cancer Inst 44:581–586.

Fisher, LB (1968) The diurnal mitotic rhythm in the human epidermis. Br J Dermatol 80:75–80.

Garcia-Sainz, M, and Halberg, F (1966) Mitotic rhythms in human cancer, reevaluated by electronic computer programs—evidence for chronopathology. J Natl Cancer Inst 37:279–292.

Gasser, RF, Scheving, LE, and Pauly, JE (1972a) Circadian rhythm in the cell division rate of the inner enamel epithelium and in the uptake of ^{3}H-thymidine by the root tip of the rat incisors. J Dent Res 51:740–746.

Gasser, RF, Scheving, LE, and Pauly, JE (1972b) Circadian rhythms in the mitotic index and in the uptake of ^{3}H-thymidine by the tongue of the rat. J Cell Physiol 80:437–442.

Goedeke, K, and Rensing, L (1974) Regulation des Zellcyclus. Naturwissenschaften 27:4–16.

Gonzalez, A, Garrido, J, and Vial, JD (1981) Epidermal growth factor inhibits cyto-skeleton changes in the surface of parietal cells. J Cell Biol 88:108–114.

Goodrum, PJ, Sowall, JG, and Cardoso, SS (1974) Characterization of the circadian rhythm of mitosis in the corneal epithelium of the immature rat. In: Scheving, LE, Halberg, F, and Pauly, JE (eds), *Chronobiology*. Tokyo: Igaku Shoin Ltd., pp. 29–32.

Gupta, BD, and Deka, AC (1975) Application of chronobiology to radiotherapy of tumor of the oral cavity. Chronobiologia 2 (Suppl. 1):125 (abstract).

Halberg, F (1959) Physiological 24-hour periodicity; general procedural consideration with reference to the adrenal cycle. Z vitamin-, hormon- u fermentforsch 10:225–296.

Halberg, F (1964) Grundlagenforschung zur Aetiologie des Karzinoms. Mkurse arztl Forbild 14:67–77.

Halberg, F (1980) Closing remarks: Chronobiology and health. In: Scheving, LE, and Halberg, F (eds), *Chronobiology: Principles and Applications to Shifts in Schedules*. Alphen aan den Rijn, The Netherlands: NATO Advanced Study Inst. Ser., Sijthoff and Noordhoff, pp. 541–562.

Halberg, F, Johnson, EA, Nelson, W, Runge, W, and Sothern, R (1972) Autorhythmometry procedures for physiologic self-measurements and their analysis. Physiol Teacher 1:1–11.

Halberg, F, Haus, E, Cardoso, SS, Scheving, LE, Kühl, JFW, Shiotsuka, R, Rosene, G, Pauly, JE, Runge, W, Spalding, JF, Lee, JK, and Good, RA (1973) Toward a chonotherapy of neoplasia: Tolerance of treatment depends upon host rhythms. Experientia 29:909–1044.

Halberg, F, Gupta, BD, Haus, E, Halberg, E, Deka, AC, Nelson, W, Sothern, RB, Cornelissen, G, Lee, JK, Lakatua, DJ, Scheving, LE, and Burns, ER (1977) Steps toward a cancer chronopolytherapy. In: *Proc. XIVth Int. Congress of Therapeutics,* Montpelier,

France, L'Expansion Scientifique Francaise, pp. 151–196.

Halberg, E, Halberg, F, Cornelissen, G, Garcia-Sainz, M, Simpson, HW, Tagaett-Anderson, MA, and Haus, E (1979a) Towards a chronopsy: Part II. A thermopsy revealing asymmetrical circadian variation in surface temperature of human female breasts and related studies. Chronobiologia 6:231–257.

Halberg, F, Nelson, W, Cornelissen, G, Haus, E, Scheving, LE, and Good, RA (1979b) On methods for testing and achieving cancer chronotherapy. Cancer Treat 63:1428–1430.

Halberg, F, Nelson, W, Cornelissen, G, Haus, E, Scheving, LE, and Good, RA (1979c) On methods for testing and achieving cancer chronotherapy. Chronobiologia 6:203–211.

Hardeland, R (1973) Diurnal variations in inducibility of hepatic tyrosine aminotransferase. Int J Biochem 4:357–364

Haus, E, Halberg, F, Scheving, LE, Cardoso, S, Kühl, J, Sothern, R, Shiotsuka, R, Hwang, DS, and Pauly, JE (1972) Increased tolerance of leukemic mice to arabinosyl cytosine with schedule adjusted to circadian system. Science 77:80–82.

Haus, E, Halberg, F, Scheving, LE, and Simpson, H (1979). Chronotherapy of cancer—a critical evaluation. Int J Chronobiol 6:67–107.

Hirata, Y, Vehihaskim, M, Nakajima, H, Fujita, T, Matsukura, S (1982) Epidermal growth factor urogastrone is present in CSF. J Clin Endocrinol 55:1174–1177.

Hrushesky, WJM (1982) Bone marrow suppression from doxorubicin and cis diamminedichloroplatinum is substantially dependent upon both circadian and circannual stage of administration. *Proceedings of NYAS Conference on Cell Proliferation, Cancer and Cancer Therapy*, in press

Hrushesky, W, Lévi, F, Halberg, F, Haus, E, Scheving, LE, Sanchez, S, Medini, E, Brown, H, and Kennedy, BJ (1980) Clinical chrono-oncology. In: Scheving, LE, and Halberg, F (eds), *Chronobiology: Principles and Applications to Shifts in Schedules*. Alphen aan den Rijn, The Netherlands: NATO Advanced Study Institutes Series, Sijthoff and Noordhoff, pp. 513–533.

Hrushesky, W, Halberg, F, Heinlen, T, Murray, C, and Kennedy, BJ (1980) Human bone marrow toxicity of adriamycin (AD) reduced by optimal circadian timing. Proc. ASCO 21:345 (abstract C-104).

Hrushesky, W, Lévi, F, Kennedy, BJ, Theologides, A, and Frenning, D (1981) Results of Circadian time-qualified chemotherapy in patients with advanced ovarian cancer. Cancer Res 22:472, abstract C-546.

Hrushesky, WJ, Borch, R, and Lévi, F (1982) A circadian time dependence of cisplatin urinary kinetics. Clin Pharm Ther 32:330–339.

Hüpe, K, and Gropp, A (1957) Über den zeitlichen Verlauf der mitoseaktivität in Gewebekulturen. A Zellforsch 46:67–70.

Killman, SA, Cronkite, EP, Fliedner, TM, and Bond, VT (1962) Mitotic indices of human bone marrow cells. I. Number and cytologic distribution of mitoses. Blood 19:743–750.

Klein, RM (1979) The third effective chemical sympathectomy on circadian variation of mitotic activity. Cell Tissue Kinet 12:649–657.

Krieger, DT, Hauser, H, Liotta, A, and Zelenetz, A (1976) Circadian periodicity of epidermal growth factor and its abolition by superior cervical ganglionectomy. Endocrinology 99:1589–1596.

Krueger, WA, Bo, WJ, and Hoopes, PC (1975) Circadian rhythm of mitotic activity in the uterine luminal epithelium of the rat: effect of estrogen. Anat Rec 183:563–566.

Kühl, JFW, Grage, TB, Halberg, F, Rosene, G, Scheving, LE, and Haus, E (1973) Ellen-effect: Tolerance of adriamycin by Bragg albino mice and Fischer rats depends on circadian timing of injection. Int J Chronobiol 1:333 (abstract).

Kühl, JFK, Haus, E, Halberg, F, Scheving, LE, Pauly, JE, Cardoso, SS, and Rosene, G (1974) Experimental chronotherapy with ara-C; Comparison of murine ara-C tolerance on differently timed treatment schedules. Chronobiologia 1:316–317.

Laerum, OD, and Aardal, NP (1981) Chronobiological aspects of bone marrow and blood cells. In: v Mayersbach, H, Scheving, LE, and Pauly, JE, (eds) Biological Rhythms in Structure and Function New York: Alan R. Liss, Inc., pp. 87–97.

Langer, R, and Rensing, L (1972) Circadian rhythm of oxygen consumption in rat liver suspension culture: changes of pattern. Z Naturforsch 27b:1117–1118.

Laurence, EB, Spargo, DJ, and Thornley, AL (1979) Cell proliferation kinetics of epidermis and sebaceous glands in relation to chalone action. Cell Tissue Kinet 12:615–633.

Lévi, F, Hrushesky, W, Haus, E, Halberg, F, Scheving, LE, and Kennedy, BJ (1980) Experimental chrono-oncology: In: Scheving, LE, and Halberg, F (eds), Chronobiology: Principles and Applications to Shifts in Schedules. Alphen aan den Rijn, The Netherlands: NATO Advanced Study Institutes Series, Sijthoff and Noordhoff, pp. 481–511.

Li, AK, Schattenkerk, ME, de Vries, JE, Ford, WDA, and Malt, RA (1980) Submandibular sialoadenectomy retards dimethylhydrazine induced colonic carcinogenesis. Gastroenterology 78:1207 (abstract).

Malholtra, SL (1964) Effect of saliva on gastric emptying. Scand J Gastro 2:95–104.

Mauer, AM (1965) Diurnal variation of proliferative activity in the human bone marrow. Blood 26:1–6.

von Mayersbach, H (1967) Seasonal influences on biological rhythms of standardized laboratory animals. In: von Mayersbach, H. (ed.), The Cellular Aspects of Biorhythms. Berlin: Springer-Verlag, pp. 87–89.

Murphy, RA, Watson, AY, Metz, J, George, W, and Forssman, WG (1980) The mouse submandibular gland: Endocrine organ for growth factors. J Histochem Cytochem 28:890–902.

Nash, RE, and Echave Llanos, JM (1971) Twenty-four-hour variations in DNA synthesis of a fast-growing and a slow-growing hepatoma: DNA synthesis rhythm in hepatoma. J Natl Cancer Inst 47:1007–1012.

Nelson, W, Zinneman, H, Selden, JA, Schaber, K, Halberg, F, and Bazin, H (1974) Circadian rhythm in Bence-Jones protein excretion by LOU rats bearing a transplantable immunocytoma, responsive to adriamycin treatment. Int J Chronobiol 2:359–366.

Panaretto, BA, Moore, CPM, and Robertson, DM (1982) Plasma concentrations and urinary excretion of mouse epidermal growth factor associated with the inhibition of food consumption and of wool growth in Merino wethers. J Endocrinol 94:191–202.

Pauly, JE, Burns, ER, Halberg, F, Tsai, S, Betterton, HO, and Scheving, LE (1975) Mealtiming dominates lighting regimen as a synchronizer of the eosinophil rhythm in mice. Acta Anat 93:60–68.

Philippens, KMH, and Scheving, LE (1979) Chronotoxic and therapeutic effects of adriamycin and Ehrlichs ascites tumor-bearing NMRI-mice. Chronobiologia 6:143 (abstract).

Philippens, KMH, von Mayersbach, H, and Scheving, LE (1977). Effects of the scheduling of meal-feeding at different phases of the circadian system in rats. J Nutr 107:176–193.

Quastler, H, and Sherman, FG (1959) Cell population kinetics in the intestinal epithelium of the mouse. Exp Cell Res 17:420–438.

Rensing, L, and Goedeke, K (1976) Circadian rhythm and cell cycle: possible entraining mechanisms. Chronobiologia 3:53–65.

Roberts, ML, Friston, JA, and Reade, PC (1976) Supression of immune responsiveness by a submandibular salivary gland factor. Immunology 30:811.

Rose, WC, Trader, MW, Laster, RW, Jr, and Schabel, SM, Jr (1978) Chronotherapy of L1210 leukemic mice with cytosine arabinoside or cyclophosphamide. Cancer Treat Rep 62:1337–1349.

Rosene, GL, and Halberg, F (1970) Circadian and ultradian rhythms in liver, breast cancer and Ehrlich ascites tumor of mice. Bull All India Inst Med Sci 4:77–94.

Rubin, NH (1981) Circadian variation in the proportion of cells in cell-cycle phases in the hamster tongue epithelium as measured by the flow microfluorometric technique. In: von Mayersbach, H, Scheving, LE, and Pauly, JE (eds), Biological Rhythms in Structure and Function. New York: Alan R. Liss, Inc., pp. 81–86.

Rubin, N, Hokanson, JA, Mayschak, JW, Tsai, TH, Barranco, SC, and Scheving, LE (1983) Several cytokinetic methods for showing circadian variation in normal murine tissues and in a tumor. Amer J Anat (in press).

Ryan, JP, and Pellecchia, D (1982) Effect of progesterone pretreatment on guinea pig gall bladder mortality in vitro. Gastroenterology 83:81–83.

Scheving, LA, Yeh, YC, Tsai, TH, and Scheving, LE (1979) Circadian-phase dependent stimulatory effects of epidermal growth factor on DNA synthesis in the tongue, esophagus and stomach of the adult male mouse. Endocrinology 105:1475–1480.

Scheving, LA, Yeh, YC, Tsai, TH, and Scheving, LE (1980) Circadian-phase dependent stimulatory effects of epidermal growth factor on DNA synthesis in the duodenum, jejunum, ileum, caecum, colon, and rectum of the adult male mouse. Endocrinology 106:1498–1503.

Scheving, LA, Scheving, LE, Tsai, TH, and Pauly, JE (1982) Circadian stage-dependent effects of insulin and glucagon on incorporation of [³H]thymidine into desoxyribonucleic acid in the esophagus, stomach, duodenum, jejunum, ileum, caecum, colon, rectum, and spleen of the adult female mouse. Endocrinology 111:308–315.

Scheving, LE, and Gatz, AJ (1955) Mitotic activity in the human epidermis. Anat Rec 12:363 (abstract).

Scheving, LE (1959) Mitotic activity in the human epidermis. Anat Rec 135:7–20.

Scheving, LE (1976) The dimension of time in biology and medicine—chronobiology. Endeavour 35(125): 66–72.

Scheving, LE (1980a) Chronobiology, a new perspective for biology and medicine. In: Saletu, E (ed), Proc. 11th Collegium Internat. Neuro-psychopharmacologicum (C.I.N.P.) Cong., Vienna, Austria, 9–14 July, 1978. Oxford: Pergamon Press Ltd., pp. 629–646.

Scheving, LE (1980b) Chronotoxicology in general and experimental chronotherapeutics of cancer. In: Scheving, LE, and Halberg, F (eds), Chronobiology: Principles and Applications to Shifts of Schedules, Alphen aan den Rijn, The Netherlands: NATO Advanced Study Institute Series, Sijtohff and Noordhoof, pp. 455–479.

Scheving, LE (1980c) Chronobiology—a new perspective in pharmacology and chemotherapy. Trends in Pharmacological Sciences, July:303–307.

Scheving, LE (1980) Chronobiological aspects of comparative experimental chemotherapy of neoplasms. In: Kaiser, HG (ed), Neoplasms—Comparative Pathology of Growth in Animals, Plants, and Man. Baltimore, Williams and Wilkins: pp. 317–331.

Scheving, LE (1981) Circadian rhythms in cell proliferation: Their importance when investigating the basic mechanism of normal versus abnormal growth. In: von Mayersbach, H, Scheving, LE, and Pauly, JE (eds), Biological Rhythms in Structure and Function. New York: Alan R. Liss, Inc., pp. 39–79.

Scheving, LE, and Burns, ER (1971) Some evidence that a consideration of the chronobiology of a cell-cycle may improve chemotherapy. In: Scharf, JH, and von Mayersbach, H (eds), Die Zeit und das Leben. Nova Acta Leopoldina 46(225):277–283.

Scheving, LE, and Pauly, JE (1967) Circadian phase relationship of thymidine-H³ uptake, labeled nuclei, grain counts and cell division rate in rat corneal epithelium. J Cell Biol 32:677–683.

Scheving, LE, and Pauly, JE (1973) Cellular

mechanisms involving biorhythms with emphasis on those rhythms associated with the S and M stages of the cell cycle. Int J Chronobiol 1:269–283.

Scheving, LE, and Pauly, JE (1974) Circadian rhythms: some examples and comments on clinical application. Chronobiologia 2:3–21.

Scheving, LE, and Pauly, JE (1977) Several problems associated with the conduct of chronobiological research. In: Scharf, JH, and von Mayersbach, H (eds), *Die Zeit und das Leben*. Nova Acta Leopoldina 46(225):237–258.

Scheving, LE, Burns, ER, and Pauly, JE (1972) Circadian rhythms in mitotic activity and ^{3}H-thymidine uptake in the duodenum; effect of isoproterenol on the mitotic rhythm. Am J Anat 135:311–317.

Scheving, LE, Sohal, G, Enna, CD, and Pauly, JE (1973) The persistence of a circadian rhythm in histamine response in guinea pigs maintained under continuous illumination. Anat Rec 175:1–6.

Scheving, LE, Cardoso, SS, Pauly, JE, Halberg, F, and Haus, E (1974a) Variation in susceptibility of mice to the carcinostatic agent arabinosyl cytosine. In: Scheving, LE, Halberg, F, and Pauly, JE (eds), *Chronobiology*. Tokyo: Igaku Shoin Ltd., pp. 213–217.

Scheving, LE, von Mayersbach, H, and Pauly, JE (1974b) An overview of chronopharmacology (a general review). J Eur Toxicol 7:203–227.

Scheving, LE, Pauly, JE, Burns, ER, Halberg, F, Tsai, T, and Betterton, HO (1974c) Lighting regimen dominates interacting meal schedules and synchronizes mitotic rhythms in mouse corneal epithelium. Anat Rec 180:447–452.

Scheving, LE, Pauly, JE, von Mayersbach, H, and Dunn, JD (1974d) The effect of continuous light or darkness on the rhythm of the mitotic index in the corneal epithelium of the rat. Acta Anat 88:411–423.

Scheving, LE, Burns, ER, Pauly, JE, Tsai, TH, Betterton, HO, and Halberg, F (1976a) Meal scheduling, cellular rhythms and the chronotherapy of cancer. In: Koishi, H (ed), *Nutrition*. Kyoto: Victory-sha Press, pp. 141–142.

Scheving, LE, Haus, E, Kühl, JFW, Pauly, JE, Halberg, F, and Cardoso, SS (1976b) Close reproduction by different laboratories of characteristics of circadian rhythms in 1-β-D-

arabinofuransylcytosine tolerance by mice. Cancer Res 36:113–1137.

Scheving, LE, Burns, ER, and Pauly, JE (1977a) Can chronobiology be ignored when considering the cancer problem? In: Neiburgs, HE (ed), *Prevention and Detection of Cancer; Pt. 1—Prevention; Vol. 1—Etiology*. New York: Marcel Dekker, pp. 1063–1079.

Scheving, LE, Burns, ER, and Pauly, JE (1977b) Coincidence in timing between the synthetic and mitotic stages of the cell cycle in liver parenchymal cells in mice bearing 8-day Ehrlich ascites tumor (EAT). In: *12th Internat. Conf. Proc. (Int. Soc. Chronobiol.)*. Milano: II Ponte, pp. 427–431.

Scheving, LE, Burns, ER, Pauly, JE, Halberg, F, and Haus, E (1977c) Survival and cure of leukemic mice after optimization of cancer treatment with cyclophosphamide and arabinosyl cytosine. Cancer Res 37:3648–3655.

Scheving, LE, Burns, ER, Pauly, JE, and Tsai, TH (1978). Circadian variation in cell division of the mouse alimentary tract, bone marrow and corneal epithelium. Anat Rec 191:479–485.

Scheving, LE, Burns, ER, Halberg, F, and Pauly, JE (1980a) Combined chronochemotherapy of L 1210 leukemic mice using B-D-arabinofur-anosylcytosine, cyclophosphamide, vincristine, methylprednisolone and cis-diamminedichloroplatinum. Chronobiologia 17(1):33–40.

Scheving, LE, Burns, ER, Pauly, JE, and Halberg, F (1980b) Circadian bioperiodic response of mice bearing a L1210 leukemia to combination therapy with adriamycin and cyclophosphamide. Cancer Res 40:1511–1515.

Sigdestad, CP, Bauman, J, and Lesher, SW (1969) Diurnal fluctuation and the number of cells in mitosis and DNA synthesis in the jejunum of the mouse. Exp Cell Res 58:159–162.

Simpson, HW (1976) A new perspective; chronobiochemistry. Essays Med Biochem 2:115–187.

Simpson, HW, and Mutch, F (1981) The fresh approach to human breast cancer. In: Bulbrook, RD, and Taylor, DJ (eds), *Commentaries on Research in Breast Disease*. New York: Allan Liss, pp. 133–164.

Simpson, HW, and Stoney, PJ (1977) A circadian variation of melphalan (L-phenylalanine nitrogen mustard) toxicity to murine bone marrow: relevance to cancer treatment protocols. Br J Haematol 35:459–464.

Skipper, HE, Schabel, FM, Jr, and Wilcox, WS

(1967) Experimental evaluation of potential anticancer agents. XXI. Scheduling of arabinosyl cytosine to take advantage of its S phase specificity against leukemia cells. Cancer Chemother Res 51:125–165.

Sothern, RB, Nelson, WL, and Halberg, F (1977) A circadian rhythm in susceptibility of mice to the anti-tumor drug, adriamycin. In: *Proceedings, XIIth Int. Conf. Int. Soc. for Chronobiology*, Washington, D.C. Milano: II Ponte, pp. 433–438.

Tähti, E (1956) Studies of the effect of x-radiation on 24-hour-variations in the mitotic activity of human malignant tumors. Acta Pathol Microbiol, Scand, Suppl. 117:166.

Takayanagi, I (1980) Effect of urogastrone mechanical activities of the stomach and intestine of the guinea-pig. J Pharm Pharmacol 32:228–230.

Todaro, GJ, De Larco JE, Fryling, CM (1982) Sarcoma growth factor and other transforming peptides produced by human cells: Interactions with membrane receptors. Fed Proceeding 41:2996–3003.

Tvermyr, EM (1969) Circadian rhythms in epidermal mitotic activity. Diurnal variations of the mitotic index, the mitotic rate and the mitotic duration. Virchows Arch; (Cell Pathol.) 2:318–325.

Voutilainen, A (1953) Ueber die 24-Stunden-rhythmik der Mitosenfrequenz in malignen Tumoren. Acta Pathol Microbiol Scand, Suppl. 99:1–104.

Yeh, YC, Scheving, LA, Tsai, TH, and Scheving, LE (1981) Circadian-phase dependent effects of epidermal growth factor on deoxyribonucleic acid synthesis in ten different organs of the adult male mouse. Endocrinology 109:644–651.

Zagula–Mally, ZW, Cardoso, SS, Williams, D, Simpson, H, and Reinberg, A (1979) Time point differences in skin mitotic activity of actinic keratoses and skin cancers. Circadian reference: plasma cortisol. In: Reinberg, A, and Halberg, F (eds), *Chronopharmacology*. New York: Pergamon Press, pp. 399–402.

5

Aspects of Human Chronopathology

Michael H. Smolensky

Often in an individual or a group of patients the manifestation of disease or the exacerbation of symptoms is predictable, exhibiting time dependencies (chronopathologies) over 24-hr, 1-month, and 1-year periods. Chronopathology may involve also alterations in the temporal structure of biological functions quantifiable by differences in the period, acrophase, mesor, and/or amplitude, preceding, following, or coincident with a change in health status. While the major emphasis of most investigations has been the substantiation of periodicities in the occurrence of symptoms or morbid events, the study of changes in the body's temporal structure associated with the commencement of illness has yet to be vigorously pursued.

Introduction

Chronopathology has been defined as the alteration of the body's temporal structure detected by quantitative changes in either the mesor, amplitude, acrophase, and/or period immediately preceding, during, or following a change in health status. This conventional definition of chronopathology, however, is not entirely satisfactory

for several reasons. First, required information pertaining to the usual and tolerable (physiological) versus intolerable (pathological) limits for the indices of temporal structure between individuals is not yet available. Second, the demarcation of health versus illness in terms of M, A, ϕ, and τ has not been explored. Third, from a clinical point of view controversy often exists, especially for certain illnesses, regarding how one decides upon the presence versus the absence of disease. Fourth, conceptually it is easier for biologists to accept the idea that in illness an alteration in organ function precedes an alteration in temporal structure than it is to contemplate that an alteration in the functioning of an organ follows a disruption of its temporal structure. Finally, the change in temporal structure in disease may be exhibited by only one or at best a limited number of biological rhythms. Therefore, a better definition of chronopathology might be (1) the rhythmic occurrence or exacerbation of illness in individuals or a group of persons and/or (2) alteration of one or more biological rhythms resulting from and/or contributing to disease. This definition implies that a deviation in temporal structure may either constitute the cause or the result of a given disease having a spatial orientation, i.e., affecting a particular organ, tissue, or group of cells located at a specific site in the body.

With regard to the present state of knowledge, chronopathologies have been identified and quantitatively described. For the most part, mechanisms remain to be uncovered and working hypotheses have yet to be formulated. Although this may be frustrating for the reader, it must be realized that even if descriptive the chronopathological approach represents an important step forward. It is postulated by many without experimental evidence that rhythmic changes *in* and/or *of* diseases are due exclusively to cyclic changes in environmental factors. Such an explanation stems from the prevailing *theory* that human physiological functions are relatively constant when growth and aging are taken into account. Presuming this to be valid, many scientists have attempted to explain the seasonal variation in both upper respiratory infection and cardiovascular disease, which peak during the winter (Smolensky et al. 1972), by the existence of seasonal changes in weather. This conventional explanation which assumes a direct causal relationship between environmental factors (such as cold, harsh weather) and these chronopathologies still awaits convincing experimental evidence. Chronopathology also involves the identification of relevant bioperiodicities in physiological functions related to rhythms in the symptoms and exacerbation of illness. In this context cyclic environmental changes such as temperature and humidity are viewed as *triggering factors* which may vary in power during different times of the day, month, or year. This conceptual approach is precisely that which has been used in elucidating the chronopathology of allergic asthma (pp. 142–148). Recognition of the temporal dimension of human disease processes suggests an etiology which may involve rhythmic changes of both environmental factors and organisms.

This chapter is not intended to represent an exhaustive review of human chronopathology. Instead, the included examples have been selected to demonstrate that illnesses and their symptoms can be rhythmic and that a chronobiologic approach results in a better understanding of disease and associated risk factors. This is achieved by discussing human chronopathologies in terms of the present knowledge of human temporal structure, especially with regard to associated or component biological rhythmicities. Although the theory and mechanisms of oscillators, e.g., the contribution of the suprachiasmatic nucleus, are pertinent to understanding the modification of rhythmic integrity in health and in certain diseases, discussion of these is beyond the scope of this chapter. Authoritative sources such as Fuller et al. (1981), Kronauer et al. (1982), Moore-Ede et al. (1982), and Suda et al. (1979) should be consulted for information on biological rhythms and their central mechanisms. Since this chapter focuses on periodicities in the occurrence and symptoms of selected human diseases, it is recommended that information on rhythmic aspects of certain health problems involving endocrine function, sleep disorders, shift work, and dyschronosis (jet lag) be obtained elsewhere (Brown and Graeber 1982; Colquhoun 1971; Colquhoun et al. 1975; Goodwin and Wehr 1981; Reinberg et al. 1981; Kripke 1981; Kripke et al. 1978; Johnson et al. 1981; Reinberg 1979b; Klein and Wegmann 1979; Krieger 1979; Weitzman 1981; Weitzman et al. 1981, 1982).

Chronopathology and Investigative Methodologies

With regard to the prominence of the body's temporal structure, it is not surprising that the manifestation and intensification of symptoms of certain diseases are rhythmic. Although clinical impressions suggest this, as verified by published descriptive accounts and case presentations, the study of chronopathologies using well-designed clinical protocols with statistical methods to test hypotheses is rather infrequent. A review of the literature reveals that a wide variety of research methods has been used to investigate chronopathologies. In some instances, physicians have recorded the number of patients experiencing a set of symptoms according to the clock hour and/or calendar date of occurrence. Others have used data from their own medical records. Occasionally, physicians have collected information during office visits by having each patient recollect the approximate time of the day, month, or year when the most recent exacerbation of disease occurred. Only on rare occasions have investigators utilized self-recording techniques and/or patient diaries to obtain relevant time-series data. With regard to more serious diseases requiring immediate medical attention such as stroke and heart disease, authors have sometimes relied upon the clock hour and calendar date of hospital admission rather than the patient's perception of when the onset of symptoms occurred simply because in retrospective studies the former information is easily accessible from hospital records. As will be discussed below, the 24-hr pattern of hospital admissions of patients having had myocardial infarction is very different from the pattern in the onset of symptoms (Stephens et al., in preparation).

The study of human chronopathologies frequently must rely on data in the form of "one time only" single events in individual patients. In this instance large and as far as possible homogeneous samples of patients are required to investigate these so-called population rhythms. This is the case for example in the research of biological rhythms in myocardial or cerebral infarction, since during one's life such an event may occur only once. On the other hand, for illnesses such as asthma and epilepsy, symptoms or exacerbations may recur frequently, thus allowing the detection of chronopathologies in individuals or groups of homogeneous patients with regard to sex, age, race, and medical history.

Whatever the source of data, certain inherent biases must be acknowledged especially when the size of the sample is small. With regard to circadian chronopathologies, the reporting of symptoms with reference to clock hour is usually done without exact information about the synchronizer schedule (sleep-wake pattern) of the individual or sample of subjects studied. Often in female subjects, data are reported without regard to the clock hour or the day of the (ovulatory or nonovulatory) menstrual cycle. For circadian rhythms, it is assumed rather than verified that the data are representative of diurnally active persons. In addition, in many reports information on the type and timing of medical treatment is rarely furnished even though medications per se as well as their timing may determine or at least influence the temporal pattern of symptoms and the exacerbation of diseases. In the case of circamensual chronopathologies in women, it is assumed that events are typical of ovulatory cycles; however, this is rarely confirmed. Also, the tendency is for investigators to group data of women with different cycle lengths over a common 28-day calendar; this is done despite the fact that cycle lengths can vary considerably, by 25% or more, from one woman to another and from this ideal. Because only a limited number of studies dealing with human chronopathologies have been published, it must be recognized that one set of findings may not be representative of other samples.

With these qualifications in mind, evidence for circadian, circamensual, and circannual rhythms in human pathological processes is presented. Most of the data for this review have been obtained from previously published clinical investigations. Although statistics are easily obtainable from various governmental agencies for the investigation of human circannual *mortality* rhythms, the emphasis here is upon morbidity even though circadian (Fig. 1) and circannual (Fig. 2) rhythms in mortality are well documented. Unless otherwise stipulated, it should be assumed that the syn-

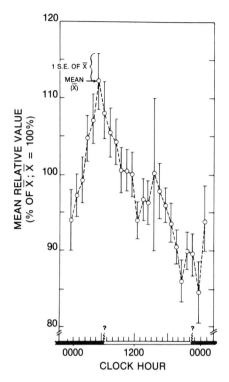

Fig. 1. The timing of 432,000 natural human deaths is not random. Death is more frequent around 0600 than it is between 1800 and 0000. The difference in mortality between the peak (0600–0700) and trough (0000–0100) is approximately 25% of the 24-hr mean, which in this graphing of relative changes over the 24 hr equals 100%. Shaded portions at the bottom of the graph suggest the assumed usual sleep span of the sample. Reproduced from Smolensky et al. 1972.

chronizer schedule is one of diurnal activity and nocturnal rest in individuals dwelling in the Northern Hemisphere.

The Chronobiology and Chronopathology of Human Birth
Circadian Rhythms and Human Birth

Evidence for circadian variation in human birth dates back to statistical reports such as those of Buek in 1829. The onset of natural labor defined by the spontaneous initiation of uterine contractions and/or the rup-

turing of fetal membranes as well as birth are not random over 24 hr. As shown in the left-hand portion of Fig. 3, the spontaneous initiation of labor for a sample of more than 280,000 pregnant women is much more frequent around midnight (0000) to 0400 than it is 12 hr later during the early afternoon. Similarly, the termination of natural labor in more than 2 million medically unassisted births is more frequent between 0000 and 1200 than it is during the remaining 12 hr. These findings suggest the physiological process of birth in diurnally active pregnant women is preferentially an early morning event.

The plots presented in the right-hand portion of Fig. 3 show the temporal distribution of medically induced birth differs from that of natural birth. Births occurring as a result of medically induced labor are more frequent between 0800 and 1500 with the crest between 0900 and 1100. The right-hand portion of this figure reveals in addition that stillbirth varies also to some degree over the 24 hr. The incidence of stillbirth is slightly greater between 1000 and 1400 than it is at other times of the day or night (Smolensky et al. 1972).

The data reported by Breart and Rumeau-Rouquette (1979) confirm the circadian rhythmicity in the onset of labor and the occurrence of birth in non-medically induced deliveries. These authors also found that the vitality of neonates as indexed by the Apgar score is dependent on the time during the day or night when spontaneously initiated birth occurs. The Apgar score (Apgar 1953, 1966; Apgar et al. 1958), devised to evaluate the physical condition of the neonate following birth, gives an indication of the need for immediate medical treatment and in addition is a predictor of survival during the first year of life. The 5 signs used to score neonatal vitality are heart rate, respiratory effort, muscle tone, reflex irritability (following cutaneous stimulation of the feet), and color. Each sign is scored by either a 0, 1, or 2 according to the criteria outlined in Table 1. The Apgar score represents a composite rating of the 5

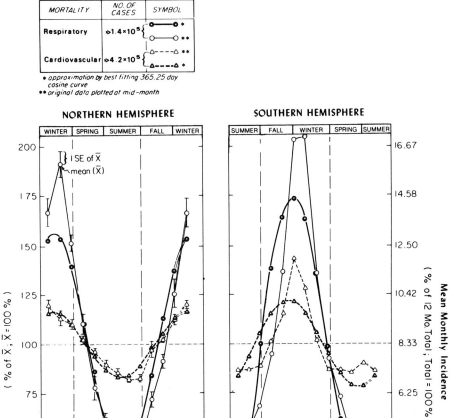

MORTALITY	NO. OF CASES	SYMBOL
Respiratory	⋙1.4×10⁵	●──● *
		○──○ **
Cardiovascular	⋙4.2×10⁵	△---△ **
		▲---▲ *

* approximation by best fitting 365.25 day cosine curve
** original data plotted at mid-month

Fig. 2. The mortality from upper respiratory (pneumonia and influenza) infection or cardiovascular (heart and cerebrovascular) disease is strongly circannually rhythmic. In both the Northern and Southern Hemispheres, highest mortality occurs during the winter. These high-amplitude circannual rhythms may result from 1 or more of the following: (1) seasonal changes in ambient conditions exclusively; (2) a circannual susceptibility rhythm arising from man's circannual temporal organization; and/or (3) seasonal differences in the nature and intensity of environmental challenge. Data are plotted as percentages of the yearly mean set equal to 100%. Reproduced from Smolensky et al. 1972.

signs and can range from 0 to 10. A score of 0–3 indicates the neonate is in very bad condition (low vitality), a score of 4–6 indicates a more or less fair condition, and one of 7–10 indicates good to excellent vitality.

Breart and Rumeau-Rouquette (1979) found that neonates with Apgar scores of 7 or less were most common in deliveries occurring between 1400 and 1500, when 7.1% of the neonates exhibited such low scores. Deliv-

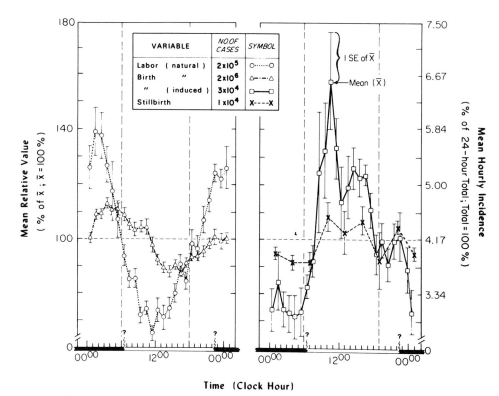

Fig. 3. Aspects of human birth are circadian rhythmic (**left:** spontaneous birth; **right:** medically induced birth). The spontaneous commencement of labor (initiation of uterine contractions and/or rupture of fetal membranes) exhibits a high-amplitude circadian rhythm; it is most frequent around 0130–0230 and is least frequent around midday. The relatively low-amplitude circadian rhythm in natural human birth peaks around 0530 with the trough in the afternoon. The 24-hr pattern of medically induced birth is differently phased with the largest number occurring between 1030 and 1530. The occurrence of stillbirth is somewhat elevated shortly before and after midday in comparison to during the early morning. Data are plotted as percentage deviations from the 24-hr mean set equal to 100%; shaded portion along the horizontal axis represents the suspected sleep span for each sample of pregnant women. Reproduced from Smolensky et al. 1972.

Table 1. *Method of Apgar Scoring.*

Biological function or sign	Score		
	0	1	2
Heart rate	Absent	Slow (less than 100)	100 or more
Respiratory effort	Absent	Weak cry; hypoventilation	Good; strong
Muscle tone	Limp	Some flexion	Well flexed
Reflex irritability	No response	Some motion	Cry
Color	Blue; pale	Body pink; extremities blue	Completely pink

Source: Apgar et al. 1958.

eries occurring during the longer intervals of either 0900 to 1300, 1600 to 2100, or 2200 to 0800 were less likely to have scores of 7 or less; the proportion during these intervals was 4.3, 4.5, and 4.0%, respectively. Differences in the frequency of neonates with Apgar scores of 7 or less between the considered intervals were statistically significant ($P < 0.05$). The authors also found a significantly ($P \leqq 0.02$) greater percentage of neonates presenting with serious medical problems when delivery was between 1400 and 1500 (3.7%); if delivery occurred during the intervals of 0900 to 1300, 1600 to 2100, or 2200 to 0800, the percentage of cases was lower—between 1.7 and 2.1%.

In summary, the available data indicate the onset of labor and, to a lesser degree, delivery when not medically assisted tend to be nocturnal in timing. Birth during the afternoon, specifically between 1400 and 1600, appears to be associated with a greater neonatal risk, i.e., increased probability of depressed neonatal vitality, medical complications, and stillbirth. The occurrence of birth in the afternoon as opposed to the early morning may be associated also with increased maternal risk (Gulyuk 1961).

Why the preferred biological time for birth coincides with the middle and later portion of the night is unknown. Most chronobiologists hypothesize that the nocturnal phasing of the circadian rhythms in labor and birth is indicative of selective pressures which were acting during our evolutionary history. Perhaps for our ancestors, whether prehominid primates or man, nocturnal birth had survival value for both individuals and species; today, this appears to be vestigial—persistence of a biological process fully developed during an earlier evolutionary stage but currently without any apparent usefulness or need (Hughes 1931). Although exogenous cyclic factors may influence the occurrence and phasing of circannual rhythms of birth in human beings, e.g., the annual cycle of photoperiod and ambient temperature affecting human sexual activity (Reinberg and Lagoguey 1978b; Smolensky et al.

1980), no convincing evidence exists to support this point of view for circadian rhythms. On the other hand, the circadian periodicity of human birth may be related to 24-hr variation in female reproductive hormones (Smolensky et al. 1972) as well as neuropeptides such as enkephalins, endorphins, and oxytocin (Dent et al. 1981).

Determination of the importance of these circadian changes is beyond exact experimental testing in human beings. This brief discussion of the possible underlying cause of the observed circadian rhythm in natural birth is presented since many human biological events, including the symptoms and occurrence of various diseases, display circadian and other periodicities for no known or readily apparent reason; frequently the physiological rationale for the observed chronopathology is obscure. Perhaps, it is for this reason that investigators search the ambient rather than the endogenous environment for cyclic events to detect time-related factors. In many cases an explanation cannot be provided for rhythmic patterns. Throughout this chapter the intent is not to purposely refrain from pursuing explanations for the presented periodicities; rather, the problem is that appropriate investigations have yet to be conducted.

Circannual Rhythms and Human Birth

Rhythms of human birth exhibit not only circadian but circannual (Aschoff 1981; Quetelet 1842; Huntington 1938; Otto 1960; Cowgill 1966a–c; Smolensky et al. 1972) and possibly circaseptan (about weekly) ones (MacFarland 1978) as well. Circannual rhythmic aspects of human birth have been summarized by Aschoff (1981), Batschelet et al. (1973), and Smolensky et al. (1972). In general, the circannual acrophase of human birth varies according to country, geographic latitude, and decade (Fig. 4).

A number of social and environmental factors are capable of creating or influencing circannual patterns of conception and

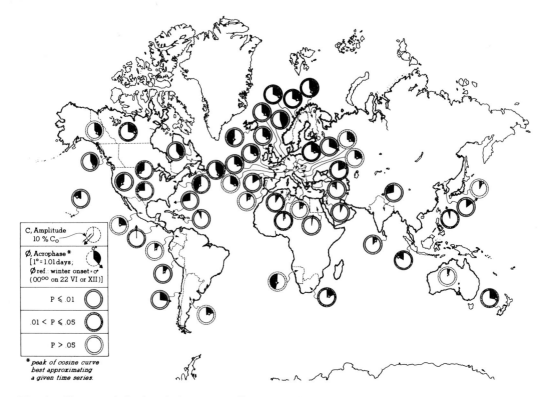

Fig. 4. Circannual rhythms in human natality summarized by the findings of separate cosinor analysis on data from 51 geographic areas representing 10.6×10^7 births. The acrophases differ between samples in association with variation in latitude north and south from the equator. Reproduced from Batschelet et al. 1973.

birth. These include in a given location culture, religion, economy, contraceptive practices, (directly or indirectly) weather (Cowgill 1966a–c), and perhaps photoperiod (Aschoff 1981). Although historically these types of factors have been cited to tentatively explain the seasonality of human birth, circannual rhythms in a number of endogenous functions related to human reproduction may be significant as well. The acrophase map in Fig. 5 indicates that human sexual activity in males and couples as well as various aspects of reproductive function or activity vary over the year (Amir 1971; Leffingwell 1892; Reinberg and Lagoguey 1978a; Reinberg et al. 1975; Udry and Morris 1967; Smals et al. 1976; Tjoa et al. 1982; Smolensky 1980; Smolensky et al. 1981a). Seasonal variation in teratospermia (percentage of abnormal sperm) and necro-

spermia (percentage of nonliving sperm) is relevant as well (Pinatel et al. 1981, 1982). In studies conducted during selected months of the year, it was found in fertile men that teratospermia and necrospermia were highest during the winter. The existence of circannual rhythms in reproductive physiology in addition to birth has suggested to some (van Cauter 1973; Parkes 1977; Smolensky 1980; Smolensky et al. 1981a; Zuckerman 1957) that human beings, although biologically capable of conceiving at any time throughout the year, may exhibit a type of autumnal breeding season during which sexual activity is increased and the chance of conception is elevated.

Circannual changes in reproductive phenomena are not restricted to human beings alone; both plant (Bünning 1963) and ani-

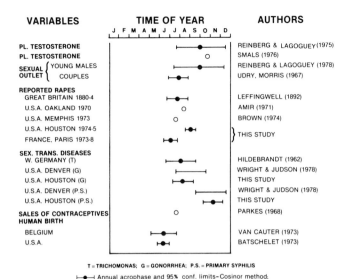

VARIABLES   TIME OF YEAR   AUTHORS

J F M A M J J A S O N D

Fig. 5. Circannual acrophase map summarizing the phasing (ϕ and 95% confidence intervals) of variables thought to be directly or indirectly associated with or related to the circannual pattern of human sexual activity during the year. From Smolensky et al. 1981a.

mal species (Benoit and Assenmacher 1970; Assenmacher and Farner 1978; Farner and Wingfield 1978; Ortavant and Reinberg 1980; Pengelley 1974) are programed in this manner. In these species, reproductive activity is influenced or triggered by the annual cycle in the duration of the daily photoperiod (Bünning 1963; Pittendrigh 1960). In man, comparable investigations on the effects and mechanisms of photoperiod are not possible either for ethical or social reasons; therefore, no direct evidence exists for the role of photoperiod on human circannual reproductive rhythms. Nonetheless, indirect evidence does exist. This includes the moderately strong dependence of the circannual acrophase of human birth on geographic latitude as reported by Batschelet et al. (1973) and Aschoff (1981). Although Aschoff (1981) found the photo- (or scoto-) period to significantly influence the circannual ϕ of human birth, in his studies the actual duration in hours and minutes of sunlight (taking into consideration cloudiness) at a given latitude seemed to be more important than the theoretically expected duration based on astronomical considerations alone. Additional indirect evidence (Parkes 1968; Smolensky 1980; Smolensky et al. 1981a) is consistent with the hypothe-

sis that man exhibits to some extent seasonal variation in breeding efficiency and activity, cycles which are presumably synchronized at least to some extent by photoperiod.

A relatively large number of investigations have been concerned with the quality rather than the quantity of human births over the year. For example, seasonal variation in neonatal birth weight has been studied by Li (1936), Hrdlicka et al. (1950), Katz (1953), Salber and Bradshaw (1952), Bivings (1934), Abels (1922), and Able (1931). In general, the birth weights of neonates delivered in the summer and autumn tend to be slightly greater on the average than of those delivered during other seasons of the year. Although in the majority of studies the differences between seasons were not statistically significant, the aforementioned trend is generally apparent even though the various investigations were conducted in different countries during different decades of the twentieth century.

Seasonal variation in spontaneous abortion and stillbirth, often due to congenital malformation, also has been studied (Kovar and Taylor 1960; Hewitt 1962; Czeizel and Elek 1967; Slatis and DeCloux 1967; Sandall 1974); however, the findings are inconsistent. Some have reported a lack of seasonal differences, whereas others have detected them. With regard to the latter, there is wide variation in the reported season of highest stillbirth frequency.

Numerous investigators have examined seasonal variation in congenital malformations. For example, the incidence of anencephaly has been reported to vary seasonally with a peak during the winter months (McKeown and Record 1951; Edwards 1961; Record 1961; Slater et al. 1964; Sandahl 1977). Publications dealing with the seasonal distribution of other kinds of congenital abnormalities such as those of the heart or lung, including patent ductus arteriosus (Rutstein et al. 1952; Polani and Campbell 1960), pulmonary stenosis (Campbell 1962), coarctation of the aorta (Miettiner et al. 1970), ventricular septal defect (Rothman and Fyler 1974; Rosenberg and Heinonen 1974; Rothman and Fyler 1976), and aortic stenosis or abnormality of the aortic or pulmonary arch (Slater et al. 1964), are not always consistent with regard to the occurrence of rhythms or the season of highest incidence.

The findings of Slater et al. (1964) have been selected for discussion here since a number of different congenital abnormalities were studied simultaneously and systematic methods of investigation were utilized. Data were obtained from physicians during a 7-year span from 1954 to 1960. The sample consisted of 9951 neonates exhibiting 1 or more congenital birth defects. The upper portion of Fig. 6 presents those congenital malformations—congenital cataract, anencephaly, spina bifida, esophageal atresia, and congenital dislocation of the hip (CDH)—which exhibited winter excess. Among these, only cataract, esophageal atresia, and CDH appear to display significant seasonal variability. The lower portion of Fig. 6 depicts those malformations—aortic or pulmonary stenosis or abnormality of the aortic or pulmonary arch, abnormality of the lower portion of the gastrointestinal tract, and partial absence or defect of the limbs—which showed a summer excess. All these appear to vary significantly with season. It is of interest to note that when the total number of congenital abnormalities per season is plotted without regard to type, only minor and insignificant seasonal variability is demonstrable. This is because the timing of the annual peak of the separate rhythms is not the same.

Of the aforementioned congenital malformations, the seasonality of congenital hip dislocation (CDH) is perhaps the most investigated. The data from several countries (Cohen 1970; Cohen 1971) of the Northern Hemisphere consistently reveal trends with a peak during the autumn—the months of September through November (Fig. 7). CHD is lowest during the spring between March and May for Sweden and Israel and during the summer between June and August for several other countries. The seasonal distribution of CDH using data from Victoria, Australia, in the Southern Hemisphere differs in timing by 6 months; in this setting the peak occurs in autumn, i.e., during the calendar months of March through May.

Although an association between seasonal variations in congenital malformations and seasonal patterns of viral or other types of infections has been inferred, there is no clear indication the latter are entirely responsible for changes in the incidence of different types of congenital malformations during the year (Stoller and Collman 1965; Cohen 1971). Huntington (1938) postulated a "basic animal rhythm" in human beings including a season of birth. Incorporating new findings, Cohen's (1971) hypothesis is compatible with Huntington's. With regard to CDH, Cohen rejects the hypotheses that seasonal patterns of infectious diseases affect the fetus and that annual cycles in weather constitute the basis for the observed variation in CDH. Cohen suggests circannual differences in gestational physiology, including those in the endocrine system of the pregnant mother, affect fetal development and thus are associated with the seasonality of certain congenital abnormalities such as CDH. In support of this hy-

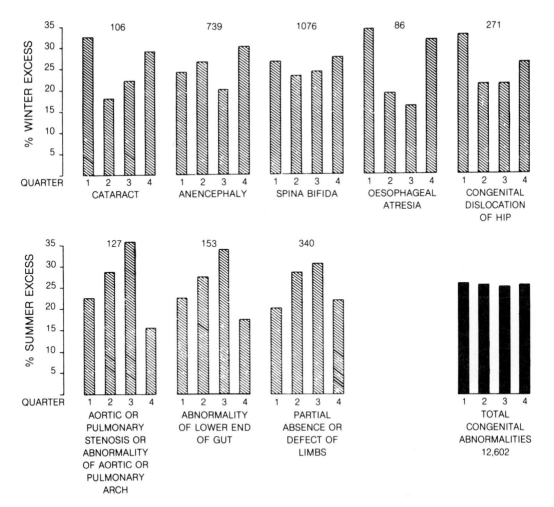

Fig. 6. Quarterly distribution of births exhibiting congenital malformations. The graphs in the upper portion of the figure present those types of congenital malformation which are more common in births occurring during the winter; the ones below present those which are more common in births during the summer. Reproduced from Slater et al. 1964.

pothesis, Kalter (1959) found cortisone, when given in the same small dosage to groups of genetically and gestationally aged similar pregnant mice during different times of the year, induced seasonally varying incidences of cleft palate. A significantly greater number of mice were born with cleft palate in those groups given cortisone between November and April than in groups treated in the same manner between May and October. These findings implicate a circannual susceptibility of the mother and/or fetus to the effects of a hormonal sub-

stance, cortisone. Dramatic circadian differences in the susceptibility of pregnant rodents/fetuses to chemically induced congenital abnormalities also have been demonstrated in the laboratory by Sauerbier (1979, 1980).

Relevant to this discussion, also, are the findings of Fröland (1967), Nielsen and Friedrick (1969), Jongbloet (1970, 1971), Nielsen et al. (1973) and Piazzini et al. (1981) who reported seasonal differences in the births of children with aneuploid chromosomes. The incidence of Kleinfelter's

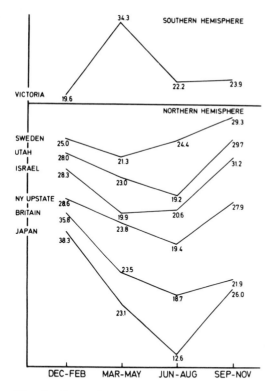

Fig. 7. Quarterly variation (by season of birth) of congenital dislocation of the hip (CDH). Irrespective of the source of data, CDH is most frequent in births occurring during the autumn and winter; this appears to be the case for the Southern as well as the Northern Hemisphere. Reproduced from Cohen 1971.

syndrome was found to be elevated in neonates delivered between March and May and also in October; the incidence was found to be reduced for those delivered at other times during the fall, summer, or winter. Deininger and Rott (1973) found a seasonal difference in the rate of spontaneous chromosomal aberration in man with a definite peak during the winter. Circannual variations in the physiology of human beings have not been studied to determine if they contribute to the observed seasonal difference in the frequency of human congenital malformations. Yet, circannual rhythmicity in a great number of biological functions, including those connected with reproduction (Fig. 5), are known (Halberg et al., 1983; Hildebrant 1962; Smolensky 1980;

Smolensky et al. 1981a) favoring the hypothesis that the efficiency of man's breeding capacity varies over the year.

The Chronopathology of Allergy

Circadian Rhythms and Hay Fever

It is generally although incorrectly assumed that hay fever symptoms are more troublesome during the day when pollens and many other antigens attain their highest ambient concentrations. However, data specific to the time of day when symptoms commence or become most bothersome are sparse. Apparently, only a single objective investigation of the 24-hr variation in hay-fever symptoms has been published (Nicholson and Bogie 1973). In this study, 246 hay-fever sufferers were queried as to the commencement and worsening of their symptoms—sneezing, coughing, wheezing, red, itchy eyes, and/or stuffy nose—with regard to specific times of the day.

Sneezing, stuffy nose, red, itchy eyes, wheezing, and coughing were most frequently troublesome in the morning from before breakfast until lunch (Fig. 8). Except for the occurrence of red, itchy eyes, the second most common interval of the day when symptoms began was during the evening and while in bed. These findings parallel those reported by Trousseau in 1865. A similar temporal distribution was found for the span during the day when patients suffered their most troublesome symptom (Fig. 9). Almost twice as many patients experienced worsening of their most troublesome symptom during the interval before breakfast and until lunch than during the span of after lunch and during the afternoon. A fairly large number of patients also described their most bothersome symptom being worst during the evening and while in bed.

Circadian Rhythms in Dyspnea and Asthma

The observation that in diurnally active patients asthma occurs during the night dates back many centuries. Although Hippocra-

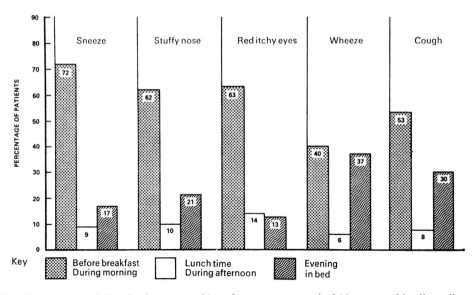

Fig. 8. Temporal variation in the onset of hay fever symptoms in 246 presumably diurnally active individuals. Except for "wheeze," the commencement of symptoms was most common before breakfast and during the morning and least so around lunchtime and during the afternoon. Reproduced from Nicholson and Bogie 1973.

tes apparently was the first to recognize the nocturnal exacerbation of asthma, it apparently was not until Aretaeus, a Greek physician in the third century A.D., that the first classical description of the nocturnal occurrence of the disease, "the evil (dyspnea) is much worse in sleep. . . ," was given (Adams 1856). Thereafter, Trousseau (1865) provided a clinical description of nocturnal asthma. Yet, it was not until the middle of the twentieth century that data were accumulated to substantiate the circadian rhythmicity of dyspnea and its dependence upon circadian variations in certain physiochemical variables (Anonymous 1983; Barnes et al. 1980, 1982; Clark and Hetzel 1977; Dawkins and Meurs 1981; Hetzel and Clark 1978, 1980; Hetzel et al. 1977a,b; Neffen et al. 1980; Prevost et al. 1980; Puchelle et al. 1975; Reinberg et al. 1963; Soutar et al. 1975, 1977; Smolensky et al. 1981b).

Figure 10 shows the magnitude of the 24-hr rhythmic variation in dyspnea and peak expiratory flow (PEF)—a measure of the patency of the upper airways—for 13 diurnally active asthmatic patients studied over a 7-day span. The patients performed self-

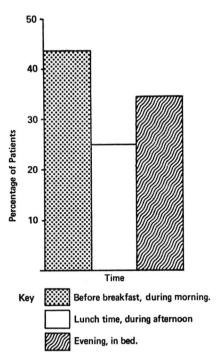

Fig. 9. Temporal variation of the worst symptom of 246 hay fever sufferers. The span from before breakfast until later in the morning was the most troublesome for this presumably diurnally active sample. Reproduced from Nicholson and Bogie 1973.

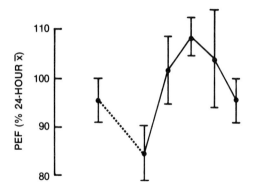

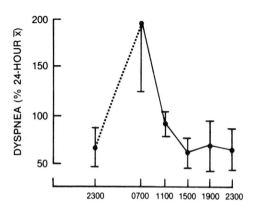

Fig. 10. Circadian variation of PEF (peak expiratory flow—a measure of airway patency) and dyspnea in 13 diurnally active (sleep, ~2300 to 0700) untreated asthmatics. The crest in dyspnea was self-rated as greatest upon arising at 0700 and least at 1500. The 24-hr pattern of PEF was 12 hours out of phase with that of dyspnea. PEF was lowest at 0700 and greatest at 1500. The data of each graph are plotted as percentages (means and standard errors) from the 24-hr average set equal to 100%. Redrawn from Reinberg et al. 1977.

ratings of dyspnea and self-measurements of PEF at 4-hr intervals during the waking span while not being treated with bronchodilator or synthetic corticosteroid medications (Reinberg et al. 1977). Dyspnea was greatest upon awakening around 0700 and lowest during the mid-afternoon around 1500. The peak-to-trough variation was great amounting to more than a 3-fold difference relative to the 24-hr mean (shown in the graph as being equal to 100%). The temporal change in the PEF was complementary; it was lowest around 0700 and greatest around 1500. The difference between the PEF at the time of the highest value, at the circadian peak, and the time of the lowest value, at the circadian trough, amounted to approximately 20% of the 24-hr mean. The magnitude of the 24-hr rhythmic variation in the PEF is not unusual for asthmatic patients and is in agreement with the findings of other investigations showing the circadian peak-to-trough difference to be as great as 20% or more of the 24-hr mesor (Smolensky et al. 1974; Smolensky and Halberg 1977; Hetzel and Clark 1980; Todisco et al. 1980). In nonasthmatic individuals, a circadian periodicity in the airway patency, e.g., when measured by PEF, is demonstrable. In comparison to asthmatic persons, the 24-hr mean is much higher (indicative of low resistance to air flow) and the peak-to-trough difference is much lower, typically being only about 5% of the 24-hr average. These findings confirm the relatively strong stability of the airway patency of healthy nonasthmatic persons over 24-hr (Smolensky and Halberg 1977). The prominence of the circadian change in airway resistance of asthmatic patients led Hetzel and Clark (1980) to consider high-amplitude changes in airway patency to be diagnostic.

The manner in which data are gathered and self-recorded appears to influence to some degree the findings of studies dealing with the 24-hr pattern of dyspnea. For example, Prevost and his colleagues (1980) investigated the temporal distribution of respiratory distress as defined by episodes of coughing, coughing up phlegm, wheezing, whistling in the chest, and shortness of breath. A sample of 286 asthmatic, bronchitic, or emphysemic patients was studied between July and October 1977 in Houston, Texas, during a consecutive 112-day span. In these diurnally active persons, the self-rated respiratory distress of breathing was most prominent during the morning between 0600 and 1200. It was lowest between 1200 and 1800. Earlier, Reinberg et al. (1963) monitored the onset and duration of asthma in 8 diurnally active patients. The exacerbation of dyspnea was always nocturnal in timing with the attacks of asthma occurring between 2300 and 0600. In other investigations involving self-ratings of dyspnea, the difficulty of breathing has been found to be greatest between the usual bedtime and awakening; in fact, many have found the airway patency of asthmatic patients to be reduced nocturnally (Balaz 1970; Bateman and Clark 1979; Clark and Hetzel 1977; Dawkins and Meurs 1981; Hetzel and Clark 1977; Hetzel et al. 1977a,b; Kales et al. 1968; Reinberg et al. 1977; Smolensky et al. 1974; Smolensky and Halberg 1977; Todisco et al. 1980).

One reason for the slight disagreement regarding the exact timing of the circadian peak of dyspnea, as found for example in the earlier study by Reinberg et al. (1963) in comparison to that by Prevost et al. (1980), may be the manner in which the data were obtained and the type of sample examined. In the study by Reinberg and his colleagues, data on the onset, intensity, and duration of dyspnea were gathered from asthmatic patients using open-ended self-reports. In the investigation by Prevost and his associates, participants (asthmatics, bronchitics, and emphysemics) indicated on a prepared data sheet when the *onset* of respiratory distress commenced with reference to 1 of 4 listed 6-hr intervals. It may be that the unfortunate selection of 0600 to separate the 6-hr intervals coinciding with the termination of nightly sleep (0000–0600) and the initiation of activity (0600–1200) made it difficult for those individuals ordinarily arising around this time to decide whether to list their attack as beginning before or after 0600. Also, the selection of 6-hr intervals rather than shorter ones, such as 1- or 2-hr intervals, made impossible the more exact determination of the temporal maximum of respiratory distress for this sample of subjects. Nonetheless, based upon the available data it appears that

dyspnea in asthmatic persons is far more common during the nocturnal and early morning span than during the afternoon and evening.

It is widely assumed without objective evidence that the nocturnal exacerbation of dyspnea in diurnally active asthmatic patients is exclusively related to external factors, for example, close contact with antigens in the bedding causing allergic reactions and postural changes leading to the pooling of fluids in the lungs and altered pulmonary dynamics at bedtime. Although external conditions undoubtedly play a role, internal chronobiologic factors typically are not taken into account or they are underestimated. In fact, they strongly contribute to the nocturnal susceptibility and timing of asthma.

Day-night variations in constituents of the ambient environment and in endogenous physiochemical processes when considered together in a holistic manner, as advocated by Haywood and McGovern (1968), help to explain the nocturnal predilection for the worsening of dyspnea and asthma. The initial concern of chronobiologists was to identify rhythmic changes in those variables known to affect bronchial patency (Reinberg et al. 1963). This involved the study of the coincidence of the circadian trough in the antiinflammatory adrenal corticosteroid secretion with the occurrence of nocturnal dyspnea. The circadian rhythm of corticosteroid secretion was suspected to be associated with this chronopathology because of the causal relationship between this hormone and bronchial patency. (It is important to recognize that agreement in phasing between two rhythmic functions, in this case the circadian trough of the rhythm in airway patency and of urinary or serum corticosteroid concentration, need not implicate a causal relationship; experimental validation is required to conclude a given physiological variable plays a role in a particular chronopathology.) The findings of earlier investigations substantiating a coincidence in time between the circadian trough of corticosteroid secretion and the occurrence of asthma suggested that the circadian periodicity in adrenocortical activity constitutes 1 of the component endogenous rhythms contributing to the nocturnal timing of this disease. Since the initial research by Reinberg et al. (1963), Reinberg and Gervais in Paris, France, and Smolensky and McGovern in Houston, Texas, for example, have continued their chronobiologic investigations on asthmatic patients, resulting in the identification of several other circadian component rhythmicities as summarized in Fig. 11.

Figure 11 shows by means of an acrophase map the timing of the circadian peak, indicated by an upward-directed arrow, and the trough, indicated by a downward-directed arrow, of several endogenous circadian component functions known to affect airway patency and/or the occur-

rence of asthma. The extended line to the right and left of each circadian acrophase or trough marker indicates the 95% confidence limits for each. In the column to the right, a directed line depicts the estimate of the circadian amplitude—a measure of the prominence of the circadian periodicity—also shown with 95% confidence limits. The peak incidence of asthma occurring during the usual nocturnal span of sleep coincides in time with the phasing of several pertinent circadian functions, i.e., (1) decreased airway patency; (2) increased pulmonary resistance; (3) decreased dynamic compliance; (4) increased bronchial reactivity to house dust, histamine, and acetylcholine (as well as increased cutaneous reactivity to histamine and several antigens); and (5) decreased circulating and/or urinary levels of bronchodilator substances—catecholamine and adrenocortical hormones (Smo-

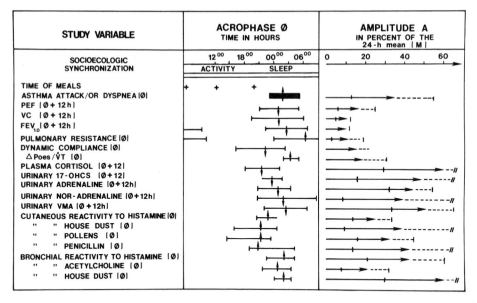

Fig. 11. Temporal variation in the peak or trough of circadian functions related to the 24-hr pattern of asthma in diurnally active patients. The arrows pointing upward indicate the timing of the circadian peaks (termed acrophases), whereas arrows pointing downward indicate the timing of the circadian troughs. A horizontal line extending to the right and left of the acrophase or trough marker represents the 95% confidence limit of each. The amplitude, a measure of the 24-hr rhythmic variability, shown in the column to the right (the length of the arrow is proportional to the circadian rhythmic variation), is expressed as a percentage of the 24-hr time series mean or mesor. The timing of the peak and trough values of these and other biological rhythms is believed to contribute to the heightened susceptibility of patients to asthma nocturnally. Reproduced from Smolensky et al. 1981b.

lensky et al. 1981b). In addition, studies by Gaultier et al. (1977) using a vagolytic agent (iapropium bromide) and a β-receptor stimulating agent (metaproteranol) indicate in day-active adolescents that airway patency and pulmonary mechanics are dominated by vagal tone during the night and by sympathetic tone during the day.

Much of the information given in Fig. 11 pertains to the endogenous circadian component rhythmicities which are thought to be associated with the observed 24-hr pattern of dyspnea and asthma and suggests why the symptoms of this disease predominate during the night. Nonetheless, until rather recently, it was thought that the circadian rhythm in dyspnea depended primarily upon 24-hr periodicities in ambient conditions. Consideration of the holistic nature of disease in general and in particular for asthma as advocated by Haywood and McGovern (1968) inspired additional investigations. A first series of studies (DeVries et al. 1962; Reinberg et al. 1971; Tammeling et al. 1977) revealed the airways of asthmatic patients to be more sensitive to chemical mediators (acetylcholine and histamine) of the allergic response during the night than during the day. A second series of studies by Gervais et al. (1977) found the bronchial response to the common environmental antigen house dust to be circadian rhythmic. In a series of investigations conducted at different times of the day and evening, Gervais and his associates demonstrated that the effect of a threshold dose of house dust (expected to induce a 15% fall in the $FEV_{1.0}$ when given by inhalation in an aerosol form to house-dust-sensitive asthmatic patients) varied greatly. It produced a much greater effect around 2300 than it did during the morning (around breakfast), afternoon, or early evening. Following the house-dust provocation at 2300, the immediate reduction in the airway patency as measured by spirometry ($FEV_{1.0}$) amounted to nearly 25% with the occurrence of wheezing and chest rales. Moreover, a significant decrement in the PEF mesor ensued during the subsequent 24-hr span after

the inhalation of the house-dust aerosol. Provocation of the same patients using the same dose of house dust and identical conditions of study at the other clock hours resulted in comparatively small decrements in the $FEV_{1.0}$ without production of dyspnea or associated symptoms (Fig. 12).

The findings summarized in Fig. 11 and those of Gervais et al. (1977) indicate not only that there exists a set of endogenous component circadian functions which favor the predisposition to asthma during the night, but that the sensitivity (and susceptibility) of the airways to environmental provocation in the form of antigens or certain chemicals is markedly circadian rhythmic. Thus, the ability of an asthmatic person to tolerate his ambient environment is dependent not only upon the type and quantity of antigen in his surroundings but also the time at which exposure occurs; what constitutes safe limits of exposure at one time of the day may well be unsafe, dangerous, or even life-threatening at another. Such findings demonstrate without question that man (and other mammals and

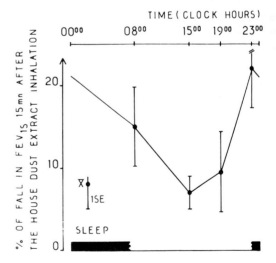

Fig. 12. Circadian changes in the airways' susceptibility to house-dust in diurnally active house-dust-sensitive asthmatic patients. The pre- to posttest difference in the $FEV_{1.0}$ at 1500 was relatively minor compared to that at 2300. Reproduced from Gervais et al. 1977.

primates) cannot be conceptualized as a passive responder who exhibits random and minor variation in endogenous state (Smolensky 1975; Smolensky et al. 1981b). Output from organisms quantified by changes in biological functions or variables need not necessarily result from alterations of the ambient environment. Even when environmental conditions are kept constant, such as in studies of asthmatic subjects when standardization of experimental conditions is achieved by the use of hypoallergenic facilities, the response of the airways, for example to the house-dust bronchial challenge, differs markedly according to the (biological) time of provocation. This is due to the inherent circadian rhythmicity in airways' susceptibility. Nonetheless, to put these findings in perspective, it must be pointed out that in asthmatic patients circadian changes such as these do not *cause* dyspnea; however, they do *contribute* to the differential, time-dependent susceptibility. From a chronobiologic perspective, the etiology of nocturnal asthma involves the temporal patterns of both endogenous and exogenous variables rather than the latter only.

Pertinent to this discussion is the observation in certain occupational settings that nonimmediate and recurrent nocturnal asthmatic reactions may follow a single daytime exposure to allergens (Burge et al. 1981; Gandevia and Milne 1970; Milne and Gandevia 1969; Mitchell 1970; Siracusa et al. 1978; Davies et al. 1976; Pepys 1976; Taylor et al. 1979; Burge et al. 1981; O'Brien et al. 1979; Pepys 1977; Pepys and Hutchcroft 1975; Pepys and Davies 1978; Taylor 1977). As first reported by Trousseau (1865), a single brief exposure to an antigen to which one is hypersensitive is capable of eliciting nocturnal dyspnea during several successive nights even without subsequent exposure to the causal agent. According to Taylor and his coworkers (1979), during the day workers suffering from recurrent nocturnal asthmatic reactions may complain only of cough or unusual breathlessness upon exertion and may even exhibit near-normal airway patency (Fig. 13). It is only at night—often for several successive nights—that moderate and sometimes severe dyspnea occurs in spite of the fact that exposure to the antigen took place only during the diurnal span of work or play.

Circamensual Rhythms and Asthma

Although dyspnea in diurnally active asthmatic patients is mainly a nocturnal event, in many women it is in addition more com-

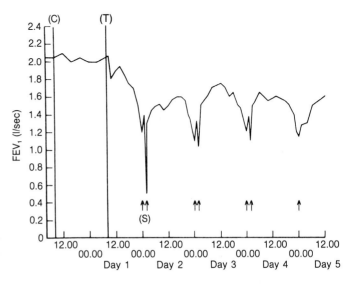

Fig. 13. Temporal variation in airway patency of 1 presumably diurnally active asthmatic patient following a single pulmonary challenge on the test day (numbered 1) with an antigen to which hypersensitivity had previously developed (budgerigar serum) through occupational exposure. Although the $FEV_{1.0}$ was close to normal during the day it was extremely low during the night, giving rise to severe episodes of dyspnea over several consecutive nights. Reproduced from Taylor et al. 1979.

mon and/or more troublesome immediately prior to and during menses. Although only a small number of clinical investigations have been published (Chiray et al. 1940; Claude and Allemany-Vall 1938; Hoseason 1938; Rossolini and Chieffi 1964; Wolfsohn and Politzer 1964), there is sufficient evidence to conclude that in many women the exacerbation of the asthmatic condition tends to be circamensually rhythmic. The findings of Wulfsohn and Politzer (1964) are exemplatory. In their study, 25 of 27 adult asthmatic women experienced exacerbation of their dyspnea during the night. This is not unexpected based upon the discussion in the previous section. In this same sample, 20 of 27 women complained that their asthma became worse premenstrually—up to 7 days before—or during menses. The findings reported by Claude and Allemany-Vall (1938) in their review of 36 cases of premenstrual and menstrual

asthma complement those of Wulfsohn and Politzer (1964). It has been theorized that this circamensual rhythmicity is associated with qualitative and quantitative changes in ovarian and adrenal hormones over the menstrual cycle (Chiray et al. 1940; Claude and Allemany-Vall 1938; Dalton 1964, 1977; Reinberg and Smolensky 1974; Reinberg et al 1974; Smolensky et al. 1973; Wulfsohn and Politzer 1964; Zondek and Bromberg 1947).

Circannual Rhythms and Asthma

In addition to circadian and circamensual periodicities in asthma, circannual ones have been frequently described (Orie et al. 1964; Tromp 1963). Figure 14 presents an example of the month-to-month variation in the occurrence of asthma over the year (Orie et al. 1964). The graph, which represents data obtained during an 11-year span from pa-

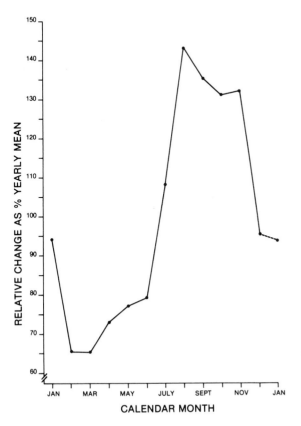

Fig. 14. Seasonal variation in asthma in the Netherlands. Over an 11-year span, asthma was on the average more frequent during the summer and fall than during the winter and spring. Data from Orie et al. 1964.

tients living in the Netherlands, shows an excess of attacks between August and November. In August the average incidence of asthma for the 11-year span was greater by about 45% than the mean number of cases over all months, which for the purpose of graphing has been set equal to 100%. For the months of February through June, there was a relatively low incidence of asthma. For example, the average incidence during the 11 years in February and March was about 35% lower than the overall mean. Undoubtedly, seasonal variation in the nature and quantity of antigens to which asthmatic persons are sensitive constitutes at least one component of the observed seasonal differences; however, up to this time relatively few studies (Grammer et al. 1981; Islam 1981; Reinberg 1971b; Reinberg and Lagoguey 1978a; Lagoguey and Reinberg 1981; Reinberg et al. 1980; Lu et al. 1980a,b; Shifrine et al. 1980a,b; Shifrine et al. 1982; Stempel et al. 1981) have evaluated the possible contribution of endogenous circannual rhythmicities such as those in catecholamines, corticosteroids, lymphocytes, and immunoglobulins to this circannual chronopathology. Failure to consider the possible role of endogenous rhythms has at least on one occasion led to an oversimplified and probably incorrect explanation for the seasonality of symptoms displayed by house-mite-sensitive allergic children. Murray et al. (1980) found a seasonal pattern in the symptoms of house-mite allergy in patients displaying this hypersensitivity only. In those patients the peak occurred during the cold months; none of the patients exhibited an aggravation of symptoms during the summer when the authors found the number of mites in mattresses to be greatest. The authors concluded that the seasonal variation in allergic complaints, which were greater during the colder months, was "possibly because that is the season when children spend more time indoors exposed to find mite debris." This may not be the correct explanation. Although the quality of the external environment is of strong significance, so it may be that circannual changes in biological functions are of equal significance in the seasonal susceptibility to house-dust-mite allergy and the resulting symptoms.

Circadian Rhythms and Atopic Dermatitis

Patients frequently complain the pruritus of atopic dermatitis worsens at night. However, objective data documenting this are limited. In a study by Borelli et al. (1966), data on the intensity of itching were gathered by frequent self-ratings over 24-hr periods. Different patients were studied on separate occasions. Patients rated their pruritus being most intense between 1900 and 2300 (Fig. 15). Pruritus also was elevated but to a lesser extent in the morning around awakening at 0700. Although a conceivable hypothesis is that pruritus is most intense at night because of a reduction in distracting influences at this time, there are no objective data to substantiate this popular explanation. It was the opinion of Borelli et al. that changes in the level of pruritus resulted from 24-hr alterations in atmospheric conditions. From a chronobiologic point of view, the temporal variation in pruritus may represent the influence of periodicities in associated component biological functions. In support of this, Cormia (1952) found the threshold for histamine-induced itching was reduced by 100-fold at midnight relative to that at 1400. In other studies, Lee et al. (1977) and Reinberg (1968) found the histamine-induced erythematous and wheal responses on the average to be two-and-one-half to three-times greater between 1900 and 2300 than between 0700 and 1100 in diurnally active allergic persons. More recently, Reinberg and Lévi (unpublished data) detected a circadian rhythm in itching induced by intradermally injected histamine. The maximum response coincided with the expected timing of the circadian peak of the histamine-induced erythematous and indurative reactions. The minimum response coincided with the circadian trough of these reactions. Overall, the findings of the considered studies are similar—the perception of

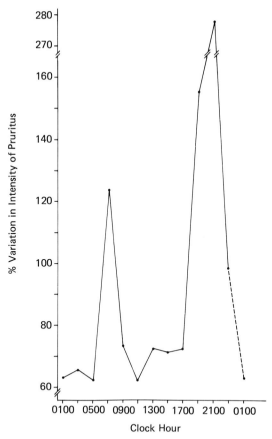

Fig. 15. Twenty-four-hour variation in the pruritus of atopic dermatitis. Group self-ratings of pruritus carried out by presumably diurnally active individuals are plotted as a percentage of the 24-hr mean (100%). During the night between 1900 and 2300 pruritus was most severe. It was moderate during most of the day, although it was somewhat troublesome around 0700. Redrawn from Borelli et al. 1966.

the itching due to histamine provocation or due to disease is greatest during the night.

Circamensual Rhythm in Urticaria

Urticaria represents a specific symptom, hives, of an atopic or immune complex disease with the causal agents varying between patients. A number of observations (Géber 1921, 1939; Leech and Kumar 1981; Guy et al. 1951; Shelley et al. 1964; Tromovitch and Heggli 1967; Farah and Shbaklu 1971) suggest certain women ex-

hibit cyclic variation in the manifestation of urticaria. An association between endocrine function and chronic urticaria has been observed. For example, in some the exacerbation is experienced only during the premenstrum or menstrum. It has been suggested that these cyclic variations are due to immunological reactions against progesterone. Our research (Smolensky et al. 1973; Reinberg et al. 1974; McGovern et al. 1977a) indicates the histamine-induced cutaneous erythematous response varies systematically throughout the menstrual cycle in regularly menstruating women not using oral contraceptives. Highest cutaneous reactivity (circadian mesor) occurs during menstruation whereas lowest reactivity occurs around midcycle. The difference in the cutaneous reactivity between the circamensual peak and trough amounts to approximately 25% of the mean of all the circadian tests conducted over the menstrual cycle. The circamensual variation in cutaneous reactivity in non-users of oral contraceptives is only about one-half to one-third that occurring over the 24-hr (circadian) time domain. In our investigation, oral contraceptive use was associated with a reduction of cutaneous reactivity to histamine and lack of circamensual rhythmicity for histamine responsiveness. With regard to the findings pertaining to the non–users of oral contraceptives, our results are in agreement with those of Bosse and Ladebeck (1972). The degree to which circamensual changes in cutaneous reactivity contributes to cyclic variations in urticaria is yet to be examined. Similarly, the exact extent to which cyclic urticaria constitutes a medical problem for women is unknown; however, the fact that most published papers contain only case reports implies it is rather uncommon.

Overview of the Chronobiology of Allergy

The examples cited in this section reveal that exacerbations of certain allergic conditions vary as periodicities of 24 hr, 28–30 days (in women), and 12 months. Although the worsening of allergic disease may take place at any time, the probability of suffering symptoms at one time of the day, menstrual cycle, or year versus another differs predictably with rhythmicity. Nonetheless, since man's activities within his environment tend to be programed temporally in association with societal, recreational, and occupational pursuits, contact with offending and provoking substances tends to be programed in time as well. Thus, allergic symptoms may become troublesome at times other than those predicted by the body's biological temporal structure and by susceptibility rhythms. In the case of recurrent nocturnal asthma, however, even though exposure to causal agents takes place during the day, the occurrence of serious episodes of dyspnea is usually restricted to the night.

From a chronobiologic point of view, *when* contact with an offending substance to which one is hypersensitive occurs, for example, in the morning or at night, may determine its "antigenicity." When house-dust-sensitive asthmatic patients are challenged by the inhalation of a house-dust aerosol (Fig. 12), the challenge is relatively well tolerated when presented in the afternoon (1500). Only a small deficit of short duration in the $FEV_{1.0}$ results. Yet, when the house-dust challenge is presented to the same asthmatic patients on another occasion under identical conditions of study, i.e., at 2300, the effect on the airways is very great. Chest rales result and the decrease in airway patency lasts for many hours (Gervais et al. 1977). From this and other examples (Tammeling et al. 1977; Reinberg et al. 1971a, DeVries et al. 1962), it is apparent that the human susceptibility to antigenic substances varies over 24 hr and apparently over the menstrual cycle as well (Ozkaragoz and Cakin 1970; Hansen-Pruss and Raymond 1942; Lee et al. 1977; McGovern et al. 1977; Reinberg 1967; Smolensky et al. 1973).

The demonstration of at least circadian rhythms in the cutaneous reactions to histamine and selected antigens and in addition in the reaction of the airways to either house dust (in house-dust-sensitive asthmatics) or to acetylcholine and histamine in asthmatic and other types of patients brings to mind the concept of circadian susceptibility-resistance rhythms initially developed by Halberg (1969) and Reinberg (1967) and later extended by Smolensky (1975). Figure 16 illustrates a homeostatic model of disease causality often presumed when evaluating the role of the environment on human health status and disease. In this presentation, the term output represents observable illnesses or symptoms. With the homeostatic model, human biological functions are assumed to be finely regulated so the internal environment is maintained relatively constant with variation being random rather than rhythmic. With this model the source of day-night or seasonal differences in symptoms and disease is sought through examining day-night or seasonal differences in the external environment exclusively. The homeostatic model precludes contemplating both the existence and contribution of predictable (rhythmic) variation in biological functions to the observed temporal patterns.

Figures 17–19 present alternatives to the homeostatic model. These models are based on chronobiologic findings from studies with antigens in human beings as well as

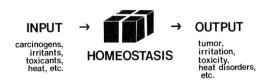

Fig. 16. The central role given the concept of homeostasis in determining the causality of disease. The human body (represented by the box) is presumed to be relatively constant in functioning; the ambient environment provides cyclically varying inputs (heat, cold, noise, chemicals, etc.) which are attended to by homeostatically controlled processes. Temporal difference in output (occurrence or exacerbation of illness), presuming constancy of the *milieu interne,* infers the source(s) of the temporal difference orginates from cyclic alteration of the ambient environment.

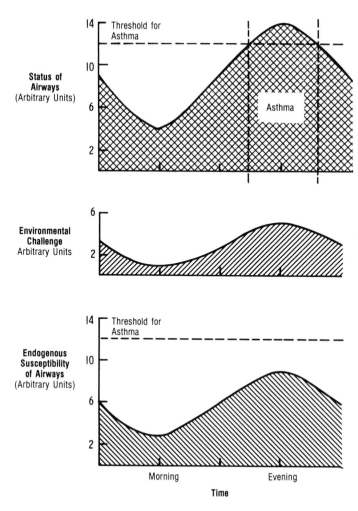

Fig. 17. At the bottom, the circadian susceptibility-resistance rhythm of the airways to house dust in diurnally active house-dust-sensitive asthmatic patients is shown. In the middle, the ambient house-dust concentration is depicted as varying over 24 hours with a peak during the evening. The upper plot indicates the likelihood of asthma during the day or night. Exposure to the ambient environment during the day would not likely result in dyspnea, whereas exposure in the evening would.

toxicants in rodents. These models suggest how cyclic or noncyclic variations in environmental quality, in this case house-dust contamination, interact with circadian susceptibility-resistance rhythms. For the purpose of discussion, the disease selected is that of immediate (as opposed to recurrent and nonimmediate) asthma. The environmental challenge in this example is the level of an environmental antigen (e.g., house dust) to which the airways of the asthmatic are hypersensitive. Figure 17 indicates a situation in which both the level of environmental challenge (house dust) and the susceptibility rhythm of the airways are cyclic over 24 hr. In this figure the phasing of each rhythm is similar with the peak of the envi-

ronmental concentration and of the biological susceptibility to dust coinciding during the night. For this situation, the likelihood of asthma resulting from exposure during the usual span of activity is relatively remote; however, the coincidence of the circadian phase of peak susceptibility and the peak of ambient house-dust concentration at night suggests exposure at this time would result in a high probability of asthma. Figure 18 illustrates the circadian variation in the environmental concentration of house dust differing in phase by 12 hours from that of airway sensitivity. In this case, it is quite likely that at no time during the 24 hr will the symptoms of dyspnea result (given a moderate level of ambient house

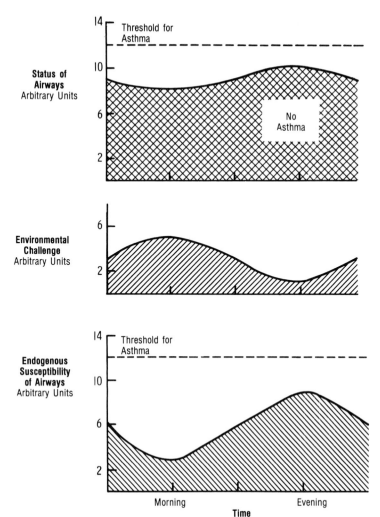

Fig. 18. At the bottom, the circadian susceptibility-resistance rhythm of the airways to house dust in diurnally active house-dust-sensitive asthmatic patients is shown. In the middle, the ambient house-dust concentration is shown as varying in a cyclic manner but differing in phase by 12 hr from the rhythm in airway susceptibility. For this situation, exposure of the asthmatic person to the ambient environment would not result in dyspnea no matter when it occurred.

dust), no matter what time exposure takes place. Finally, Figure 19 depicts the existence of the same circadian susceptibility-resistance pattern for house dust with a nonvarying environmental concentration of house dust. In this example, exposure of house-dust-sensitive asthmatic patients during the early and middle hours of activity will most likely not result in dyspnea. On the other hand, exposure to the same environmental concentration later in the evening will more likely result in asthma. In considering the aforementioned three models it is evident that it is critical not only to appreciate the influence of cyclic patterns in the concentration of the envi-

ronmental challenge but to appreciate as well the existence of circadian patterns of biological susceptibility-resistance. The examples put forth here are based upon research conducted by Gervais et al. (1977) for house-dust-sensitive asthmatics as well as by others (Tammeling et al. 1977; Reinberg et al. 1971a; DeVries et al. 1962) using nonspecific irritants such as histamine and acetylcholine. The findings suggest that the important variables to consider from the point of view of environmentally induced illness are not only the nature and quantity of the environmental contamination but *the time when* exposure occurs with regard to the phasing of circadian resistance-suscep-

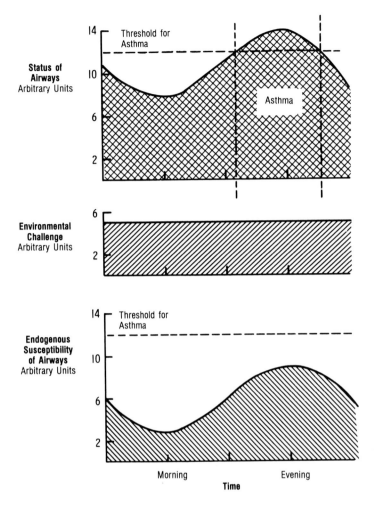

Fig. 19. At the bottom, the circadian susceptibility-resistance rhythm of the airways to house dust in diurnally active house-dust-sensitive asthmatic patients is shown. In the middle, the ambient house-dust concentration is shown as non-varying over 24 hr. For this situation, exposure to the ambient environment during the morning and afternoon would not likely result in asthma. Only during a relatively short span in the evening would exposure to the ambient environment possibly provoke asthma.

tibility rhythms. What may be well tolerated by human beings at one time of the day may not be at another. The importance of circamensual susceptibility-resistance rhythms for diseases occurring preferentially at different times of the menstrual cycle or circannual susceptibility-resistance rhythms of women and men over the year has been postulated but as yet not proven.

Cardiovascular Chronopathology

Textbooks on cardiovascular physiology and pathology fail to consider chronobiologic aspects. Except for the variables of heart rate and blood pressure, only in a limited number of published papers has the time of day or time of year been consid-

ered. A large number of publications have dealt with seasonal differences in cardiovascular disease, noting for the most part winter peaks. Others have been concerned with the association of myocardial infarction (MI) with the consumption of large meals or participation in strenuous activities. Actually temporal variation in cardiovascular functions and diseases is rather prominent (Smolensky et al. 1976). However, it is unknown to what extent biological rhythms in cardiovascular and certain other bodily functions significantly contribute to temporal patterns of cardiovascular disorders.

Since the 1950s, a large number of reports have been published substantiating circannual rhythms in human mortality due to lesions of the vascular system or due to MI (Haberman et al. 1981; Ramirez-Lassepas et al. 1980; Reinberg et al. 1973; Smolensky et al. 1972). Too, a small number of reports have produced evidence for circadian differences in cardiac or cerebrovascular mortality (Bock and Kreuzenbeck 1966; Reinberg et al. 1973; Smolensky et al. 1972, 1976). Although data on cardiac and vascular mortality are rather easily accessible from governmental departments of vital statistics, especially for examining circannual patterns, data pertaining to 24-hr and seasonal differences in *morbidity* are considerably more difficult to obtain. With respect to 24-hr morbidity rhythms, the nature of certain data sets requires careful examination in that the clock-hour totals may represent to a greater extent the timing of hospital admissions rather than the timing of attacks. The two events can be separated by an unknown number of hours or even days. Moreover, discrepancies between the findings of investigations of circadian cardiovascular morbidity rhythms may result from artifacts due to imprecision in the recording of the clock hour of the onset of symptoms and also to a disregard for the synchronizer pattern of the individuals constituting the available sample of patients. Nonetheless, several published reports infer that cardiovascular morbidities exhibit rather high-amplitude circadian and circannual variations.

Circadian Rhythms and Myocardial Infarct

Differences in the occurrence of heart attacks in groups of patients with reference to clock hour have been studied, although only by a relatively small number of physicians and researchers, primarily since the middle of the twentieth century (Bock and Kreuzenbeck 1966; Churina et al. 1975; Eltringham and Dobson 1979; Gyárfás et al. 1976; Johansson 1972; Kaufmann et al. 1981; Master 1960; Master and Jaffe 1952; Master et al. 1937, 1952; Mey-

ers and Deuar 1975; Pell and D'Alonzo 1963; Stephens et al., in preparation). Initially, time-qualified MI morbidity (and mortality in the case of sudden death) data were tabulated to examine the temporal association between infarct and the type and level of activity preceding or coinciding with the morbid event. Typically, the number of cases in each study has been rather small, usually less than 400 to 500. One of the earliest American physicians to report a temporal pattern of morbidity in myocardial infarct over 24 hr in a sufficiently large sample of patients was Master and his colleagues (1937; 1952; 1960). Their data representing MIs in a sample of 1229 patients indicated large temporal variation with a peak around 1000 (Fig. 20).

Since the earlier investigation by Master and his colleagues, the results of several others have been published. However, in some it is not always clear whether the authors reported the clock hour totals of hospital admissions for MI or their occurrence as indicated by the patients. Figure 21 (Smolensky and Kennelly, unpublished data), the temporal distribution of hospital admissions, and Fig. 22 (Stephens et al., in preparation), the temporal pattern of medically substantiated MI, for 1497 and 1209 patients, respectively, show that neither the hospital admissions for MI nor the MI attacks, themselves, are randomly distributed over time. Moreover, the temporal patterns of each differ. The lowest number of hospital admissions for MI took place during the morning between 0600 and 0800; the greatest number took place during the afternoon around 1400. The temporal distribution of the onset of MI, based on the commencement of associated symptoms in 1209 of these patients, varied significantly from that of hospital admissions. Specifically, the waveform for the onset of MI is biomodal with a major peak around 0900 and a secondary one 12 hr later. The number of attacks which occurred between 0800 and 1000 was approximately twice that occurring between 0400 to 0600 or between

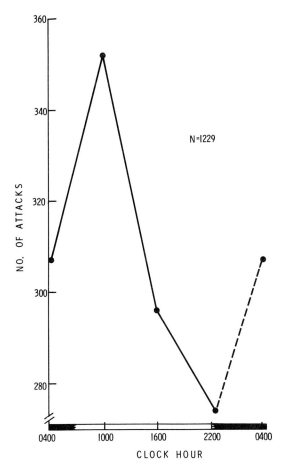

N=1229

Fig. 20. Data for 1229 myocardial infarctions summarized as the number of attacks per 6-hr span reveal a peak during the morning around 1000 and a trough around 2200. The dark shading along the horizontal axis indicates the alleged, although not verified, sleep span of the sample. Data from Master 1960.

emergency room admission data for studying human chronopathologies is inappropriate and misleading.

The detection of a prominent morning peak in the occurrence of MI by Stephens (in preparation) is consistent with the finding of others, such as Master (1960), Gyárfás (1976), and Churina et al. (1975). In the past, the timing of elevated numbers of MI has been discussed from an epidemiologic point of view with emphasis on exogenous factors such as workload, meal timing, and weather. However, the temporal pattern of MI may represent both exogenous as well as endogenous periodic influences. Although temporal changes in workload, physical effort, and emotional pressure over the 24-hr span cannot be ignored, neither can the circadian rhythmicity in pertinent endogenous functions be ignored (Reinberg et al. 1973; Smolensky et al. 1976; Yasue et al. 1978, 1979). Figure 23 by means of an acrophase map shows that several cardiovascular-related functions or indices are circadian rhythmic (Smolensky et al. 1976). The information depicted in this figure, while revealing a circadian organization of various cardiovascular processes, indicates that a number of critical functions have yet to be studied for periodicities. At this time, circadian rhythms are known for heart rate and certain dynamic aspects of cardiac function such as the preejection period index (PEPI), the left ventricular ejection time index (LVETI), and the indexed duration of left ventricular systole (QS$_2$I). The circadian acrophase of the latter differs by 12 hr from the ϕ of urinary catecholamine excretion. With respect to the 24-hr time domain, it is not surprising that the acrophase of the circadian rhythm of blood catecholamine concentration is phase-related to the circadian ϕ of heart rate and the trough (ϕ + 12 hr) of the circadian rhythm of myocardial ejection time (Wertheimer et al. 1972). Circadian rhythms have been demonstrated also for blood (systolic, diastolic, and pulse) pressure, cardiac output, stroke volume, capillary resistance, and

1800 and 2000. In addition to confirming the major finding of Master and colleagues, i.e., the existence of a 24-hr pattern in MI with a peak in the morning, the data of Smolensky, Kennelly and Stephens reveal the inappropriateness of depending on hospital records for investigating chronopathologies. The temporal pattern of hospital admissions for MI is not at all comparable to that for the onset of MI. The obvious implication is that the use of hospital or

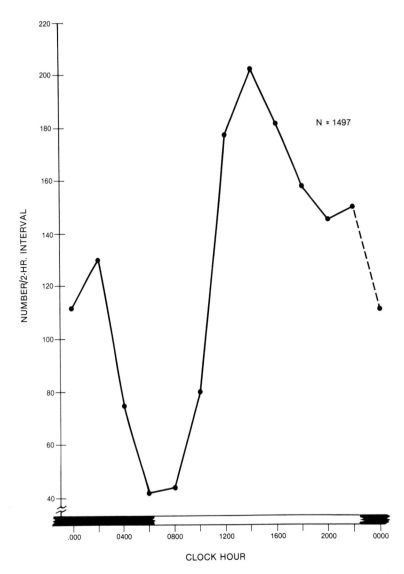

Fig. 21. Twenty-four-hour distribution of 1497 hospital emergency room admissions for the treatment of myocardial infarction in Cape Town, South Africa. The pattern is circadian rhythmic with a peak early in the afternoon and a trough around 0600. Shadings along the horizontal axis approximate the suspected sleep span for the sample. Unpublished data of M.H. Smolensky and B. Kennelly.

other cardiovascular variables (Smolensky et al. 1976). It is doubtful that any one of these particular circadian variables is associated directly and specifically with the observed temporal patterns in MI. Nonetheless, the acrophase map (presented as a review of known circadian rhythmic changes in cardiovascular measures and functions) shows that variability in cardiac function is not random over time. It is likely that several circadian biosystems are involved with cardiac efficiency as well as vulnerability.

The results of two other types of investigations—the first indicating temporal differences in the capacity of healthy human beings for physical effort and the second indicating temporal differences in the oc-

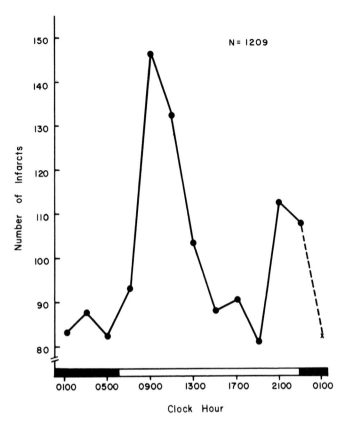

N = 1209

Fig. 22. The temporal distribution of myocardial infarction (MI) is non-random; MIs are more common around 0900 and 2100 than 0500 and also 1500–1900. The shaded portion of the horizontal axis shows the presumed sleep span for the sample of patients. Data from Stephens et al., in preparation.

currence of cardiac arrhythmias in heart patients—appear to be pertinent to understanding the observed temporal patterns in MI. With regard to the first type of study, Bier and Rompel-Purckhauser (1979) found physical training by means of treadmill-induced 130 beat/min pulse rate was best tolerated as far as producing optimal work capacity when timed from one day to the next around 1700. Minimum effectiveness of the training was found when it was scheduled at 0900. These findings are consistent also with those of Ilmarinen et al. (1980) who reported the recovery heart rate 5 min following a standardized exercise load was higher after a test conducted between 0700 and 1000 than after being conducted between 1900 and 2200. These findings differ from those of Voigt et al. (1967) who found the daily performance-pulse index (the ratio of the change of pulse rate to the increase in work output) during bicycle ergometry to

be greatest in the afternoon between 1600 and 1800 and lowest between 0200 and 0400. The latter findings are in agreement also with those of Klein et al. (1966) and Davis and Sargent (1975).

Overall, the findings from healthy samples suggest the occurrence of circadian rhythms of cardiopulmonary efficiency and tolerance for physical effort. Perhaps, the morning crest in MI coinciding closely in time with the rather abrupt shift from the inactive state of sleep to a high level of physical and emotional activity represents a type of circadian intolerance of predisposed persons for physical work or activity at this time. From an ethical and medical perspective, a laboratory investigation designed to research circadian rhythmicity in the susceptibility of predisposed patients to arrhythmias or MI is dangerous. Thus, although it is feasible to investigate the circadian susceptibility of volunteering asth-

160   Michael H. Smolensky

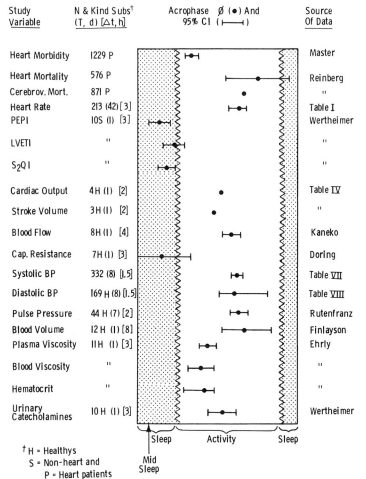

Study Variable	N & Kind Subs[†] (T, d) [Δt, h]	Acrophase ∅ (●) And 95% CI (⊢——⊣)	Source Of Data

Fig. 23. The circadian φ and 95% CL (the latter given only when circadian rhythmicity is documented at P ≦ .05) for human cardiovascular functions of diurnally active samples of healthy subjects. Although φs are provided for heart morbidity and mortality as well as cerebrovascular mortality, no cause and effect relationships are implied among the cardiovascular rhythms listed and those in morbidity and mortality (see original publication for sources of data). Reproduced from Smolensky et al. 1976.

matic patients to bronchial provocation, a procedure conducted under careful medical supervision in the clinic to substantiate diagnosis, this is not the case for MI. Nonetheless, because of a lack of relevant data the question of when to prescribe physical activity or exercise, in addition to how much, as a rehabilitative medical treatment must be examined. In this regard, Yasue et al. (1979) found Prinzmetal's variant angina patients incapable of completing a prescribed physical exercise load in the morning but capable of completing it rather easily when scheduled later in the afternoon.

With regard to the second type of studies, Bouvrain et al. (1977), Brisse et al. (1979), Christ and Hoff (1975), Sensi et al.

(1980), and Steinbach et al. (1978) found temporal differences in the occurrence of cardiac arrhythmias over the 24-hr period. However, only Brisse and her colleagues (1979) studied sufficiently large samples of cardiac patients. Brisse et al., by means of 24-hr Holter investigations, found that atrial and ventricular arrhythmias were more frequent between 0600 and 0900 and again about 12 hours later. This pattern in the frequency of arrhythmias resembles that of MI as described in Fig. 22. Additional 24-hr Holter investigations are required to evaluate the occurrence of temporal differences in the nature as well as number of arrhythmias to achieve a better understanding of the importance of such with regard to the temporal variation in MI.

Circadian Rhythms and Angina Pectoris

Angina pectoris is characterized by chest pain associated with transient episodes of myocardial ischemia resulting from an imbalance between oxygen supply and tissue demand. One type referred to as exercise-induced or exertional angina is believed to result from an elevated myocardial oxygen requirement in patients exhibiting a fixed stenosis of the large coronary arteries. The symptoms of another type, Prinzmetal's variant angina, occur not during exertion but primarily during nocturnal rest and apparently result from spasm of the coronary arteries (Prinzmetal et al. 1959; Nowlin et al. 1965; Kuroiwa 1978). According to Prinzmetal (1959) this form of angina, characterized by the episodic cyclic waxing and waning of ST-segment elevations as detectable from ECG records, is not necessarily coincident with chest pain. Kuroiwa (1978) found cyclic variation in this ST-segment anomaly in 31 of 58 (63%) of his patients. During sleep, episodes of ST-wave segment elevation were exhibited at intervals of 3 to 5 seconds. The manifestation of this ECG anomaly is thus ultradian rhythmic with as many as 12 to 20 or more episodes of ST-segment elevation/min. Data from 38 diurnally active Prinzmetal's variant patients studied by Kuroiwa (1978) reveal a circadian rhythm in the ultradian pattern of this ST-segment anomaly with the peak incidence between 0200 and 0400. Relatively few patients displayed this ECG anomaly after sleep or during the afternoon (Fig. 24).

The temporal etiology of this cardiac disorder has been further investigated by Yasue and his associates (1978, 1979) using an exercise challenge and angiography at different times of the day to visualize the patency of the coronary arteries. In their investigation, 13 patients with Prinzmetal's variant angina were subjected to treadmill exercise early in the morning between 0500 and 0800 and again in the afternoon between 1500 and 1600 on the same day. In the morning tests, patients were requested to walk for 3 min at a rate of 2.5 mi/hr on a grade of 12%. In the afternoon tests, patients were to walk longer and faster—for 4.5 min at a rate of 3 mi/hr also at a 12% grade. Attacks of angina associated with ST-segment elevations were induced in all 13 patients when the exercise was scheduled between 0500 and 0800. In contrast

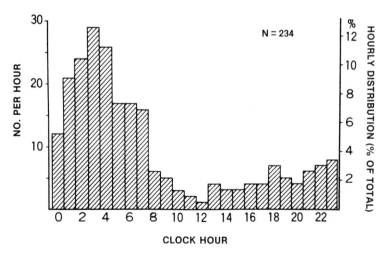

Fig. 24. Circadian variation in the occurrence of 234 (cyclic) episodes of ST-segment elevation in a sample of diurnally active patients suffering from Prinzmetal's variant angina. The number of episodes of ST-segment anomalies per hour, which in themselves display ultradian periodicity, is greatest during the sleep span with the peak around 0300. Few episodes of cyclic ST-segment anomaly are detected throughout the daytime span of activity. Reproduced from Kuroiwa 1978.

only 2 of the 13 patients exhibited ST-segment alterations when exercised in the afternoon in spite of the fact that the treadmill speed and duration of exercise were greater. The difference in the response to morning versus afternoon exercise was at least in part due to the temporal difference in the tone of the large coronary arteries. The tone was higher, i.e., the patency was smaller, during the morning than during the afternoon. Consistent with this finding was the observation that the effect of nitroglycerin on the patency of the large coronary arteries was always greater when taken in the morning, when the tone of the vessels was high, than when taken in the afternoon when the tone of the large coronary arteries was so low the medication was ineffective. Thus, temporal variation in the vasomotor tone of the large coronary arteries appears to explain at least partially the 24-hr susceptibility of the vasculature of the coronary arteries to vasospasm and the resulting temporal variability in the symptoms and electrocardiographic anomalies characteristic of Prinzmetal's variant angina.

The results of Yasue et al. (1978, 1979) are intriguing for another reason. The findings indicate without doubt that the effectiveness of nitroglycerin as a cardiac medication, at least for this type of patient, is clearly not the same in the morning and afternoon. The medication is highly effective in changing the patency of the large coronary arteries in the morning; it is predictably less effective in the afternoon because of the temporal pattern in the vasomotor tone of the large coronary arteries. The extent to which these findings are applicable to patients having other types of cardiac disease is not known but worthy of exploration considering the large number of patients now taking this medication.

Circadian Rhythms and Cerebral Infarction

Circadian rhythms in cerebral infarction have been postulated previously (Toole 1968; Kendell and Marshall 1963; Marshall 1977) based on reports of circadian rhythms in systolic and diastolic blood pressures (Smolensky et al. 1976). However, until recently data from a sufficiently large sample of patients have been unavailable to properly evaluate whether the occurrence of cerebral infarction is circadian rhythmic. Marshall in 1977 was the first to report a circadian rhythm in cerebral infarction (CI) with the highest incidence at 0300 and the lowest at 1500 (Fig. 25). The amplitude of this circadian chronopathology in groups of male and female patients is quite large with the number of cases at the peak more than twice that at the trough.

The coincidence in time in diurnally active persons between the circadian peak of cerebral infarction at 0300 and the trough of the circadian rhythm in diastolic and systolic blood pressure as found in studies of patients as well as healthy persons (Smolensky et al. 1976) is striking. In diurnally active persons, the peak in systolic and diastolic blood pressure generally occurs between the middle and late afternoon with slight deviation between individuals depending upon the exact activity-sleep routine (Tables 2 and 3). Although many explanations have been offered—e.g., reduced blood pressure occurring during sleep, regional changes in the distribution of blood within the brain, and the effects of posture and head-turning on the flow of blood through the vertebral and carotid arteries (Toole 1968; Townsend et al. 1973)—to explain the predilection for CI during nocturnal rest, none are adequate.

Circadian Rhythms and Spontaneous Intracerebral Hemorrhage

Marshall (1977) appears to have been the first to accumulate a relatively large sample of cases for studying the temporal variation in cerebral hemorrhage, although his data failed to show a significant 24-hr rhythmicity. Rigorous investigations by Ramirez-Lassepas et al. (1978), however, did reveal a prominent circadian difference in the onset of spontaneous intracerebral hemorrhage (SICH). The data for their study con-

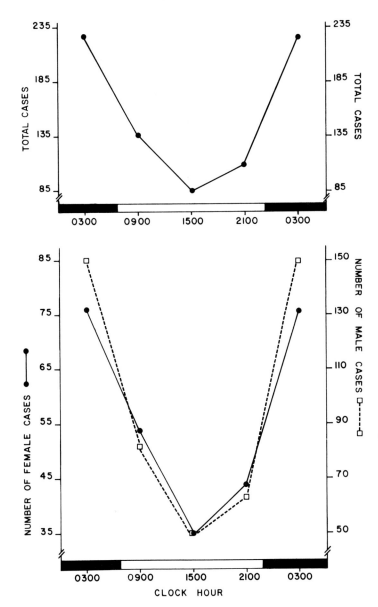

Fig. 25. Circadian rhythm in the occurrence of cerebral infarction (morbidity). In both presumably diurnally active males and females a cerebral infarction was considerably more common at night around 0300 than during the afternoon at 1500. Shaded portion at bottom shows the presumed usual sleep span. Data from Marshall 1977.

sisted of the time of the perceived onset of SICH for 118 consecutive cases collected during a 6-year span. Diagnosis was established by laboratory investigations showing hemorrhagic or xanthochromic cerebrospinal and angiographic demonstration of an intracerebral avascular mass in the absence of aneurysm in 9, by computerized axial tomography in 22, and by postmortem examination in 87 cases. The data and timing of the onset of symptoms were carefully recorded for the purpose of evaluating the existence of circadian as well as circannual rhythmicity. Figure 26 (E. Haus, personal communication) presents the 24-hr pattern of SICH in a sample of 100 patients for which the clock hour of the SICH event was accurately ascertained. A much higher than expected number of patients experienced SICH between 1730 and 2130. Only a small number experienced SICH between 0130 and 1330 in this sample of presumably diurnally active patients. Cosinor analysis of these data revealed a statistically signifi-

Table 2.   *Circadian Rhythm in Human Systolic Blood Pressure.*

Number and Type of Subjects (no. days) [Δt, hours]	P (rhythm detection)	Mesor: M[a] (M ± SE)	Amplitude: A[a]	Acrophase: Φ[b]	First Author
			(95% confidence limits)		
12H (14) [1.5][c]	<.05	NG	2.1 (0.8 to 3.4)	13^{56} (11^{56} to 17^{36})	Levine[73]
7H (NG)	<.005	118.8 ± 4.4	8.4 (4. to 12.3)	15^{50} (12^{56} to 21^{32})	Reinberg[92]
18H (1) [2]	<.05	121.8 ± 2.2	14.6 (10.4 to 18.8)	13^{28} (12^{56} to 14^{04})	Gautherie[29]
7S (1) [2]	<.05	131.5 ± 3.0	17.9 (15.8 to 20.0)	13^{12} (12^{52} to 13^{36})	Gautherie[29]
8E (1) [2]	<.05	117.0 ± 2.2	13.0 (12.0 to 14.0)	13^{44} (13^{12} to 14^{16})	Gautherie[29]
3V (3) [2]	<.05	112.0 ± 3.7	11.1 (9.1 to 13.2)	13^{56} (13^{10} to 14^{12})	Gautherie[29]
7H (1) [4]	—[d]	100%	8.9 (4.5 to 13.3)[c]	12^{48} (10^{56} to 14^{40})	Richardson[100]
13H (10) [1.5][c]	<.005	119.0 ± 2.0	5.4 (1.8 to 10.0)	12^{36} (09^{28} to 15^{28})	Kanabrocki[58]
12H (10) [1.5][c]	<.001	117.7 ± 3.7	4.5 (2.9 to 6.0)	14^{44} (13^{32} to 16^{28})	Kanabrocki[58]
25H (1) [0.1]	<.001	146.0 ± 0.8	6.2 (4.0 to 8.4)	08^{40} (07^{20} to 10^{24})	Gross[31]
5H (1) [1]	<.005	120.8 ± 0.8	4.2 (1.8 to 6.6)	10^{32} (08^{20} to 12^{40})	Bidoggia[8]
120H (1) [1]	<.001	125.2 ± 0.4	5.5 (3.5 to 7.5)	12^{20} (11^{36} to 13^{04})	Zulch[142]
10H (NG)	<.01	123.0 ± 2.6	2.2 (0.8 to 3.6)	17^{28} (15^{04} to 21^{48})	Levine[72]
1H (21) [1.5][c]	.009	122.9 ± 0.8	3.0 (1.2 to 4.8)	18^{24} (15^{05} to 23^{52})	Sothern[122]
7H (1) [4]	.002	NG	8.4 (4.5 to 12.3)	12^{20} (09^{28} to 14^{04})	Reinberg[93]
7D (1) [4]	.006	NG	5.9 (2.6 to 9.1)	12^{00} (10^{48} to 13^{04})	Reinberg[93]
35H (4–100) [1.5][c]	<.001	100%	0.8 (0.4 to 1.2)[c]	16^{56} (14^{36} to 19^{52})	LaSalle[69]
6U (6) [2]	<.001	109.2 ± 0.5	7.4 (6.0 to 7.8)	13^{24} (12^{40} to 14^{08})	Rutenfranz[105]
7X (9) [2]	<.001	106.3 ± 0.7	11.1 (9.3 to 12.9)	13^{08} (12^{32} to 13^{38})	Rutenfranz[105]
4Y (7) [2]	<.001	107.4 ± 0.7	9.9 (7.9 to 11.9)	13^{32} (12^{44} to 14^{20})	Rutenfranz[105]
3Z (5) [2]	<.001	102.9 ± 0.8	9.0 (6.6 to 11.4)	12^{26} (11^{26} to 13^{26})	Rutenfranz[105]
18X (~8) [2]	<.001	106.8 ± 0.6	5.7 (4.1 to 7.3)	13^{20} (12^{16} to 13^{44})	Rutenfranz[105]
6Y (~9) [2]	.003	103.9 ± 0.6	4.2 (2.6 to 5.8)	13^{52} (12^{28} to 15^{20})	Rutenfranz[105]
9R (10) [~3]	<.001	145.9 ± 17.4	6.4 (2.4 to 10.4)	19^{24} (14^{08} to 21^{44})	Scheving[107]
10L (10) [3]	<.02	130.0 ± 4.0	3.1 (0.6 to 5.6)	19^{30} (14^{34} to 23^{14})	Enna[23]
29C (1) [0.1]	<.001	154.1 ± 0.9	6.4 (3.9 to 8.9)	11^{22} (09^{56} to 12^{56})	Gross[31]
36I (1) [0.1]	<.001	160.6 ± 1.0	6.3 (3.4 to 9.2)	10^{38} (08^{56} to 12^{22})	Gross[31]
10M (1) [0.1]	<.001	176.0 ± 0.8	7.2 (5.2 to 9.4)	08^{50} (07^{42} to 09^{58})	Gross[31,]
1P (42) [1.5][c]	<.01	160.0 ± 0.9	9.8 (8.4 to 11.4)	11^{36} (10^{48} to 12^{20})	Levine[71]
9P (1) [1]	<.001	166.9 ± 1.0	7.9 (5.1 to 10.7)	11^{28} (10^{12} to 12^{48})	Bidoggia[8]

[a] M and A given in mmHg except when mesor = 100%, then A given in %M.

[b] Acrophase, Φ, referenced to designated or estimated midsleep time and given as a delay in hours and minutes.

[c] Data obtained during the waking hours only for designated T.

[d] P > .05 but signal to noise ratio (A/SE) ⩾ 0.33.

NG, not given.

Subjects: H, healthy normotensive; C, carotid ischemia; N, equilibrate healthy; M, carotid and vertebrobasilar ischemia; P, hypertensive patients; I, vertebrobasilar ischemia; R, older (x̄ age = 80.4 years) but healthy; L, leprosy; S, sympathicotonics; V, vagotonics; D, restricted diet, healthy.

Analyses by LSS (least squares spectral) and cosinor.

Note: See Smolensky et al. (1976) for source of citations shown in table.

cant circadian rhythmicity in both males and females with the acrophase for the former at 1748 (with the 95% confidence limits being 1516 to 2016) and 1728 (1548 to 1912) for the latter. Although the underlying temporal features of this circadian chronopathology have not been elucidated, Ramirez-Lassepas et al. (1978) point out that the peak incidence of SICH coincides closely with the circadian peak of blood pressure observed in normal and hypertensive individuals.

Circadian Rhythms and Hypertension

Although hypertension is considered one of the most prevalent diseases of modern civilization, the diagnostic criteria are not universally agreed upon by physicians and

Table 3. *Circadian rhythm in Human Diastolic Blood Pressure.*

Number and Type of Subjects (no. days) [Δt, hours]	P (rhythm detection)	Mesor: M^a (M ± SE)	Amplitude: A^a (95% confidence limits)	Acrophase: Φ^b	First author
13H (10) [1.5][c]	<.02	75.0 ± 2.0	4.7 (0.8 to 8.5)	21^{28} (18^{56} to 01^{08})	Kanabrocki[58]
12H (10) [1.5][c]	.001	77.7 ± 2.3	1.9 (0.4 to 3.5)	16^{44} (14^{08} to 22^{28})	Kanabrocki[58]
18H (1) [2]	<.05	73.7 ± 9.6	4.3 (2.7 to 5.9)	12^{00} (11^{00} to 13^{00})	Gautherie[29]
7S (1) [2]	<.05	80.5 ± 5.5	5.5 (5.2 to 5.8)	11^{24} (11^{04} to 11^{44})	Gautherie[29]
8E (1) [2]	<.05	71.0 ± 6.0	3.8 (3.0 to 4.6)	12^{20} (12^{00} to 12^{36})	Gautherie[29]
3V (3) [2]	<.05	65.0 ± 5.0	2.8 (2.1 to 3.5)	12^{48} (12^{28} to 13^{08})	Gautherie[29]
25H (1) [0.1]	.001	87.7 ± 0.7	3.2 (1.2 to 5.2)	09^{36} (07^{28} to 11^{52})	Gross[31]
7H (1) [4][c]	—[d]	100%	13.4 (10.1 to 16.5)[c]	12^{24} (10^{44} to 14^{04})	Richardson[100]
10H (1) NG	<.01	83.0 ± 3.0	2.7 (2.5 to 3.8)	20^{40} (18^{28} to 04^{16})	Levine[72]
1H (21) [1.5]	.009	75.5 ± 0.6	3.4 (2.0 to 4.8)	08^{52} (07^{03} to 10^{31})	Sothern[122]
48H (16–64) [1.5]	<.001	70.0 ± NG	2.6 (1.4 to 4.0)	04^{40} (01^{36} to 12^{52})	Halberg[38]
6U (6) [2]	.001	81.8 ± 0.3	3.8 (3.4 to 4.3)	13^{52} (12^{00} to 13^{44})	Rutenfranz[105]
7X (7) [2]	.001	75.3 ± 0.3	4.1 (3.7 to 4.5)	13^{16} (12^{36} to 14^{00})	Rutenfranz[105]
4Y (7) [2]	.001	77.0 ± 0.4	4.8 (4.2 to 5.4)	13^{32} (12^{40} to 14^{28})	Rutenfranz[105]
3Z (5) [2]	.001	75.5 ± 0.6	6.0 (5.1 to 6.9)	12^{22} (11^{26} to 13^{26})	Rutenfranz[105]
6Y (~9) [2]	.008	73.2 ± 0.4	2.3 (1.8 to 2.9)	22^{20} (20^{52} to 00^{16})	Rutenfranz[105]
9R (10) [~3][c]	<.01	NG	4.1 (1.5 to 6.6)	20^{24} (16^{00} to 21^{36})	Scheving[107]
1P (42) [1.5][c]	<.01	91.4 ± 0.4	2.8 (2.0 to 3.5)	12^{00} (10^{40} to 13^{20})	Levine[71]
9P (1) [1]	<.05	101.3 ± 0.6	2.0 (0.3 to 6.7)	15^{44} (12^{32} to 18^{56})	Bidoggia[8]
29C (1) [0.1]	.001	91.5 ± 0.5	3.8 (2.3 to 5.3)	10^{06} (08^{38} to 11^{38})	Gross[31]
36I (1) [0.1]	.001	98.2 ± 0.8	4.7 (2.4 to 7.0)	09^{18} (07^{54} to 10^{38})	Gross[31]
10M (1) [0.1]	.001	96.3 ± 0.6	4.3 (2.5 to 6.1)	08^{18} (06^{46} to 09^{50})	Gross[31]

[a] M and A given in mmHg except when mesor = 100%, then A given in %M.

[b] Acrophase, Φ, referenced to designated or estimated midsleep time and given as a delay in hours and minutes.

[c] Data obtained during the waking hours only for designated T.

[d] P > .05 but signal to noise ratio (A/SE) ⩾ 0.33.

NG, not given.

Subjects: H, healthy normotensive; I, vertebrobasilar ischemia; V, vagotonics; P, hypertensive patients; M, carotid and vertebrobasilar ischemia; N, equilibrate healthy; R, older (x̄ age = 80.4 yrs) but healthy; C, carotid ischemia; S, sympathicotonics. Age of children: U, 3–4 years; X, 7–10 years; Y, 11–13 years; Z, 15 years.

Analyses by LSS (least squares spectral) and cosinor.

Note: See Smolensky et al. (1976) for source of citations shown in table.

researchers. Conventionally, a systolic pressure of 140 mmHg or a diastolic pressure of 90 mmHg is the agreed upon demarcation between normotension and hypertension in adults. Although it has been suggested that the diagnosis of hypertension should be based on elevated blood pressures on at least 2–3 consecutive clinical visits, there are no criteria as to the time or the duration during the 24 hr that the pressures must be elevated to substantiate the diagnosis.

Diastolic and systolic blood pressures exhibit both random as well as predictable circadian and other rhythmic patterns (Bartter et al. 1976; Smolensky et al. 1976). In general, the blood pressure of day-active individuals tends to be greater during the afternoon and evening than the morning. Either due to random fluctuations or to circadian rhythms, elevated blood pressure values beyond the generally accepted limits of normotension are from time to time observed even in healthy persons free of cardiovascular or other illness (Pickering 1972; Pickering et al. 1982; Halberg et al. 1974). Because sometimes rather large-amplitude circadian changes in blood pressure may occur even in health, pressures above 140/90 mmHg occasionally can be expected. With recognition of biological rhythms in blood pressure, Bartter et al. (1976) suggested the term *mesor-hypertension,* meaning the elevation over the entire 24-hr span

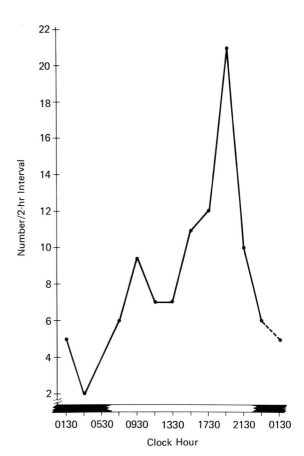

Fig. 26. The occurrence of spontaneous intracerebral hemorrhage (SICH) is not evenly distributed over the 24 hr. In a sample of 100 cases for which the time of the event was known, the susceptibility was considerably greater between 1730 and 2130 than between 2330 and 1330. Shaded portion at bottom depicts the presumed usual sleep span. Illustration provided by E. Haus as a personal communication.

of systolic and diastolic pressure beyond conventionally considered safe levels such as 140/90 mmHg. According to Halberg and his colleagues (1974) mesor-hypertension, referring either to significant transient or lasting elevation in the systolic and/or diastolic circadian rhythm-adjusted mean (mesor, see Chap. 2), represents a validated statistically significant difference in the 24-hr blood pressure level relative to a patient's previously established baseline mesor obtained while healthy or relative to a range of mesor values of an appropriate reference group.

The timing of high and low values of diastolic and systolic blood pressure during the 24-hr period does not occur at random (Smolensky et al. 1976). Biological functions have a precise temporal structure. In the case of blood pressure, the vasomotor tone, stroke volume, and blood volume among other factors influence blood pressure. Adrenal hormones both from the medula and cortex also exhibit strong influences. Since the secretion of these hormones is circadian rhythmic, biological functions dependent on these adrenal hormones should be expected to be circadian rhythmic as well. Figure 27 (Reinberg 1979a, 1980) by means of an acrophase map presents the temporal coordination of some of these functions. For heart rate (lower portion of figure) there is an almost exact phase coupling to the rhythm of urinary catecholamines, an observation made previously (Wertheimer 1972; Smolensky et al. 1976). The ϕ of systolic pressure appears to be more precisely coupled to the ϕ of urinary aldosterone, whereas the ϕ of diastolic pressure seems to be more closely linked to the ϕ of plasma renin activity. The ϕ of both systolic and diastolic blood pres-

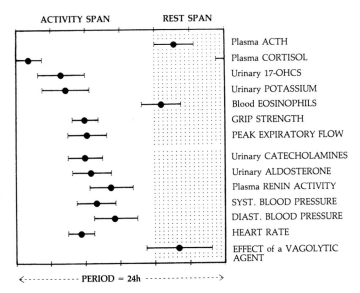

ACTIVITY SPAN   REST SPAN

Plasma ACTH
Plasma CORTISOL
Urinary 17-OHCS
Urinary POTASSIUM
Blood EOSINOPHILS
GRIP STRENGTH
PEAK EXPIRATORY FLOW

Urinary CATECHOLAMINES
Urinary ALDOSTERONE
Plasma RENIN ACTIVITY
SYST. BLOOD PRESSURE
DIAST. BLOOD PRESSURE
HEART RATE
EFFECT of a VAGOLYTIC
AGENT

<-------------- PERIOD = 24h --------------->

Fig. 27. The circadian acrophase (●) and the 95% CL (shown by the extension of a line to either side of the φ) are indicated for several adrenal hormones and adrenal-influenced rhythmic functions. The φs for these rhythms are not random in occurrence. Instead, there is a strong phase coupling— between urinary catecholamine and aldosterone concentration and heart rate and systolic blood pressure on the one hand and between plasma renin activity and diastolic blood pressure on the other. The upper portion of the figure illustrates the temporal organization of the pituitary-adrenal axis and also the effects of adrenocortical hormone rhythmicity on the component rhythms of blood eosinophils and urinary potassium. The circadian rhythms of grip strength and peak expiratory flow are influenced by 24-hr variation in the secretion of hormones from the adrenal cortex and medulla. The greatest effect of a vagolytic agent (iapropium bromide) is approximately 12 hr out of phase with the rhythm of urinary catecholamine concentration. Reproduced from Reinberg 1979a.

sure exhibits a relatively close temporal co-incidence with that of the rhythm of urinary catecholamines, although the phase coupling seems to be somewhat stronger for systolic than diastolic blood pressure.

The temporal occurrence of the acrophases for blood pressure and heart rate appears to be determined largely by circadian rhythms in the production of hormones from the adrenal medulla and cortex. Rhythms in these hormones create a precise temporal order in certain functions (upper portion of Fig. 27). The plasma levels of ACTH reach a peak several hours prior to the acrophase of the rhythm in plasma cortisol and urinary aldosterone. The rhythmicity in cortisol, in particular, gives rise to circadian changes in several different cortisol-dependent variables. Thus, the φ of the plasma cortisol rhythm

precedes that of the rhythm of urinary 17-OHCS (cortisol metabolite) as well as potassium excretion; it is completely out of phase with the circadian rhythm in blood eosinophil numbers as expected since corticosteroids generally inhibit mitotic activity. The circadian rhythm of grip strength, only in part dependent on cortisol, exhibits an appreciable phase delay from the φ of plasma cortisol; it is more closely timed to the φ of the rhythm in urinary catecholamines. The peak expiratory flow (PEF), affected by both catecholamines and cortisol, reveals a phase coincidence with the former and a phase delay from the latter. The acrophases of the rhythms in PEF (indicating highest bronchial patency), heart rate, and diastolic and systolic pressure are approximately 12 hr out of phase with the circadian rhythm in the effectiveness of a vagolytic agent. The temporal patterns of these 2 strong circadian adrenal oscillator systems—defined by concentrations of cortisol and catecholamines—give rise to 24-hr periodicities in numerous dependent variables throughout the body.

Circannual Rhythms and Cardiovascular Morbidity

Circannual rhythmicity in cardiovascular morbidity as well as mortality has been rather well documented (Reinberg 1973; Reinberg et al. 1973; Smolensky et al. 1972; Tromp 1963). With regard to heart attacks, most authors have ascribed the seasonal variation (morbidity and mortality) to differences in weather, i.e., temperature, relative humidity, and/or precipitation. However, circannual rhythms in heart attacks are known even in settings where the seasonal alteration in the environment is rather moderate, such as in Hawaii (Smolensky et al. 1972). Figure 2 presented the seasonal distribution of mortality from cardiovascular disease for data collected from geographic locations in the Northern (left-hand portion of the figure) and Southern (right-hand portion of the figure) Hemispheres. These data, which were accumulated as part of an extensive literature review (Smolensky et al. 1972), show independent of hemisphere the occurrence of high-amplitude circannual variations with a winter peak. Figure 28 presents the circannual acrophases for each of the separate time series making up the curves shown in Fig. 2 and provides in addition the ϕs for cardiac morbidity. Shown as well are the acrophases of time series dealing with respiratory morbidity (primarily upper respiratory infections such as colds, influenza, and pneumonia) and mortality. The acrophases relating to cardiovascular morbidity occur primarily during the winter months between December and February in the Northern Hemisphere. A few time series (from cities in Louisiana, Texas, and Egypt) each consisting of a small number of cases exhibit summer acrophases. In the Southern Hemisphere, only a few studies of

seasonal variation in cardiovascular morbidity are known. Each exhibits a winter acrophase.

Although a popular hypothesis is that the circannual variation in heart disease results from seasonal patterns of weather, perhaps other factors such as those related to the body's circannual biological time structure and/or a circannual susceptibility-resistance rhythm are involved. Although the extent to which the phasing of critical circannually organized physiological functions contributes to the seasonal variation in the susceptibility to cardiovascular accidents is yet to be investigated, the fact that in both the Northern and Southern Hemispheres the peak in cardiovascular disease occurs during the winter need not implicate weather as the only significant etiologic factor in this circannual chronopathology. It may be that several component circannual biological rhythms are involved. In the Northern and Southern Hemispheres, the phasing of these rhythms could differ by 6 months due to phase differences between the hemispheres in the primary synchronizers of circannual rhythms.

Circannual rhythms in many different types of biological functions at different levels of organization are known. Acrophase maps shown in Figs. 29 and 30 represent the findings of Cosinor analyses on data reported in previous publications. The data for these maps thus are representative of investigations conducted by various authors using unique methodologies applied to separate groups of differently aged subjects dwelling in different geographic locations in the Northern Hemisphere. Interpretation of the information provided in these particular charts, although useful in formulating hypotheses or reviewing the scope of the circannual temporal structure, is restricted because of the multitude of unknown and uncontrolled influences. Certainly, the great number of variables which are known to exhibit circannual rhythmicity as demonstrated by the comprehensive reviews of Hildebrandt (1962, 1973), De-Rudder (1952), Tromp (1963), and Hal-

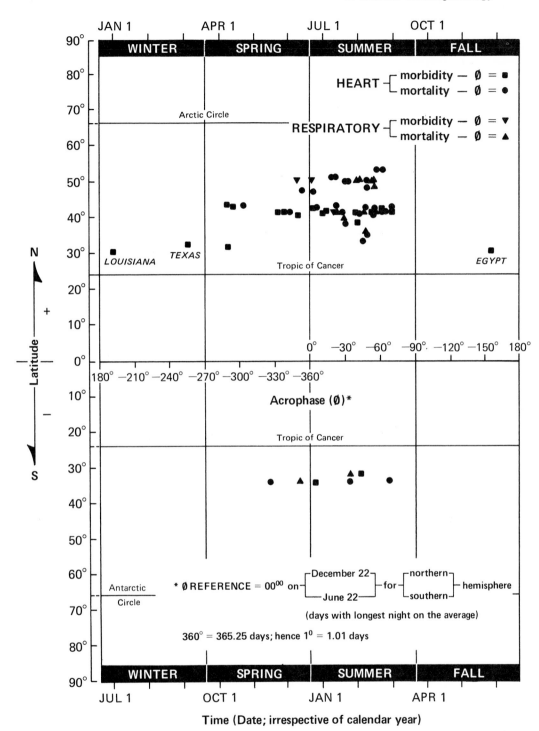

Fig. 28. Circannual acrophases (φ) of time series on cardiovascular morbidity (and mortality as well as respiratory morbidity and mortality) are not randomly distributed over the year. In both the Northern and Southern Hemispheres, the φs occur primarily during the winter with the exception of a few time series (Louisiana, Texas, and Egypt) made up of a relatively small number of cases; these latter exhibit summer or autumn φs. Reproduced from Smolensky et al. 1972.

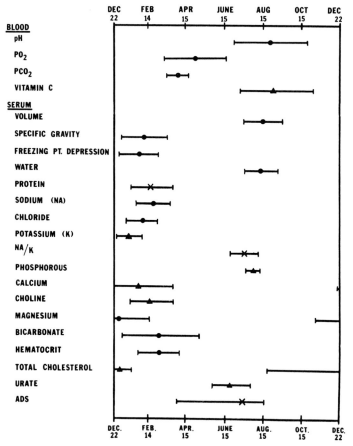

Fig. 29. The φs and 95% CL for several constituents of the blood and serum which have been demonstrated to be circannually rhythmic. The data were accumulated by a literature search and reanalyzed for circannual rhythms by Cosinor. The different symbols which are used to denote the acrophases also serve to indicate the prominence of the rhythm, i.e., the circannual amplitude expressed relative to the circannual mesor. Generally, every entry represents a separate study; investigations were conducted in various locations in the Northern Hemisphere.

berg et al. (1983) or by study of specific variables (Brennan, 1982; Letellier and Desjarlais 1982) support the concept of a circannual organization of biological functioning. Nonetheless, not yet established is the degree to which such circannual changes are dependent on seasonal changes in ambient conditions.

Acrophase charts when representative of various samples dwelling at different geographic locations and studied by different protocols are not always useful for predicting temporal events. On the other hand, when the information contained in such charts is representative of a well-controlled study on a stable sample of subjects intensively investigated while residing in a single geographic setting it is much more useful. In

this regard the information in Fig. 31 reveals circannual rhythmicity in many different plasma and urinary constituents (Lagoguey and Reinberg 1981; Reinberg 1979a, 1980; Reinberg and Lagoguey 1978a,b). The investigation of these circannual rhythms followed a precise and well-controlled chronobiologic methodology. A small group of 5 young adult healthy men were studied at approximately 2-month intervals. On the dates of study the subjects reported to the laboratory early in the morning and remained there until the following morning. During these 28-hr spans, 4-hr samplings of blood and urine (complete integrated sequential voidings) were conducted. Under these conditions, circannual rhythms were detected for 9 plasma hormones, 6 urinary

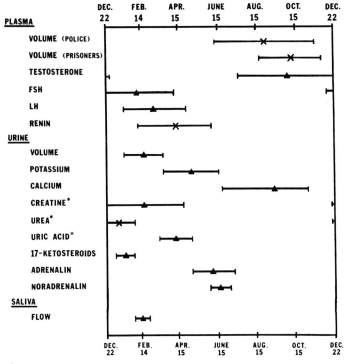

Fig. 30. The φs and 95% CL for several constituents of the plasma and urine plus salivary flow. See legend to Fig. 29 for further details.

*DATA ANALYZED AS EXCRETION PER NIGHT

SYMBOLS ●, X, ▲ DENOTE Ø AND A WHERE ● = A < 5% M.; X = 5% M. ≤ A ≤ 10% M.; ▲ = A > 10% M.; ┝──┥ = 95% C.I. FOR Ø.

constituents (of which 4 represent hormones or hormone-metabolites), and 2 other variables—sexual activity and body weight (studied by self recordings throughout the year). Although circadian rhythms were consistently detected for most variables throughout the year, circadian rhythmicity in certain variables (as a group phenomenon) was lacking. This was the case for FSH (throughout the year), testosterone (during March), and LH (from January to June) (Lagoguey and Reinberg 1981). Circadian rhythms on the other hand were regularly detected in plasma cortisol, prolactin, thyroxine, GH, TSH, and renin activity. Moreover in these studies involving transverse samplings, systematic circannual modifications of the circadian acrophase were detected (Lagoguey and Reinberg 1981), a finding previously reported for the circannual rhythm of serum corticosterone of mice housed under rigor-

ously controlled conditions with L(0600–1800):D(1800–0600) with food and water available ad libitum (Haus and Halberg 1970). Circamensual modulation of circadian rhythms in women has been detected as well (Smolensky et al. 1973; Proccacci et al. 1974).

The circannual temporal organization revealed by the acrophase charts (Figs. 29–31) suggests the possibility of endogenous rhythmic components of seasonal differences in cardiovascular morbidity and mortality; this could be similar in nature, although differing in period, to the circadian temporal organization contributing to nocturnal asthma. Although it has been reported that human serum cholesterol levels vary over the year with a peak during the winter or spring (Antonis et al. 1965; Doyle et al. 1965; Fyfe et al. 1968; Green et al. 1963; Paloheimo 1961; Thomas et al. 1961; Watanabe and Aoki 1956) in the Northern

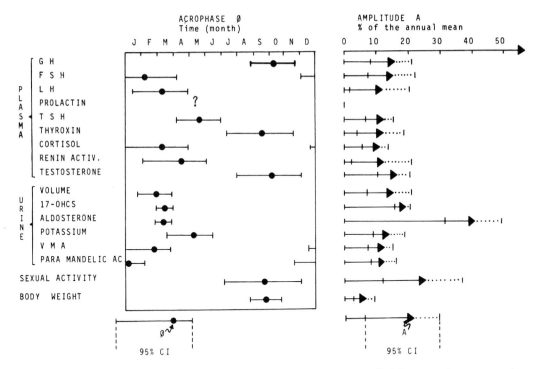

Fig. 31. Circannual rhythms of 5 healthy young Parisian males studied in a precise manner (see text). The circannual ϕ and A (expressed as a percentage of the annual mean) are indicated with their 95% CL. The A is quite large for the circannual rhythm of urinary aldosterone but relatively small for body weight. The As of the other rhythms are moderate. No circannual rhythm was detected in plasma prolactin. Reproduced from Reinberg and Lagoguey 1978a.

Hemisphere, the statistical significance of such changes has been questioned (Rippey 1981). In any event, this seasonal variation does not in itself appear to be sufficient to contribute to the increase in heart and vascular disease during winter in those at risk. According to Reinberg and Lagoguey (1978a,b), the coincidence in time between elevated cardiovascular disease and the circannual ϕs of certain adrenal hormone rhythms is striking. Not only might the circannual rhythms of aldosterone and plasma renin activity be involved, but also those of adrenalin and noradrenalin (Reinberg and Lagoguey 1978a; Descovitch et al. 1974). Nonetheless, the speculation that increased cardiovascular morbidity and mortality during the winter are expressions of our temporal organization, although intriguing as a hypothesis, has yet to be appropriately explored. Similarly, the speculation that these rhythms represent the impact of seasonal differences in exogenous conditions, e.g., cold, harsh weather, as most often suggested, has yet to be rigorously investigated as well.

The Chronobiology of Epilepsy

Circadian Rhythms

Temporal differences in the onset of epileptic seizures over 24 hr were apparently first recognized by Beau in 1836 and thereafter by Féré in 1888. Since then, the development of EEG recordings led to the determination of epilepsy by specific electrical events rather than clinical manifestations only as in earlier studies. The manifestations of epileptic seizures, whether studied by EEG and/or symptoms, have been shown to exhibit ultradian, circadian, and circamensual rhythms (Engle et al. 1952; Halberg 1953; Halberg and Howard 1958; Griffiths and Fox 1938; Gowers 1901; Langdon-Down and Brain 1929; Patry 1931; Hopkins 1933; Magnussen 1936; Kamraj-Mazurkiewicz 1971). Several investigators have classified their patients according to the usual timing during the day or night of their seizures. For example, Gowers (1901), Langdon-Down and Brain (1929), and Patry (1931) recognized three different types of adult patients. Those exhibiting a majority of their attacks during the daytime were termed "diurnal" in type. Those experiencing a majority of seizures during the night were classified as "nocturnal" in type. Patients showing neither a diurnal nor nocturnal pattern were referred to as "diffuse" in type. Griffiths and Fox (1938) also identified an additional category—an "awakening" type to identify those experiencing seizures just after arising from nightly rest.

In general, the diurnal type is most common, whereas the nocturnal type is least so. As many as 40% of epileptic patients may be diurnal in type. On the other hand, no more than 25% are likely to be nocturnal in type (Halberg 1953). Although it is feasible to categorize patients in the aforementioned manner, there appears to be a tendency for epileptic patients to lose their diurnal or nocturnal specificity with aging so that seizures may occur both during the day and night. Thus, results of studies on the temporal patterns of epileptic seizures are likely to be influenced by the age distribution of samples. At best, the study of circadian rhythms in epilepsy is made difficult because of the existence of several types of patients. When patients are studied for 24-hr variations in the occurrence of seizures, combining data from the different types of patients confounds the true description and/or detection of rhythmicity as a group phenomenon.

In investigating rhythms in epileptic seizures, knowledge of the synchronizer schedule is fundamental as it is for the study of any periodicity. The point is illustrated by data published by Halberg and Howard (1958) for an epileptic patient who continually resided in one institution from 1932 until 1944, when sleep was scheduled from approximately 2100 until 0600, and thereafter from 1945 to 1952 when sleep was from 0300 until 1100 (Fig. 32). Between 1932 and 1944, the diurnal seizures were exhibited primarily between 0600 and 1930. After transfer to a different work shift and adopting a new sleep-activity schedule, the occurrence of seizures was still greater during the hours following awakening; however, with regard to clock hour they were displaced in the same direction and amount of time that the sleep-wakefulness schedule had been changed such that seizures were now most common between 1200 and 1930. This example demonstrates once again the importance of qualifying temporal patterns in disease processes in individuals or groups of patients with regard to the synchronizer schedule of sleep and activity.

Although some attempt has been made to explain the etiology of the temporal variation in epileptic seizures (Halberg 1953), nothing definite is known. Several investigators have theorized that certain events related to the commencement and termination of sleep are important. In this regard, Magnussen (1936) found awakening (morning) type epileptics, when made to nap after their noontime meal, experienced additional seizures after awakening later in the early afternoon. Although these findings cite the importance of sleep-related processes, much remains to be learned about the many factors which contribute to the 24-hr patterns in epileptic seizures.

Circamensual Rhythm

The observation that epileptic seizures vary over the menstrual cycle dates back at least to Gowers, who in 1885 seemingly was the first to mention an association between menses and epilepsy. Since then a rather

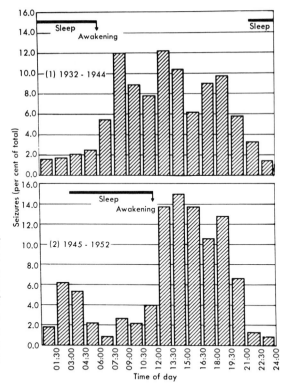

Fig. 32. Circadian pattern in the initiation of epileptic seizures in 1 (diurnal type) patient studied longitudinally over several years while residing in the same institution. The temporal distribution with regard to the clock hour of the seizures changed following transfer to a different work-rest pattern when the sleep schedule was delayed from ~2100–0600 to ~0300–1100. Reproduced from Halberg and Howard 1958.

large number of reports on so-called catamenial epilepsy have been published. In their comprehensive review, Newmark and Penry (1980) found that the published incidence of menses-associated epilepsy varied between investigators. Some reported the incidence of catamenial epilepsy to be as high as 35 to 60%, whereas a lesser number reported it as low as 5%. Based on the relatively numerous reports on the topic, it is probable that between 25 and 50% of epileptic women exhibit exacerbation during menses.

Data from Laidlaw (1956) are representative of the circamensual pattern of epilepsy in women. Laidlaw studied 50 female institutionalized epileptic patients by examining records for the calendar date of seizures in relationship to menstrual cycle day. In an attempt to minimize the effect of differences in menstrual cycle length, Laidlaw categorized his data with regard to the number of days before or after menses that seizures occurred. Separate analyses were

conducted on samples of women whose menstrual cycle lengths were nonvarying in duration and those who exhibited inconsistency. Overall, the 50 women experienced more than 23,500 seizures. Figure 33 reveals an almost 2-fold elevation in the number of seizures on the first day of menses (labeled as menstrual day 1) as compared to the seventh day (−7) prior to menses. There was a secondary peak in the incidence of seizures around the time of the expected, although not confirmed, ovulation around day −14. The temporal pattern in seizures did not differ between the two samples of women. In both groups, the increase in the incidence of seizures commenced rather precipitously 3–4 days before menstruation and continued to be high thereafter throughout menses. Although it has been hypothesized that the premenstrual rise in the incidence of epileptic seizures is related to the reproductive hormone progesterone, controversy continues to exist concerning the temporal etiology of

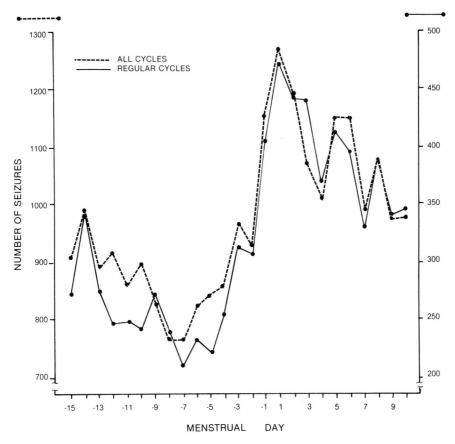

Fig. 33. In this sample of 50 institutionalized menstruating women, the incidence of epileptic seizures varied with the phase of the menstrual cycle. The incidence during menstruation was nearly twice what it was 7 days prior to menses. Similar patterns were exhibited independent of the regularity or irregularity in the menstrual cycle duration. Data from Laidlaw 1956.

this circamensual chronopathology (Thiry et al. 1954; Backstrom 1976; Hall 1977).

The Chronobiology of Infectious Diseases

Circadian Rhythms

Fever is a prevailing symptom of most infectious diseases; yet, the demarcation of hyperthermia or for that matter the demarcation of hypothermia from normothermia is not well founded. It is stated in many medical textbooks and recent papers (Kluger 1979; Manerv 1979) that the average human body temperature is 37 ± 0.5°C (1 ±

SE) with "small fluctuations around this mean." Even when textbooks have acknowledged the circadian rhythm of body temperature, the applied and theoretical significance of its existence to medicine has never been adequately explored. Accordingly, it is stated that hyperthermia commences at a body temperature of 37.5°C (or at 38°C with 95% CL), whereas hypothermia commences at or below 36.5 or 36°C. These definitions are obsolete, since they are not time qualified (Halberg and Reinberg 1967). A better quantification of hypothermia and hyperthermia including fever can be attained by using as a reference system for a given person an individualized temperature circadian chronogram derived during health. In this manner, a body temperature measurement made at a given clock hour can be compared to a time-qualified reference to determine whether it is within the time-specified normal range with a given level of confidence (Levine et al. 1979). An infectious state considered apyretic by a conventional single and/or non–time-qualified measurement may be associated with an alteration in the waveform and/or other parameter such as the mesor, amplitude, and/or acrophase of the temperature rhythm. Thus, a chronobiologic approach serves to better quantify body temperature changes and is helpful for establishing criteria of health and disease.

With regard to infectious agents and circadian rhythms, early experiments on rodents revealed the prominence of 24-hr rhythms in the response of animals to bacterial endotoxins and other infectious agents (Halberg et al. 1955; Halberg et al. 1960; Halberg and Stephens 1958; Feigin et al. 1969, 1972, 1978; Shackelford and Feigin 1973; Wongwiwat et al. 1972). In a series of studies on human beings by Hejl (1977), it was noted that the commencement of fever, used by the author to denote the onset of an infectious disease, was time dependent with respect to the scales of 24 hr, 1 year, and in women the menstrual cycle. In Hejl's studies, only acute cases with marked fever above 37°C were considered. Routine diagnostic criteria were applied to determine the type of infection, i.e., bacterial or viral. Information on the clock hour and calendar date when the fever signaled the commencement of the infection was provided by the patient. Data for studying the distribution of infectious disease over the menstrual cycle were derived from non-oral contraceptive users who kept menstrual-cycle calendars. Overall, the gathered data represented information from 2044 persons, 1498 men and 546 women, between 14 and 74 years of age residing in a small Czechoslovakian town.

Figure 34 presents the temporal distribu-tion of the commencement of fever due to bacterial or viral infection. The onset of fever resulting from bacterial infection oc-curred predominantly during the morning between 0500 and 1200. On the other hand, the onset of fever resulting from viral infection predominated during the late afternoon and evening between 1500 and 2200.

Circamensual Rhythms

Figure 35 presents the temporal distribution of fevers associated with the onset of bacterial or viral infection during the menstrual cycle for the sample of 546 women. Fevers indicative of bacterial infection were found to be most likely during the second quarter of the menstrual cycle around ovulation; they were less likely during the third quarter of the menstrual cycle. The temporal pattern in the onset of fevers signaling the occurrence of viral infection was more or less the reverse of that for bacterial infection; viral infections were much more common during the premenstrum and menstrum with a secondary peak around ovulation.

Overall, the graphs depicting the onset of infectious disease during 24 hr and the menstrual cycle reveal rather high-amplitude circadian and circamensual rhythms in viral disorders. In comparison, the rhythms in the onset of bacterial infection over the same time scales are of relatively low amplitude. Just as it is for other chronopathologies, it is difficult to explain Hejl's findings. It might be suspected for a significant number of those comprising the sample that the time spent at work by adults or at school by children interfered with the vigilance of determining exactly when symptoms began as well as the ability to monitor body temperature. With regard to the 24-hr rhythms, it is likely that a greater frequency of infectious symptoms might be detected in the morning before school and work or in the evening when one is most likely to be at home and when daily commitments would be less likely to detract from one's vigi-

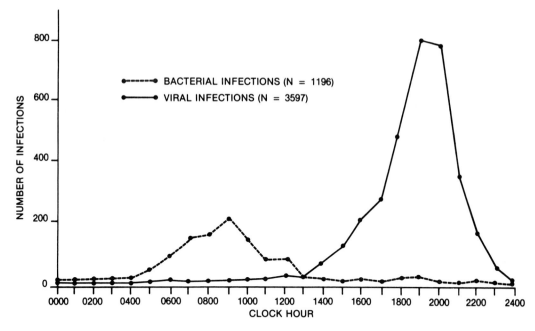

Fig. 34. The onset of bacterial and viral infection signaled by fever exhibits different temporal patterns. Fevers due to bacterial infection are more common during the morning, whereas those from viral infection are more common during the evening in presumably day-active individuals. Reproduced from Hejl 1977.

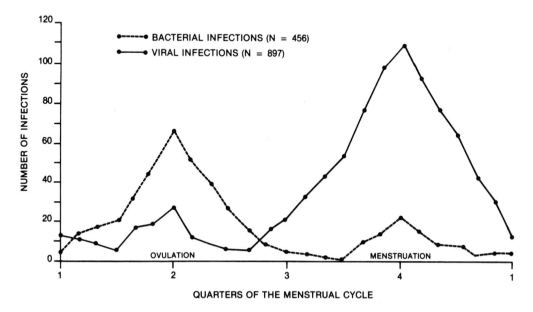

Fig. 35. In women, bacterial infection signaled by fever is more likely around ovulation, whereas viral infection signaled by fever is more likely around menstruation. Reproduced from Hejl 1977.

lance. As a matter of fact, fevers signaling the onset of bacterial or viral infection were most often noted during the morning and evening hours. Since Hejl's publication represents the first report of such circadian and circamensual variations in human beings, these interesting findings must await confirmation.

Circannual Rhythms

Circannual rhythms in the occurrence of infectious diseases in human beings have been well described since being discussed (as seasonal differences) by Hippocrates in his aphorisms approximately 400 years before the birth of Christ. An earlier review (Smolensky et al. 1972) found the morbidity and mortality from infectious diseases was greatest during the winter and least during the summer in both the Northern and Southern Hemispheres (Figs. 2 and 28). Circannual rhythmicity in the incidence of infectious diseases, mainly upper respiratory infections—cold, flu and pneumonia—is quite prominent and is of high amplitude. As a matter of fact, annual changes in the risk of infectious diseases are conventionally accepted as clinical background for both their diagnosis and prevention.

Circannual changes in the incidence of infections other than upper respiratory ones are frequently observed in populations of school-aged children, for example, in chicken pox, mumps, rubeola, and rubella. Monthly tabulations provided by the Center for Disease Control in the United States, summarized in *Morbidity and Mortality Weekly Reports*, clearly and consistently reveal from one year to the next such patterns. For the most part, each of the aforementioned childhood infectious diseases exhibits high-amplitude circannual patterns with peaks during the spring or summer. Conventional explanations for the circannual patterns of these infectious diseases take into consideration variables other than endogenous 1-year biological rhythms (e.g., Fine and Clarkson 1982). Nonetheless, the latter are known to occur (Figs.

29–31) even for rubella antibody titers (Rosenblatt et al. 1982).

Although infectious diseases like chicken pox, mumps, rubella, and rubeola become epidemic at certain times of the year in children (Figs. 36 and 37), the incidence of these diseases in adults is rather uncommon. A class of infections epidemic especially among young adults is the venereal diseases of syphilis and gonorrhea. Examination of data from Houston, Texas, for the span between January 1970 and May 1979 reveals the occurrence of high-amplitude circannual periodicities with acrophases late in the year (Smolensky et al. 1981a). With regard to gonorrhea, which exhibits a relatively short delay between exposure and symptoms, the peak occurs early in August; the trough occurs in March (Fig. 38). The circannual pattern in primary syphilis is less sinusoidal in form; nonetheless, it is evident that on the average the monthly incidence in Houston, Texas, between August and December is greater than between January and July. The findings of circannual rhythms in sexually transmitted diseases (STD) with a peak in gonorrhea during August and a peak in primary syphilis a few months later are remarkably similar to those described by others (see Figs. 5 and 37) such as Wright and Judson (1978) for Denver, Colorado and the Center for Disease Control for the USA (*Mortality and Mortality Weekly Reports*, 1980/1981), as well as for other locales such as Israel (personal communication, Israel Ashkenasi) and Gabone near the equator (personal communication, Vincent 1981).

The acrophases of the rhythms in STD fit well with the peak of the circannual rhythm in human sexual activity. In particular, based upon the expected increase in sexual activity of males (Reinberg and Lagoguey 1978b) and married couples (Udry and Morris 1967) in late summer or the autumn, it is reasonable to envision increased sexual activity in the general population resulting in elevated numbers of STD during the later part of the year. The overt and painful clinical manifestation of gonorrhea

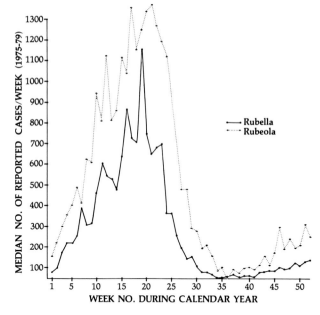

Fig. 36. Seasonal variation in infectious diseases of children and young adults. Although there were occasionally large differences in the week-to-week reports for the United States and its territories for new cases of rubella and rubeola—perhaps indicative of shortcomings of the reporting procedures—the median number of cases over the 5-year span of 1975–1979 for these primarily childhood communicable diseases was tremendously greater during the first than the last 6 months of the year. Remarkably few cases of rubella and rubeola were reported after week 30. Data from *Mortality and Morbidity Weekly Reports* 1980/1981.

would tend to induce more immediate medical consultation and diagnosis. Thus, the acrophase of this circannual rhythm is likely to coincide in time with the reported circannual acrophase of sexual activity. On the other hand, primary syphilis, requiring 3–4 weeks for the development of symptoms, in addition to the fact that they are less obvious than those of gonorrhea, is likely to be later detected. Thus, it is not

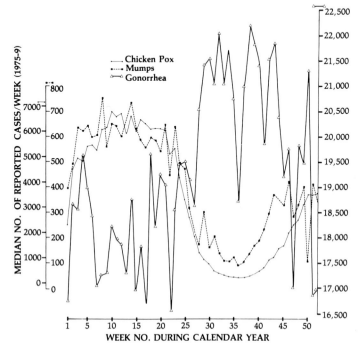

Fig. 37. Seasonal variation in infectious diseases of children and young adults (also see the legend to Fig. 36). For chicken pox and mumps relatively few cases were reported between weeks 30 and 42. The circannual pattern for gonorrhea, primarily although not solely a disease of young adults, was completely out of phase with that of the communicable childhood diseases of rubella, rubeola, chicken pox and mumps. Increased numbers of cases of gonorrhea were reported between weeks 28 and 45 with the greatest numbers during week 38. Data from *Mortality and Morbidity Weekly Reports* 1980/1981.

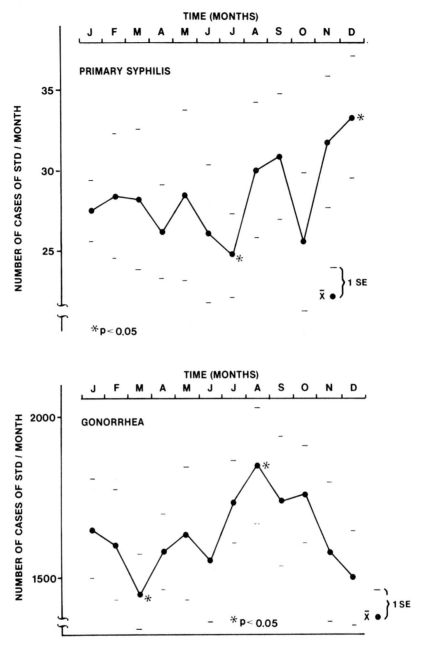

Fig. 38.   Monthly occurrence in Houston, Texas, of primary syphilis and gonorrhea over the span January 1970–May 1979. The plot of primary syphilis, perhaps because of a relatively low number of cases, is nonsinusoidal and exhibits a series of peaks and troughs. The major peak in December is significantly different from the trough in July. For gonorrhea the plot is more sinusoidal; the peak in August is significantly different from the trough in March. Reproduced from Smolensky et al. 1981a.

unexpected that the peak in the occurrence of primary syphilis occurs several months after the reported circannual peak in sexual activity.

With regard to STD, until otherwise disproved, it is necessary to acknowledge the possibility these circannual rhythms might represent seasonal differences in (1) immunosurveillance and/or (2) pathogen virulence. Circannual rhythms in serum IgA as well as seasonal changes in serum IgG have been reported previously (Bratescu and Teodorescu 1981; Lu et al. 1980a; Reinberg et al. 1977). Yet the magnitude of change in these was quite small. Apparently, there are as yet no studies of circannual rhythms in the immune status of the human genitourinary tract. Similarly, with regard to human infectious disorders, no research has been conducted specifically to evaluate the possible existence of circannual rhythms in pathogen virulence. Although circannual rhythms in human upper respiratory morbidity and mortality have been repeatedly documented (Smolensky et al. 1972) with peaks in the winter or spring, it is unclear what factors constitute the etiologic phenomena for the increased incidence at these times and what these circannual rhythms represent, i.e., chronosusceptibilities resulting from temporal variation in pathogen virulence, transmission, immunity, and so on. The seasonality of the venereal diseases of primary syphilis and gonorrhea seems to depend at least in part on the seasonality of human sexual activity. However, it may depend on other circannual variations as well, including the possibility of changes in immune surveillance during the year. For example, analyses of blood samples (Reinberg et al. 1977) gathered every other month (on a circadian basis) from healthy young Parisians (6 men and 3 women) revealed circannual rhythms in blood leukocytes (annual ϕ, December; 95% CL from October to January), IgA (ϕ, November; 95% CL from September to January), IgM (ϕ, September; 95% CL from August to September), and IgG (ϕ, July; 95% CL from early July to late August). Findings comparable to these were detected by Lu et al. (1980a) in studies done in Houston, Texas.

Circadian Temperature Rhythms and Breast Cancer

The circadian temperature rhythm of a cancerous breast in comparison with that of the contralateral healthy breast becomes altered (Gautherie and Gros 1977; Halberg et al. 1977, 1979; Mansfield et al. 1970, 1973; Simpson 1977; Smolensky 1973) as shown in Fig. 39. Spectral analysis of continuous recordings of either surface or deep breast temperature has shown that noncancerous breasts exhibit rhythms with predominant periods (τ) of 24 hr and 7 days. A tumorous breast, on the other hand, often exhibits non–24-hr rhythms, i.e., predominant periodicities of approximately 20, 40, and 80 hrs. In other words, the temperature pattern of the cancerous breast undergoes a transformation from a circadian to an (about 20-hr) ultradian organization with other prominent τs at integer multiples of the 20-hr one. A corresponding switch from circadian to ultradian rhythmicity in the mitotic rhythm of cells of cancerous breasts also has been reported (data from Voutilainen 1953 and Tähti 1956 reanalyzed by Halberg and Reinberg 1967).

Changes in the surface temperature rhythm of cancerous breasts appear to have application in clinical oncology as a diagnostic tool. Continuous monitoring of the breast surface temperature is currently being evaluated as a means of detecting breast cancer and of rapidly evaluating the efficacy of its treatment. For these purposes, Simpson (1977) has developed a "thermobra" which allows the automatic and continuous recording of breast surface temperature.

Glaucoma

Circadian Rhythms

Circadian rhythms in the intraocular pressure of normal and glaucomatous eyes have been reported by many authors (Boyd and

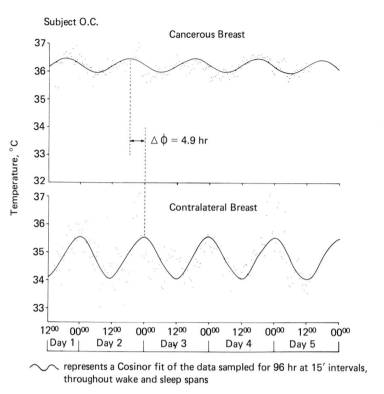

Subject O.C.

Cancerous Breast

Contralateral Breast

$\triangle \phi = 4.9$ hr

Temperature, °C

12⁰⁰ 00⁰⁰ 12⁰⁰ 00⁰⁰ 12⁰⁰ 00⁰⁰ 12⁰⁰ 00⁰⁰ 12⁰⁰ 00⁰⁰
| Day 1 | Day 2 | Day 3 | Day 4 | Day 5 |

∿ represents a Cosinor fit of the data sampled for 96 hr at 15′ intervals, throughout wake and sleep spans

Fig. 39. Two prominent rhythmometric characteristics differentiate the thermoregulatory aspects of the cancerous (CaBr) and the contralateral healthy breast in this diurnally active postmenopausal patient. First, the temporal temperature pattern of the CaBr exhibits a difference in period (τ) from that of the healthy breast, with the CaBr having a $\tau < 24.0$ hr and the healthy one having a $\tau \cong 24.0$ hr. It is because of this difference in τ that a $\Delta\phi$ of 4.9 hr is demonstrable by Cosinor by day 2 of the temperature monitoring. Second, the mesor (the rhythm-adjusted 24-hr mean determined by the Cosinor method) of the CaBr is considerably greater, ~1.5°C, than that of the healthy contralateral breast. Although this example represents only 1 patient, other reports support the existence of these rhythmometric alterations ($\Delta\phi$ and ΔM) in cancerous breasts. Reproduced from Phillips, MJ, et al. Characterization of breast skin temperature rhythms of women in relation to menstrual status. Acta Endocrinologica 96:350–360, 1981.

McLeod 1964; Boyd et al. 1962; Duke-Elder 1952; Henkind and Walsh 1981; Rowland et al. 1981; Ferrario et al. 1982; Katavisto 1965; Langley and Swanljung 1951; Newell and Krill 1965). In non-glaucomatous eyes the intraocular pressure represents a balanced inflow and outflow of aqueous humor. Aqueous inflow resulting from secretions of the ciliary body passes between the lens and iris through the pupil into the anterior chamber of the eye where it is subsequently removed through a trabecular network in the angle and finally into the canal of Schlemm. Exit canals carry the aqueous humor into the episcleral venules posterior to the corneal margin. The control of the inflow and outflow of the aqueous humor is subject to variations including rhythmic ones. Random as well as predictable circadian variations are detectable. In normal eyes of diurnally active persons, the circadian rhythm of intraocular pressure tends to be of low amplitude (bottom portion of Fig. 40) with the pressure being least during the night and greatest during the morning between 0800 and 1200.

Glaucoma is an ocular disease in which tissue damage results from elevated intraocular pressure; the condition can be either acute or chronic. The symptoms commonly include eye pain, impaired and occasionally blurred vision (primarily in the acute form),

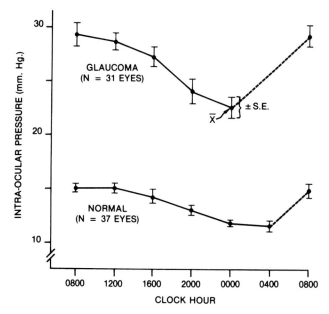

Fig. 40. The circadian rhythm of intraocular pressure exhibited by presumably diurnally active healthy persons is of low amplitude and mesor. The circadian rhythm of intraocular pressure exhibited by diurnally active patients with glaucoma in comparison has an elevated mesor and high amplitude. There is no acrophase difference between the 2 groups. Data from Boyd and McLeod 1964.

colored rainbows, and headache. The circadian variation of intraocular pressure in 31 glaucomatous eyes illustrated in the upper portion of Fig. 40 reveals that the 24-hr mean and amplitude are considerably greater than those of healthy eyes. The increase in intraocular pressure in persons with glaucoma, according to Boyd and McLeod (1964), results from the decreased facility of outflow for intraocular fluid. It can result also from the hypersecretion of aqueous humor. Although the majority of investigators have found the circadian patterns of intraocular pressure to be similarly phased among patients, Katavisto (1965) and Ferrario et al. (1982) have reported differences between patients for the timing during the 24-hr period of highest intraocular pressures.

Circamensual Rhythms

Dalton (1964, 1967, 1973, 1976, 1977) investigated the influence of menstruation on many disorders including glaucoma. Figure 41 presents her findings for the distribution of ocular symptoms in women with diagnosed closed-angle and simple chronic glaucoma. An analysis of 356 episodes of

ocular symptoms over 106 menstrual cycles revealed 49% to have occurred during an 8-day interval—4 days before and 4 days after the commencement of menses. The circamensual variation in symptoms was much more apparent in those cases with closed-angle glaucoma (representing acute episodes of elevated intraocular pressure) than in those with simple chronic glaucoma (in whom elevated intraocular pressure was a chronic condition). However, in both types of glaucoma the occurrence of the peak in ocular symptoms was always during the same 8-day span. According to Dalton (1967, 1977), circamensual changes in the quantity and quality of reproductive hormones, especially progesterone, constitute an important component of the temporal etiology of increased ocular symptoms around menses in predisposed women.

Chronopathology and Pain

A common symptom of many human diseases is pain. In earlier writings the mention of exacerbation of pain during the night is common. However, the scientific and standardized investigation of temporal (diurnal and nocturnal) variation in the

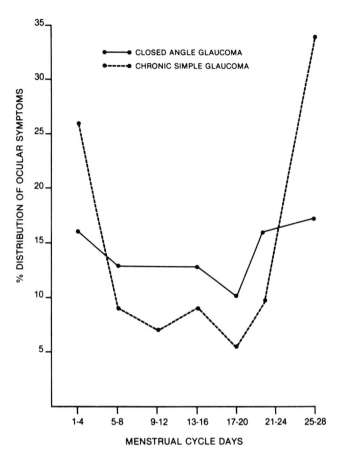

Fig. 41. The symptoms of closed angle and chronic simple glaucoma vary over the menstrual cycle in regularly menstruating women with the peak during menses. Although the pattern for the former is of relatively low amplitude, that for chronic simple glaucoma is of high amplitude. Data from Dalton 1967.

sensory threshold to painful stimuli apparently was not initiated until the early part of this century, commencing apparently with the investigations of Grabfield and Martin (1913) and Martin et al. (1914). Thereafter, both circadian (Jores and Frees 1937; Kleitman and Ramsaroop 1946; Pöllmann and Harris 1978; Pöllmann and Hildebrandt 1979; Proccacci et al. 1972, 1974; Rogers and Vilkin 1978; Strempel 1977) as well as circamensual (Arcangeli et al. 1960; Buzzelli et al. 1968; Proccacci et al. 1972) rhythms in the threshold to pain have been reported in healthy subjects. Of particular interest are circadian and circamensual rhythms in the occurrence of pain, e.g., in patients who suffer from recurring headaches, intractable pain, toothache, and arthritis. In general, diurnally active healthy individuals exhibit a lowered threshold to pain-inducing (heat, cold, or faradic) stimuli during the hours typically associated with nocturnal sleep and an elevated threshold during the afternoon. In the subsequent sections examples of ultradian, circadian, and circamensual patterns in pain are presented.

Circadian Rhythms in Pain and Duodenal Ulcer

The occurrence as well as the timing of pain during the day or night was used around the turn of this century to make the differential diagnosis of duodenal ulcer. According to the prominent surgeon Moynihan (1910a,b), patients complained during the early history of their disease that duodenal pain "comes usually two hours or little more after food has been taken." Immediately after a meal there is relief from pain;

however, within 2–6 hr the pain returns. According to Moynihan, if the pain begins earlier than 2 hrs after mealtime, 2 conditions are possible: "either an active ulcer has contracted recent adhesions to the abdominal wall or the liver; or stenosis is beginning to develop" (Moynihan, 1910a). Since many of Moynihan's patients indicated their pain commenced when feeling hungry, Moynihan suggested the term "hunger pain" to describe this symptom. Again, according to Moynihan (1910a): "The pain, as a rule, is noticed, at first, only or chiefly after the heaviest meal of the day; if a large meal is taken between 1 P.M. and 2 P.M., the pain will come with unvarying regularity at, or near, 4 P.M. For a long period this may be the only time of day when discomfort is felt. . . . With progression of the disease, the pain becomes more frequent, occurring usually about two hours following each meal." In addition, according to Moynihan (1910a,b), "It is a characteristic feature of pain that it wakes the patient in the night and constantly the time of waking is said to be 2 o'clock."

Between 1909 and 1910 a marked controversy existed among surgeons and clinicians regarding the exact timing of the pain from duodenal ulcer, both with regard to mealtimes and its occurrence during the night (Hutchison and Moynihan 1909; Moynihan and Childe 1909; Saundby et al. 1909). This controversy, which was puncuated by scandalous statements and allegations of medical incompetence, arose in part from misconceptions about the rhythmic events of peristalsis and pain threshold and an incomplete understanding about the temporal-spatial processes of gastric emptying during and following food consumption. Although modern diagnostic techniques and instrumentation confirm the differential diagnosis of duodenal ulcer, thus making the "timing" of duodenal pain less important for determining diagnosis than was the case earlier in the century, it is only within the last decade or so that the significance of circadian changes in the duodenum have been related to ulcerogenesis.

Investigations by Moore and Englert (1970), Feurle et al. (1972), Pounder et al. (1977), Tonnesen (1974), and Puscas et al. (1979) established the existence of circadian rhythmicity in gastric acidity. Even before this the data of Illingworth et al. (1944a,b) inferred the existence of circannual, circaseptan, and circadian (Fig. 42) differences in the perforation of peptic ulcers in patients. Moreover, Dubrasquet et al. (1971) and later Carandente et al. (1978) used experimental rodent models for investigating circadian aspects of ulcerogenesis.

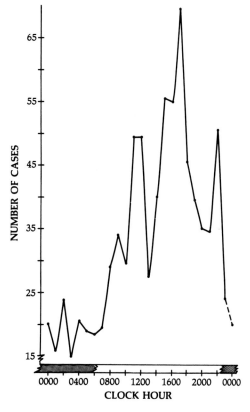

Fig. 42. Circadian rhythm in the occurrence of perforated peptic ulcer in 884 presumably diurnally active patients consuming breakfast at ~0700–0730, lunch at ~1200, and supper at ~1730–1800. The frequency of 951 perforations (cases) was greatest during the afternoon around 1700 and least during the usual hours of sleep. The shading along the horizontal axis indicates the presumed sleep schedule of the patients. Data from Illingworth et al. 1944b.

With respect to human beings, Tarquini (1978) and Tarquini et al. (1977) reported differences in the circadian rhythms of gastric acid secretion, mitosis of the duodenal cells, and the thickness of the duodenal mucosa between patients having duodenal ulcer and healthy controls. Although circadian rhythmicity of gastric acid concentration was detected by Tarquini in both groups, the timing of the acrophase in patients was less exact resulting, when considered as a group phenomenon, in a longer duration of elevated acid production over the 24 hr. An additional difference between the 2 groups was the substantiation of circadian rhythmicity of gastric hormone secretion in controls but not in patients with duodenal ulcer. According to Tarquini (1978), there are major differences between patients and healthy controls with regard to the temporal integration of duodenal rhythms. In patients there is a prolonged duration of time between the circadian span of heightened gastric acid secretion and the circadian span of increased duodenal mucosal thickness, and there is an absence of a circadian periodicity of gastric hormone secretion. In healthy controls the duration of elevated gastric acid secretion over the 24-hr period is shorter than it is in patients. Moreover, the circadian peak of this rhythm follows that of the circadian rhythms of serum gastrin and duodenal mucosal thickness by at least several hours. Thus, in healthy controls the circadian peak of gastric acid secretion is phase delayed by only a short duration from the circadian peak of the rhythm in mucosal thickness, so the maximum secretion of gastric acid occurs at a time when the duodenum is best protected by a thickened mucosal lining (Tarquini 1978). In patients, maximum acid production takes place in an environment of temporally reduced mucosal thickness. Other chronobiologic differences have been noted between the 24-hr patterns of prostaglandin E (PGE) production of healthy persons and patients with duodenal ulcer. In healthy controls there is a phase difference of about 8 hrs between the crest of the temporal pattern in gastric acidity and PGE. In patients there is a disruption of the PGE secretory pattern and also a disruption of its phase relationship to the cycle of gastric acid secretion (Tonnesen et al. 1974). Although some interesting and important chronobiologic differences have been described, circadian changes in this clinical disorder are presumably related to a large set of component rhythms and oscillator systems, rather than only the few thus far objectively identified.

Circadian, Circaseptan, and Circamensual Rhythms and Headache

Although head pain is a commonly experienced symptom in those who suffer migraine, cluster, and muscle headache, biological rhythms in their occurrence have not been well studied (Dexter and Weitzman 1970; Kunkle et al. 1972; Kunkle 1964; Osterman et al. 1980, 1981; Ostfeld 1963; Waters and O'Connor 1971). In one investigation (Waters and O'Connor 1971), 117 women recorded in diaries the onset of every migraine and muscle headache for up to 6 consecutive months. In the study by Ostfeld (1963), 114 patients seeking treatment over a 4-year span were surveyed by recall. The findings of Ostfeld and Waters and O'Connor are given in Fig. 43. Wolff in 1963, apparently using clinical impressions, reported migraine and to a lesser degree muscle headaches begin during the night, sometimes awakening the patient from sleep. The data from Ostfeld (1963) confirm this clinical impression for migraine. However, the data from Waters and O'Connor (1971) indicate a slightly different circadian pattern for migraine as well as muscle headaches, since they found them more common between awakening in the morning until noontime. These latter findings are in agreement with those of Osterman et al. (1980) who found that (migraine and nonmigraine) headaches were more common between 1000 and 1800 than between either

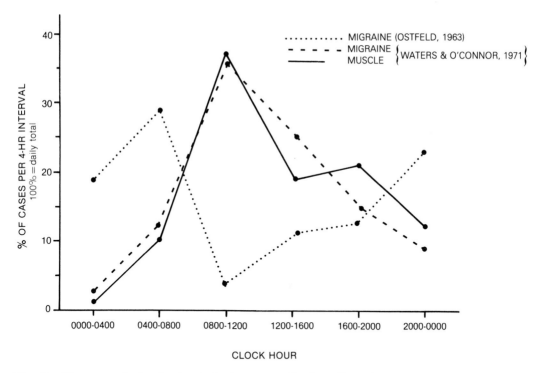

Fig. 43. The onset of migraine headache in presumably diurnally active persons appears to be most likely between 0400 and 1200; the commencement of muscle (contraction) headache appears to be more likely after awakening from sleep. Data from Ostfeld 1963 and Waters and O'Connor 1971.

1800 and 0200 or 0200 and 1000. Differences between the findings of the various studies with regard to the time-dependent occurrence of migraine headache are difficult to explain. Presumably they represent differences between the experimental methodologies and/or characteristics of the patients sampled. It is possible also that the difference results from the timing of medications or disparities in the sleep-wakefulness patterns of the patients investigated. Since information on these was not provided, it is difficult to interpret the differences in findings.

Temporal (24-hr) patterns in the onset of cluster headaches have been noted by several investigators (Harris 1926; Harris 1936; Ekbom 1947, 1970; Symonds 1956; Kunkle et al. 1972). In the study by Symonds (1956) more than 65% of the patients suffering from cluster headache exhibited a nocturnal commencement of each bout. Ekbom (1970), studying a large sample of patients,

obtained identical results; more than 60% of the bouts of cluster headache started between 2300 and 0600 with many patients describing their attacks commencing with remarkable precision 1–2 hr after the onset of sleep, around 0100 to 0200.

Two groups of investigators, Waters and O'Connor (1971) and Osterman et al. (1980), studied 7-day patterns in the occurrence of headaches. Waters and O'Connor (1971), in their survey of 2933 women, found the frequency of migraine most common over the weekend (Saturday and Sunday). The fewest number of headaches were experienced on Mondays. Nonmigraine headaches did not exhibit a cyclic 7-day pattern, although there was an unequal distribution during the week with Mondays being most headache free. Osterman et al. (1980) found a statistically significant difference between the daily incidence of migraine headaches with the highest frequency on Thursdays and Fridays and the lowest frequency on Mondays. Although the original consideration of Osterman et al. (1980) was the association of changes in weather with temporal patterns of headaches, the authors found no causal relationship between their reported 7-day variation in headaches and the ambient conditions. Perhaps the circaseptan (about 7-day) variation in the incidence of headache represents emotional pressures associated with work and family activities over the week. Although circaseptan rhythms in biological functions are known, they tend to be of relatively low amplitude. Nonetheless, the possibility of an endogenous rhythmic component in the occurrence of headaches over 7 days cannot be dismissed.

Circamensual rhythmicity in migraine headache is rather well recognized both in the clinic as well as in the literature (Green 1967; Dalton 1973, 1976; Kashiwagi et al. 1972; Dalessio 1973; Pöllmann and Harris 1978). Figure 44 presents the data from Dalton (1973), 512 headaches experienced by 52 regularly menstruating women not taking oral contraceptives. Of the total, 36% of the headaches were experienced

during the 4-day span before menses, while an additional 30% were experienced during menses. The prominent circamensual rhythmicity in migraine was detectable also in oral contraceptive users. In a group of oral contraceptive users and exusers, the incidence of migraine during the premenstrum and menses was more than twice that expected had its occurrence been randomly distributed over the menstrual cycle (Dalton 1973, 1976, 1977).

Circadian Rhythms and Toothache

Pöllmann and Harris (1978) studied the onset of continuous pain caused by dental caries in 543 patients primarily between the ages of 18 and 25 years. It was hypothesized, based on the authors' earlier finding of a circadian rhythm in pain threshold with a minimum between the evening and early morning hours in diurnally active persons, that tooh pain would more likely be perceived as beginning during this span than it would at other times of the day or night. Although some patients experienced toothache after meals (Fig. 45), the majority ex-

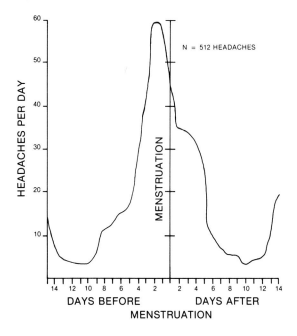

Fig. 44. Data obtained from a group of regularly menstruating women confirm the well-known prominence of migraine headache during or just prior to menses. Reproduced from Dalton 1967.

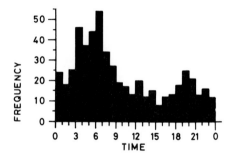

Fig. 45. The commencement of tooth pain (toothache) from dental caries in 543 diurnally active patients occurs not only after meals to some extent, but much more prominently during the early morning hours. Reproduced from Pöllmann and Harris 1978.

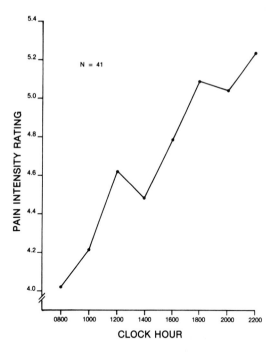

N = 41

Fig. 46. Circadian changes in the intensity of intractable pain in diurnally active patients has not been well studied. In 41 patients volunteering to subjectively self-rate their intractable pain, intensity was found to steadily increase during the day, reaching a peak just prior to bedtime. Reproduced from Folkard 1976.

perienced the painful onset of toothache during the early morning hours between 0300 and 0800. Presumably this rhythm at least in part represents the circadian variation of human pain sensitivity (Pöllmann and Harris 1978; Pöllmann, 1982).

Diurnal Variation in the Intensity of Intractable Pain

Temporal patterns in the level of intractable pain during the day and night have not been often investigated. Folkard (1976) and Glynn et al. (1975) studied 54 patients suffering from intractable pain using self-reports and visual analog scales every 2 hr during the waking span for 7 consecutive days. Complete records obtained from 39 of the patients indicated an increase in the intensity of the pain throughout the day after awakening with the peak around 2200, the latest clock hour that self-ratings were done each day by the patients (Fig. 46). The temporal pattern in the level of intractable pain was not appreciably altered by the use of analgesics; nor was it affected by the patient's activity level, e.g., patients remaining at home and those working outside the home during the day displayed comparable variation over time.

Circadian Rhythm in the Pain of Rheumatoid Arthritis

The symptoms and signs of rheumatoid arthritis vary within and between days (Scott 1960; Delbarre 1979; Kowanko et al. 1981, 1982a,b; Harkness et al. 1981, 1982). Although the major symptoms of this common disease are pain, stiffness, and inflammation, systematic investigation of the temporal variation in these have been carried out only on a few occasions (Delbarre 1979; Kowanko et al. 1981, 1982b; Harkness et al. 1981, 1982). Circamensual and circannual studies using quantitative endpoints have never been conducted. The data of Kowanko et al. (1981, 1982a) are germaine to the discussion of circadian rhythms in the pain of rheumatoid arthritis.

Figure 47 presents the data of a patient who self-monitored his rheumatoid arthritic symptoms 6 times daily (at approximately 3-hr intervals) during the waking span for 3 consecutive days while being treated with a nonsteroid antiinflammatory medication (100 mg flurbiprofen, Froben) daily at 1300 and 2300. From one day to the next, pain was consistently self-rated higher in the morning after awakening than in the afternoon and evening. In phase with this circadian pattern in subjectively rated pain was circadian variation in joint stiffness as well as inflammation, the latter monitored by the cumulative sum of the circumference of 10 finger joints. These rhythms differed in phase by approximately 12 hr from the circadian changes of left- and right-hand grip strength; highest grip strength was demonstrable when the subjective ratings of stiffness and pain as well as joint circumference were least.

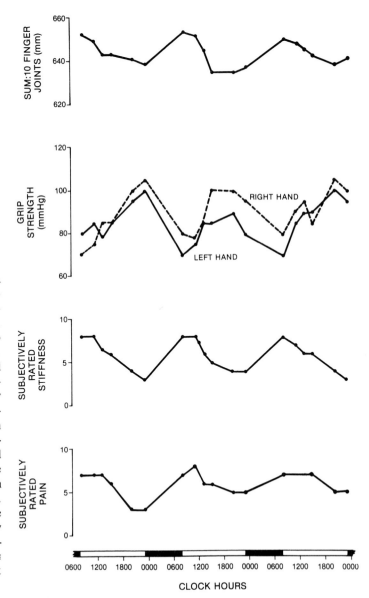

Fig. 47. Data obtained from a diurnally active rheumatoid arthritic patient conducting self-assessments of pain, stiffness, joint circumference, and grip strength several times daily. The patient was being treated with antiinflammatory medication (flurbiprofen) twice daily (1300 and 2300). The data reveal circadian rhythmicity with the temporal patterns of subjectively rated pain, stiffness, and grip strength differing in phase by approximately 12 hr from that of joint circumference. The units for grip strength are expressed in mmHg; they may be transformed into Pascals using the conversion 1 mmHg ≅ 133 P. Data from Kowanko et al. 1981.

Table 4. *Circadian Rhythm in the Symptoms and Signs of Rheumatoid Arthritis.*

Studied Variable (units)	Mesor: M (M ± SE)	Circadian Amplitude: A (95% confidence limits)	Circadian Acrophase: φ (95% confidence limits)	Rhythm detection (P)
Self-rated pain (10-point scale)	5.6 ± 0.2	1.6 (1.1 to 2.2)	1020 (0824 to 1212)	<.001
Self-rated stiffness (10-point scale)	5.7 ± 0.2	2.2 (1.7 to 2.7)	0900 (0752 to 1012)	<.001
Sum: 10 finger joints (mm)	644.3 ± 0.7	7.9 (5.3 to 10.6)	0716 (0604 to 0848)	<.001
Grip strength right hand (mmHg)	90.4 ± 1.5	11.5 (6.7 to 16.7)	2032 (1840 to 2256)	<.001
Grip strength left hand (mmHg)	85.0 ± 1.6	9.8 (41. to 16.2)	1932 (1724 to 2244)	<.001

Note: One patient medicated daily at 1300 and 2300 with flurbiprofen.

Data collected six times daily during waking for three consecutive days analyzed by single cosinor.

Findings kindly provided by Dr. Roy Pownall (Chronotherapeutics Research Group, City Hospital, Hucknall Road, Nottingham NG5 1PD, England) as a personal communication.

Table 4 presents the Cosinor analyses of the data from this patient. Circadian rhythms were substantiated (P < 0.001) for each symptom and measurement with the acrophases for joint circumference, stiffness, and pain occurring more or less in phase between 0700 and 1030. The acrophase of the rhythm in grip strength of the left and right hands was approximately 12 hr out of phase with those of the other circadian rhythms. Table 5 presents the data of another investigation (Kowanko et al. 1981) in which 15 patients were studied while taking flurbiprofen at 1300 and 2300 daily for 14 days. Circadian variations in joint circumference (inflammation) were, as expected, greatest in the morning around 0700. The circadian variation in grip strength of both hands was, as was the case for the subject presented in Fig. 47 and Table 4, about 12 hr out of phase with the other studied rhythms.

It should be pointed out that in these particular studies the patients were investigated while receiving antiinflammatory medication twice daily, once in the early afternoon (1300) and again in the evening (2300). It is apparent from both Tables 4 and 5 and Fig. 47 that the amplitude of the investigated circadian rhythms is not large. The antiinflammatory medication most likely affected the studied symptoms thereby creating the possibility that the observed circadian changes in joint size, grip

Table 5. *Circadian Rhythm in Grip Strength and Joint Circumference.*

Studied variable (units)	Mesor: M	Circadian Amplitude: A (95% confidence limits)	Circadian Acrophase: φ (95% confidence limits)	Rhythm detection (P)
Sum: 10 finger joints (mm)	593	4.1 (1.3 to 6.9)	0654 (0407 to 0724)	<.05
Grip strength right hand (mmHg)	130	5.5 (2.4 to 8.8)	1635 (1359 to 1905)	<.05
Grip strength left hand (mmHg)	131	6.3 (2.0 to 10.7)	1719 (1547 to 1915)	<.05

Note: N = 15 except for variable of joint circumference where N = 14; patients taking flurbiprofen daily at 1300 and 2300.

Data from Kowanko et al. 1981.

strength, joint stiffness, and pain were moderated. With regard to the measurement of joint circumference, not all the joints measured were arthritic; thus, the amplitude values must be considered as conservative estimates of the circadian variability, since the nonaffected joints probably exhibited only slight changes over 24 hr. Since appropriate investigations with as well as without medications have yet to be published, much remains to be learned about circadian and other periodic aspects of rheumatoid arthritic disorders. This discussion of rhythms in arthritis is not offered with the intention of documenting the obvious, i.e., circadian variations in joint size, stiffness, and pain in arthritic patients; rather, it is made to stimulate the accumulation of baselines before intervention trials with various medications aimed at moderating symptoms and manifestations of this painful and sometimes crippling disease. Although rheumatoid arthritis is a relatively common disorder, information on the magnitude of circadian variation in relevant end points from a large sample of patients is lacking.

Circadian Rhythm in the Pain of Osteoarthritis of the Hip and Knee

Pain and stiffness were self-rated by patients suffering from stable osteoarthritis of the hip or knee (stages II and III) in an investigation by Job et al. (1981). Diurnally active patients were studied both while taking placebo and indomethacin (50 mg/24 hr) during a 4-week span to evaluate the chronotherapeutic effects of this nonsteroid antiinflammatory agent taken once daily either at 0800, 1200, or 2000. A statistically significant circadian rhythm with afternoon acrophases characterized the data of both pain and stiffness regardless of whether the patients were given placebo or indomethacin. A statistically significant decrease in symptoms was achieved when indomethacin was given at 1200. Similar results have been obtained by Lévi et al. (1982, unpublished data) with a rather large

number of patients (over 400) in a chronobiologic investigation.

The greatest level of pain due to osteoarthritis in diurnally active patients occurs 12 hrs later than that due to rheumatoid arthritis. This difference can be tentatively explained by the fact that in osteoarthritis one deals with mechanically induced pain resulting from friction within the altered joints. Physically induced pain—using heat, cold, or faradic stimuli as reported by Pöllmann (1982), Pöllmann and Harris (1978), Pöllmann and Hildebrandt (1979), and Proccacci et al. (1974)—exhibits a nocturnal acrophase. In patients with rheumatoid arthritis, inflammatory phenomena predominate in the morning. The morning stiffness and associated pain in rheumatoid arthritis not only result from decreased movement during nocturnal sleep but from the decreased level of corticosteroids circulating in the blood and in the tissue during the night.

A finding of particular relevance is that the timing of the circadian acrophase of pain and stiffness may vary between patients suffering from osteoarthritis of the knee or hip (Lévi et al., unpublished data); this was the finding of a study on 68 patients using a visual analog scale for the self-rating of symptoms. If it is true in a majority of patients given placebo that pain and stiffness predominate in the afternoon while for others symptoms predominate in the morning, this must be taken into account from a chronotherapeutic point of view. Using a sustained-release form of indomethacin (Chronoindocid), Lévi et al. (personal communication) demonstrated that the circadian acrophase of both pain and stiffness must be monitored in each *individual* in order to determine the circadian timing of the worsening of symptoms and to thus determine the optimum administration time for this antiinflammatory medication. The timing of the medication must be done on an *individual* basis since, although for a majority of patients tolerance and best effect are achieved by an evening administration, for some a morning administration is best. Using an individualized chronotherapy, Lévi et al. found it possible to increase by 50% the efficiency of and by 94% the tolerance (with regard to side effects) to indomethacin. This example shows that a chronopathology can be individualized; this must be considered in optimizing therapy.

From a physiopathological point of view it is interesting to consider that the peak time of pain, whether induced experimentally or occurring spontaneously (Pöllmann 1982), usually coincides with the trough of the circadian rhythm of a natural endogenous analgesic chemical substance in the plasma–β-endorphin (Dent et al. 1981; Wesche and Frederickson 1981). It could well be that the circadian rhythm in the secretion of this chemical (among others yet to be found) contributes to the observed circadian changes of pain threshold. Other components could involve circadian changes in brain function, as suggested by Pöllmann (1982) in studies involving the circadian rhythmicity of the pain-reducing effect of a placebo. With regard to control measurements, placebo given at noon lowered pain by 40 ± 5%, whereas when given at midnight it lowered pain only by 10 ± 3%.

Chronobiology and Progressive Dystonia

Siehr (1899), Bury (1902), and Hunt (1917) described case studies of progressive dystonia in young children exhibiting diurnal fluctuations in symptoms. Since those early reports, Nasu et al. (1958), Schenck and Kruschke (1975), Hardvogl and Stögmann (1976), Segawa et al. (1976), Yamamura et al. (1973), and Ouvrier (1978) have noted the dystonic syndrome characterized by marked diurnal fluctuations in symptoms. Various authors have categorized this apparently hereditary childhood disease differently terming it paralysis agitans of early onset (Yamamura et al. 1973; Bury 1902; Siehr 1899), juvenile paralysis agitans (Nasu 1958), progressive atrophy of the globus pallidus (Hunt 1917), or progressive

dystonia with marked diurnal fluctuations (Hardvogl and Stögmann 1976; Segawa 1976; Ouvrier 1978). In general, the term dystonia refers to an abnormal degree of fixity caused by sustained muscular contraction. In the clinical context, the term includes abnormalities of movement superimposed on an often unusual posture resulting from simultaneous excessive contraction of agonist and antagonist muscle groups. The symptoms of patients described by each of the aforementioned authors are similar; they appear insidiously in childhood with the patients initially displaying dystonic postures and unusual movement of one limb, usually the leg. The symptoms progress so that usually within 5 years the ipsilateral arm and the other leg and arm become affected. In most cases the legs are more affected than the arms. According to Segawa (1976) and Ouvrier (1978), the characteristic feature of this disorder is the "remarkable diurnal fluctuation" in symptoms. They tend to be mild or even absent early in the morning, after arising from nightly sleep, or sometimes after a daytime nap, but are always more aggravated toward the evening.

Conclusion

Chronopathologies most likely result from cyclic variations in the ambient environment and from periodicities in certain critical biological functions (Reinberg 1982; Reinberg and Lagoguey 1978). With regard to the latter, bioperiodicities are detectable at all levels of organization from the eukaryote to man. This ubiquitous characteristic is considered by many biologists as a significant aspect of the adaptability of species and of the adaptive plasticity and capacity of individuals (Sargent 1967). During evolution, organisms developed within an ambient environment which changed drastically and predictably over time in a rhythmic manner with periods related to the rotation of the earth around its axis—every approximately 24 hr—and around the sun—every approximately 365.25 days. There were other periodic influences, such as lunar ones as well. It is likely that endogenous, genetically transmitted rhythms exhibiting these and other periods have been maintained throughout generations of plants and animals because they confer a selective advantage. (Bioperiodic phenomena which are genetic in origin are not only restricted to 24 hr, 28 days, or 365.25 days; ones of approximately 90 min, 3 hr, and 7 days among others have been detected which do not correspond to any known cosmic periodicities.)

From a theoretical point of view it is more economical for an organism to be genetically programed to anticipate cyclic demands based upon predictably occurring synchronizer signals from the ambient environment than it is to rely upon immediate adjustments and responses to one set of environmental conditions which is repeated every day and another set which is repeated every night. In vertebrate species synchronized to environmental light-dark cycles, for example, hormones of the adrenal cortex which exert strong effects on energy metabolism exhibit large-amplitude circadian rhythms with a trough during the middle of sleep and a peak prior to awakening. The activities of hepatic cells are programed for glycogen deposition during rest and glycogen breakdown into glucose commencing prior to the onset of activity (see Chap. 3).

The adaptation of species to cyclic changes in the ambient environment presumably involves the integration of endogenous rhythms of approximately the same periods at all hierarchial levels of biological organization. In particular, it seems that circadian and circannual bioperiodicities and perhaps others have been reinforced as an adaptive strategy in the evolution of species. This explanation for the ubiquity of rhythms in life cannot be demonstrated experimentally; however, it is a working hypothesis of most chronobiologists.

Sargent (1967), a human ecologist, viewed the temporal structure of biological functions as an important attribute of the adaptive capacity of individuals to meet and survive environmental demands and challenges. The organization of biological processes over 24 hr, the year, and so on, consists of self-sustaining oscillators of the same periods which are interconnected with a hierarchy and influenced by a set of synchronizers. This temporal organization in human beings is more readily recognized over the 24-hr span perhaps because of the apparent wide variation in activity over a relatively short interval of time. Except for those employed in shift work, man is active during the day and at rest during the night. The existence of a circannual temporal organization in human beings as opposed to hibernating animals is not as easily recognized or accepted since the seasonal difference in activity does not appear to be so great. Yet since the Stone Age, human beings have maintained a rather high level of activity during the warmer months when hunting, fishing, and agricultural activities were easily accomplished than during the winter months when activity was at its nadir, as is still readily apparent today in agricultural areas of the world. Circannual rhythms in biological functions including those of metabolism (see Chap. 7) conceivably are associated with seasonal differences in human activity levels. However, some may represent biological reactions to seasonal variations in the environment. It could well be that circadian and circannual rhythms in the occurrence and exacerbation of human disease represent in part the contribution of underlying rhythmic changes which became fixed during evolution. Thus, for allergic asthma, an example of a disease that is strongly circadian rhythmic, several component endogenous 24-hr bioperiodicities can be identified which contribute to the nocturnal exacerbation of bronchial reactivity of diurnally active patients. Some of the identified component rhythms, such as those of catecholamines and cortisol, are closely linked to the temporally differing metabolic requirements of activity during the day and rest during the night.

Circannual changes in endocrine function may be associated with the etiology of seasonal differences in human morbidity. For example, there is a striking coincidence between the circannual peak in the incidence of influenza and pneumonia and the phasing of the circannual rhythm of adrenal activity with a peak in the spring. Circannual rhythms in immune status, at least somewhat influenced by the annual cycle of adrenal function, also have been substantiated (Bratescu and Teodorescu 1981; Lu et al. 1980a, 1980b; Reinberg et al. 1971; Shifrine et al. 1980a, 1980b, 1982). The detection of circannual rhythms in these and other functions, perhaps genetically programed and synchronized by seasonal differences in human activity or photoperiod, does not imply the existence of a cause-and-effect relationship; however, such rhythms may contribute to the timing of chronopathologies over the year. The emphasis on endogenous rhythmic factors is not intended without due recognition of the importance of temporal differences in ambient conditions which may favor the occurrence of disease during a particular season.

Circamensual differences in the occurrence or exacerbation of illness in women seemingly result from quantitative and qualitative changes in endocrine function during the menstrual cycle. A majority of investigators noting a heightened likelihood of exacerbation during the premenstrum and menses suggest the importance of the hormone progesterone. However, other endocrine and physiologic rhythms having circamensual periods may be contributory even if the latter are themselves dependent on changes in the level and type of circulating reproductive hormones during the menstrual cycle (Reinberg and Smolensky 1974).

This discussion has dealt largely with the theoretical and hypothetical aspects of human chronopathologies. However, these hypotheses can be tested in the future as were those developed earlier concerning the chronopathology of allergic asthma (McGovern et al. 1977). The physiological rhythmic components of this circadian chronopathology have been investigated

leading to a more complete understanding of its pathogenesis and treatment. In the beginning of this chapter, chronopathology was defined as the (1) rhythmic occurrence or exacerbation of illness in individuals or in groups of persons and/or (2) alteration of one or more biological rhythms resulting either from and/or contributing to disease. The focus of this chapter has been on the first aspect since as yet a large background of information is not available on the second. However, significant chronobiologic strides are being made with regard to the second, for example, concerning delayed-onset sleep (Weitzman 1981; Weitzman et al. 1981, 1982), breast cancer (Smolensky 1973; Simpson 1977; Halberg et al. 1977, 1979; Gautherie and Gros 1977), emotional illness (Goodwin and Wehr 1981; Brown and Graeber 1982) and endocrine disorders (Krieger et al. 1981). The significance of alterations in biological rhythms to human disease brings to mind the thoughts of Ehret et al. (1978): "A creature with all its systems in strong synchrony has somehow learned how to 'put it all together' so that the multiple environmental amenities and the multitude of inner appetites mesh in a satiable circadian harmony. Such fortunate creatures are rewarded by functional proficiency and longevity." Recognition of the chronobiologic features of human diseases opens new avenues to researching their etiology. It also brings into consideration new approaches to treating illness, taking into account not only the chronopathology of disease but also the chronopharmacology of medications (Chap. 7).

References

Abel, H (1931) Seasonal variations in weight of newborn. Z Kinderheilk 52:31–40.

Abels, H (1922) Über die Wichtigkeit der Vitamine für die Entwicklung des menschlichen fötalen und mütterlichen Organismus. Klin Wochenschr 1:1785–1787.

Adams, F (ed. and trans.) (1856) The Extant Works of Aretaeus, the Cappadocian. London: Printed for the Sydenham Society.

Amir, M (1971) *Patterns in Forcible Rape*. Chicago: University of Chicago Press.

Anonymous (1983) Asthma at night. Lancet 1:220–222.

Anonymous (1910) Discussion on duodenal ulcer. Clin J R Soc Med, pp. 378–384.

Antonis, a, Bersohn, I, Plotkin, R, Easty, DL, and Lewis, HE (1965) The influence of seasonal variation, diet, and physical activity on serum lipids in young men in Antarctica. Am J Clin Nutr 16:428–435.

Apgar, V (1953) A proposal for a new method of evaluation of the newborn infant. Curr Res Anesth Analg 32:260–267.

Apgar, V (1966) The newborn (Apgar) scoring system. Pediatr Clin North Am 13(3):645–650.

Apgar, V, Holaday, DA, James, LS, and Weisbrot, IM (1958) Evaluation of the newborn infant—second report. JAMA 168(15):1985–1988.

Arcangeli, P, Furian, R, and Milano, M (1960) La percezione del tatto e del dolore nelle varie fasi del ciclo menstruale. Rass Neurol Veg 14:461–473.

Aschoff, J (1981) Annual rhythms in man. In: Aschoff, J (ed), *Biological Rhythms, Handbook of Behavioral Neurobiology*. New York: Plenum 4:475–487.

Assenmacher, IA, and Farner, DS (1978) *Environmental Endocrinology*. Berlin: Springer-Verlag.

Backstrom, T (1976) Epileptic seizures in women related to plasma estrogen and progesterone during the menstrual cycle. Acta Neurol Scand 54:321–347.

Baier, H, and Rompel-Purckhauer, C (1979) Circadian variation of the effect of physical training. Chronobiologia 6:77.

Balaz, V (1970) Diurnal periodicity of dyspnea in bronchial asthma. Vnitr Lek 16:1007–1016.

Barnes, P, Fitzgerald, G, Brown, M, and Dollery, C (1980) Nocturnal asthma and changes in circulating epinephrine, histamine, and cortisol. N Engl J Med 303:263–267.

Barnes, PJ, Fitzgerald, GA, and Dollery, CT (1982) Circadian variation in adrenergic responses in asthmatic patients. Clin Sci 62:349–354.

Bartter, FC, Delea, C, Baker, W, Halberg, F, and Lee, J-K (1976) Chronobiology in the diagnosis and treatment of mesor-hypertension. Chronobiologia 3:199–213.

Bateman, JRM, and Clark, SW (1979) Sudden death in asthma. Thorax 34:40–44.

Batschelet, E, Hillman, D, Smolensky, MH, and Halberg, F (1973) Angular-linear correlation coefficient for rhythmometry and circannually changing human birth rates at different geographic latitudes. Int J Chronobiol 1:183–202.

Beau, M (1836) Recherches statistics pour servir à l'histoire de l'épilepsie et de l'hystérie. Arch Gen Med 11:328–352.

Benoit, J, and Assenmacher, I (1970) *La photorégulation de la reproduction chez les oiseaux et les mammifères*. Paris CNRS 172:1.

Bivings, L (1934) Racial, geographic, annual and seasonal variations in birth weights. Am J Obstet Gynecol 27:725–728.

Bock, KD, and Kreuzenbeck, W (1966) Spontaneous blood-pressure variations in hypertension. The effect of antihypertensive therapy and correlations with the incidence of complications. In: Gross, F (ed), *Ciba Symposium on Hypertensive Therapy, Principles, and Practices*. New York: Springer-Verlag, pp. 224–241.

Borelli, S, Chlebarov, S, and Flach, E (1966) Atopic neurodermatitis, and the problem of its 24-hour rhythm and its dependence on weather and climate. Munch Med Wochenschr 108:474–480.

Bosse, K, and Ladebeck, HE (1972) Die kutane Histaminreaktion in Korrelation zum Cyclus der Frau. Z Haut Geschlechtskr 47:365–370.

Bouvrain, Y, Coumel, P, and Leclercq, JF (1977) Arrhythmias and chronobiology. Arch Mal Coeur 70:781–787.

Boyd, TAS, and McLeod, LE (1964) Circadian rhythms of plasma corticoid levels, intraocular pressure and aqueous outflow facility in normal and glaucomatous eyes. Ann NY Acad Sci 117:597–613.

Boyd, TAS, McLeod, LE, Hassard, DTR, and Patrick, A (1962) Relation of diurnal variation of plasma corticoid levels and intraocular pressure in glaucoma. Can Med Assoc J 86:772–775.

Bratescu, A, and Teodorescu, M (1981) Circannual variations in the B cell/T cell ratio in normal human peripheral blood. Allergy Clin Immunol 68(4):273–280.

Breart, G, and Rumeau-Rouquette, C (1979) Rhythmes spontanés et rythmes induits dans le déclenchement et le déroulement du travail et de l'accouchement. J Interdiscipl Cycle Res 10:195–205.

Brennan, PJ, Greenberg, G, Miall, WE, and Thompson, SG (1982) Seasonal variation in arterial blood pressure. Br Med J 285:919–922.

Brisse, B, Bender, F, Gradaus, D, Gülker, H, Schwippe, G, Bramann, H, and Kuhs, H (1979) Circadian changes of heart rate and arrhythmias. Chronobiologia 6:81.

Brown, FM, and Graeber, RC (1982) *Rhythmic Aspects of Behavior*. Hillsdale, N.J.: Lawrence Erlbaum Assoc.

Buek, HW (1829) Nachrichten von dem Gesundheitszustand der Stadt Hamburg. In: *Gersons und Julius Magazin der Ausländischen Litterature der Gesammten*. Hamburg: Heilkunde, pp. 347–354.

Bünning, E (1963) *Die Physiologische Uhr*. Berlin: Springer-Verlag.

Burge, PS, Edge, G, Hawkins, R, White, V, and Newman-Taylor, AJ (1981). Occupational asthma in a factory making flux-covered solder containing colophony. Thorax 36:828–834.

Bury, JS (1902) Two cases of paralysis agitans in the same family in which improvement followed the administration of hyoscine. Lancet 1:1097.

Buzzelli, G, Procacci, P, Voegelin, MR, and Bozza, G (1968) Changes in the cutaneous pricking pain threshold during the menstrual cycle. Arch Fisiol 66:97–106.

Campbell, M (1962) Factors in the aetiology of pulmonary stenosis. Br Heart J 24:625–632.

Carandente, F, Halberg, E, and Halberg, F (1978) Circadian periodicity and stomach ulcer. An animal experiment model for the detection of rhythm factors in the genesis of civilization diseases. Fortschr Med 96:983–988.

Chiray, M, Mollard, H, and Duret, M (1940) Asthma and variation of ovarian hormone secretions. Presse Med 48:201–203.

Christ, JE, and Hoff, HE (1975) An analysis of the circadian rhythmicity of atrial and ventricular rates in complete heart block. J Electrocardiol 8:69–72.

Churina, SK, Ganelina, IE, and Vol'Pert, EI (1975) Pattern of the incidence of acute myocardial infarct within a 24-hour period. Kardiologiia 15:115–118.

Clark, TJH, and Hetzel, MR (1977) Diurnal variation of asthma. Br J Dis Chest 71:87–92.

Claude, F, and Allemany Vall, R (1938) Asthma and menstruation. Presse Med 46:755–759.

Cohen, P (1970) Seasonal variation of congenital malformations. J Interdiscipl Cycle Res 3:271–274.

Cohen, P (1971) Seasonal variations of congenital dislocation of the hip. J Interdiscipl Cycle Res 2:417–425.

Colquhoun, WP (1971) *Biological Rhythms and Human Performance*. London: Academic Press.

Colquhoun, WP, Folkard, S, Knauth, P, and Rutenfranz, J (eds) (1975) *Experimental Studies of Shiftwork*. Opladen: Westdeutscher Verlag.

Cormia, FE (1952) Experimental histamine pruritus. I. Influence of physical and psychological factors on threshold reactivity. J Invest Dermatol 19:21–34.

Cowgill, UM (1966a) Historical study of the season of birth in the city of York, England. Nature 209:1067–1070.

Cowgill, UM (1966b) Season of birth in man. Contemporary situation with special reference to Europe and the southern hemisphere. Ecology 47:614–623.

Cowgill, UM (1966c) Season of birth in man: The northern new world. Kroeber Anthr Soc Pa 35:1–9.

Czeizel, E, and Elek, E (1967) Seasonal changes in the frequency of fetal damages and fertility. Gynaecologie 164:89–95.

Dalessio, DJ (1973) Hormonal levels linked to migraine during the menstrual period. Headache 13(1):29–31.

Dalton, KD (1964) *The Premenstrual Syndrome*. Springfield, Ill.: Thomas.

Dalton, K (1967) Influence of menstruation on glaucoma. Br J Ophthalmol 51:692–695.

Dalton, K (1973) Progesterone suppositories and pessaries in the treatment of menstrual migraine. Headache 12:151–159.

Dalton, K (1976) Migraine and oral contraceptives. Headache 15:247–251.

Dalton, KD (1977) *The Premenstrual Syndrome and Progesterone Therapy*. Chicago: Yearbook Medical.

Davies, RJ, Green, M, and Schofield, NM (1976) Recurrent nocturnal asthma after exposure to grain dust. Am Rev Respir Dis 114:1011–1019.

Davis, CTM, and Sargent, AJ (1975) Circadian variation in physiological responses to exercise on a stationary bicycle ergometer. Br J Industr Med 32:110–114.

Dawkins, KD, and Muers, MF (1981) Diurnal variation in airflow obstruction in chronic bronchitis. Thorax 36:618–621.

Deininger, BR, and Rott, HD (1973) Cytogenetic studies on the seasonal variations in the rate

198   Michael H. Smolensky

of spontaneous chromosomal aberrations in
man. Acta Genet Med Gemellol 22:19–26.

Delbarre, F (1979) Chronobiology in the service
of public health. In: Reinberg, A, and
Halberg, F (eds), *Chronopharmacology*. Oxford: Pergamon Press, pp. 15–34.

Dent, RR, Guilleminault, C, Albert, LH,
Posner, BI, Cox, BM, and Goldstein, A (1981)
Diurnal rhythm of plasma immunoreactive
beta-endorphin and its relationship to sleep
stages and plasma rhythms of cortisol and
prolactin. J Clin Endocrinol Metab 52:942–
947.

DeRudder, B (1952) *Der Grundriss einer Meteo-
robiologie des Menschen: Wetter und Jahres-
zeiteneinflüsse*. Berlin: Springer-Verlag.

Descovitch, GC, Montalbetti, N, Kuhl, JFW,
Rimondi, S, Halberg, F and Ceredi, C (1974)
Age and catecholamine rhythms. Chrono-
biologia 1:163–171.

DeVries, K, Goei, JT, Booy-Noord, H, and
Orie, NGM (1962) Changes during 24 hours in
the lung function and histamine hyperreactivity of the bronchial tree in asthmatic and bronchitic patients. Int Arch Allerg Appl Immunol
20:93–101.

Dexter, JD, and Weitzman, ED (1970) The relationship of nocturnal headaches to sleep stage
patterns. Neurology 20:513–518.

Doyle, JT, Kinch, SH, and Brown, DF (1965)
Seasonal variation in serum cholesterol concentration. J Chronic Dis 18:657–664.

Dubrasquet, M, Sergent, D, Lewin, M, and
Bonfils, S (1971) Relationship between circadian rhythms, spontaneous activity, and re-
straint ulcer in the rat. In: Pfeiffer, CJ (ed),
Peptic Ulcer. Copenhagen: Munkgaard, pp.
105–112.

Duke-Elder, S (1952) The phasic variations in
the ocular tension in primary glaucoma. Am J
Ophthalmol 35:1–21.

Edwards, JH (1961) Seasonal incidence of congenital disease in Birmingham. Ann Hum
Genet 25:89–93.

Ehret, CF, Groh, KR, and Meinert, JC (1978)
Circadian dyschronism and chronotypic
ecophilia as factors in aging and longevity. In:
Samis, HV, and Capobianco, S (eds), *Aging
and Biological Rhythms*. New York: Plenum
Press, pp. 185–214.

Ekbom, KA (1947) Ergotamine tartrate orally in
Horton's "histaminic cephalgia" (also called
Harris's "ciliary neuralgia"). Acta Psychiatr
Neurol (Suppl) 46:106–113.

Ekbom, KA (1970) Patterns of cluster headache
with a note on the relations to angina pectoris
and peptic ulcer. Acta Neurol Scand 46:225–
237.

Eltringham, RJ, and Dobson, MB (1979) Cardio-
respiratory arrests—a diurnal variation? Br J
Anaesth 51:72.

Engle, R, Halberg, F, and Gurly, R (1952) The
diurnal rhythm in EEG discharge and in circulating eosinophils in certain types of epilepsy.
Electroencephalogr Clin Neurophysiol 4:115–
116.

Farah, FS, and Shbaklu, Z (1971) Autoimmune
progesterone urticaria. J Allergy Clin Immunol 48:257–261.

Farner, DS, and Wingfield, JC (1978) Environmental endocrinology and the control of annual reproductive cycles in passerine birds.
In: Assenmacher, I, and Farner, DS (eds), *Environmental Endocrinology*. Berlin: Springer-
Verlag, pp. 44–51.

Feigin, GA, Fraser, RC, and Peterson, NS
(1978) Sex hormones and the immune response. II. Perturbation of antibody production by estradiol 17B. Int Arch Allergy Appl
Immunol 57:488–497.

Feigin, RD, Middelkamp, JN and Reed, C (1972)
Circadian rhythmicity of mice to sublethal
coxsackie B₃ infection. Nature (New Biol)
240:57–58.

Feigin, RD, San Joaquin, VH, Hamond, MW,
and Wyatt, RG (1969) Daily periodicity of susceptibility of mice to pneumococcal infection.
Nature 224:379–380.

Féré, C (1888) De la fréquence des accés d'épilepsie suivant les heures. CR Soc Biol 40:740–
742.

Ferrario, VF, Bianchi, R, Giunta, G, and
Roveda, L (1982) Circadian rhythm in human
intraocular pressure. Chronobiologia 9:33–
38.

Feurle, G, Ketterer, H, Becker, HD, and
Creutzfeldt, W (1972) Circadian serum gastrin
concentrations in control persons and in patients with ulcer disease. Scand J Gastroenterol 7:177–183.

Fine, PEM, and Clarkson, JA (1982) Measles in
England and Wales—1: An analysis of factors
underlying seasonal patterns. Int J Epidemiol
11:5–25.

Folkard, S (1976) Diurnal variation and individual differences in the perception of intractable
pain. J Psychosom Res 20:289–301.

Fröland, A (1967) Seasonal dependence in birth

of patients with Klinefelter's syndrome. Lancet 2:771.

Fuller, CA, Lydic, R, Sulzman, FM, Albers, HE, Tepper, B, and Moore-Ede, MC (1981) Circadian rhythm of body temperature persists after suprachiasmatic lesions in the squirrel monkey. Am J Physiol 241:R385–R391.

Fyfe, T, Dunnigan, MG, Hamilton, E, and Rae, RJ (1968) Seasonal variation in serum lipids, and incidence and mortality of ischaemic heart disease. J Atheroscler Res 8:591–596.

Gandevia, B, and Milne, J (1970) Occupational asthma and rhinitis due to Western red cedar (*Thuja plicata*), with special reference to bronchial reactivity. Br J Ind Med 27:235–244.

Gaultier, C, Reinberg, A, and Girard, F (1977) Circadian rhythms in lung resistance and dynamic lung compliance of healthy children. Effects of two bronchodilators. Resp. Physiol. 31:169–182.

Gautherie, M, and Gros, C (1977) Circadian rhythm alteration of skin temperature in breast cancer. Chronobiologia 4:1–17.

Géber, H (1921) Einige Daten zur Pathologie der Urticaria menstruationalis. Dermatol Zochenschr 32:143–150.

Gervais, P, Reinberg, A, Gervais, C, Smolensky, MH, and DeFrance, O (1977) Twenty-four-hour rhythm in the bronchial hyperreactivity to house dust in asthmatics. J Allergy Clin Immunol 59:207–213.

Géuber, J (1939) Densensitization in the treatment of menstrual intoxication and other allergic symptoms. Br J Dermatol 51:265–268.

Glynn, CJ, Lloyd, JW, and Folkard, S (1975) The diurnal variation in perception of pain. Proc R Soc Med 69:369–372.

Goodwin, F, and Wehr, T (eds) (1981) *Circadian Rhythms in Psychiatry*. California: Boxwood Press.

Gowers, WR (1885) *Epilepsy and Other Chronic Convulsive Diseases: Their Causes, Symptoms and Treatment.* New York: William Wood & Co.

Gowers, WR (1901) *Epilepsy and Other Convulsive Diseases: Their Causes, Symptoms and Treatment,* 2nd ed. Philadelphia: P. Blakeston's Son and Co.

Grabfield, GP, and Martin, EG (1913) Variations in the sensory threshold for faradic stimulation in normal human subjects. I. The diurnal rhythm. Am J Physiol 31:300–308.

Grammer, L, Levitz, D, Roberts, M, Pruzansky, JJ, and Zeiss, CR (1981) Seasonal variation of IgE antibody specific for ragweed antigen E (IgE-a-AgE) from the basophil surface in patients with ragweed pollenosis. Int Arch Allergy Appl Immunol 66:179–188.

Green, KG, Inman, WHW, and Thorp, JM (1963) Multicentre trial in the United Kingdom and Ireland of a mixture of ethyl chlorophenoxyisobutyrate and androsterone (Atromid). A preliminary report. J Atheroscler Res 3:593–616.

Greene, R (1967) Menstrual headache. Res Clin Stud Headache 1:62–73.

Griffiths, GM, and Fox, JT (1938) Rhythm in epilepsy. Lancet 2:409–416.

Gulyuk, NG (1961) Seasonal and diurnal rhythms of labor in women. Relation of some complications in labor to the daily rhythm of labor activity. Akush Ginekol 37:45–49.

Guy, WH, Jacob, FM, and Guy, WB (1951) Sex hormone sensitization (corpus luteum). Arch Dermatol 63:377–378.

Gyárfás, I, Csukas, A, Horvath-Gaucli, I (1976) Analysis of the diurnal periodicity of acute myocardial infarction attacks. Santé Publique (Bucur) 19:77–84.

Haberman, S, Capildeo, R, and Rose, FC (1981) The seasonal variation in mortality from cerebrovascular disease. J Neurol Sci 52:25–36.

Halberg, E, Halberg, F, Cornelissen, G, Garcia-Sainz, M, Simpson, HW, Taggett-Anderson, MA, and Haus, E (1979) Toward a chronopsy: II. A thermopsy revealing asymmetrical circadian variation in surface temperature of human female breasts and related studies. Chronobiologia 6:231–257.

Halberg, F (1953) Some physiological and clinical aspects of 24-hour periodicity. Lancet (Minneapolis) 73:20–32.

Halberg, F (1964) Organisms as circadian systems; temporal analysis of their physiologic and pathologic responses, including injury and death. In: *Medical Aspects of Stress in the Military Climate.* Walter Reed Army Institute of Research. Washington, D.C.: Walter Reed Army Medical Center, pp. 1–36.

Halberg, F (1969) Chronobiology. Ann Rev Physiol 31:675–725.

Halberg, F, Gupta, BD, Haus, E, Halberg, E, Deka, AC, Nelson, W, Sothern, RB, Cornelissen, G, Klee, J, Lakatua, DJ, Scheving, LE, and Burns, ER (1977) Steps toward a cancer chronopolytherapy. In: *14th Therapeutic*

200   Michael H. Smolensky

Int. Cong., Montpellier, 1977. Paris: Expansion Scientifique, pp. 151–196.

Halberg, F, Haus, E, Ahlgren, A, Halberg, E, Strobel, H, Angellar, A, Kuhl, JFW, Lucas, R, Gedgaudas, E, and Leong, J (1974) Blood pressure self-measurements for computer health assessment and the teaching of chronobiology in high schools. In: Scheving, LE, Halberg, F, and Pauly, JE (eds), *Chronobiology*. Tokyo: Igaku Shoin, pp. 372–378.

Halberg, F, and Howard, RB (1958) 24-hour periodicity and experimental medicine; examples and interpretations. Postgrad Med 24:349–358.

Halberg, F, Johnson, EA, Brown, BW, and Bittner, JJ (1960) Susceptibility rhythm to *E. coli* endotoxin and bioassay. Proc Soc Exp Biol Med 103:142–144.

Halberg, F, Lagoguey, M, and Reinberg, A (1983) Human circannual rhythms over a broad spectrum of physiological processes. Int J Chronobiol (in press).

Halberg, F, and Reinberg, A (1967) Rythmes circadiens et rythmes de basses fréquences en physiologie humaine. J Physiol (Paris) 59:117–200.

Halberg, F, Spink, WW, Albrecht, P, and Gully, RJ (1955) Resistance of mice to brucella somatic antigen, 24-hour periodicity and the adrenals. J Clin Endocrinol Metab 15:887.

Halberg, F, and Stephens, AN (1958) Twenty-four-hour periodicity in mortality of C-mice from *E. coli* lipopolysaccharide. Fed Proc 17:439.

Hall, SM (1977) Treatment of menstrual epilepsy with a progesterone-only oral contraceptive. Epilepsia 18:235–236.

Hansen-Pruss, OC, and Raymond, R (1942) Skin reactivity during the menstrual cycle. J Clin Endocrinol Metab 2:161–166.

Hardvogl, M, and Stögmann, W (1976) Hereditäre progressive Dystonie mit Tagesschwankungen (abstract). Jahrestag Ost Ges Kinderheilkd Millstatt 24:9.

Harkness, JAL, Panayi, GS, Richter, MB, Van de Pette, K, Unger, A, and Pownall, R (1981) Circadian variation in disease activity in rheumatoid arthritis. Ann Rheum Dis 40:529.

Harkness, JAL, Richter, MB, Panayi, GS, Van de Pette, K, Unger, A, Pownall, R, and Geddawi, M (1982) Circadian variation in disease activity in rheumatoid arthritis. Br Med J 284:551–554.

Harris, W (1926) *Neuritis and Neuralgia*. London: Oxford University Press.

Harris, W (1936) Ciliary (migrainous) neuralgia and its treatment. Br Med J 1:457–460.

Haus, E, and Halberg, F (1970) Circannual rhythm in level and timing of serum corticosterone in standardized inbred mature C-mice. Environ Res 3:81–106.

Haywood, TJ, and McGovern, JP (1968) So-called "nonspecific" factors in allergic disease. Ann Allergy 26:299–304.

Hejl, Z (1977) Daily, lunar, yearly, and menstrual cycles and bacterial or viral infections in man. J Interdiscipl Cycle Res 8:250–253.

Henkind, P, and Walsh, JB (1981) Diurnal variations in intraocular pressure. Chronic open angle glaucoma. Preliminary report. Trans Ophthalmol Soc NZ 33:18–20.

Hetzel, MR, and Clark, TJH (1978) Clinical importance of circadian factors in severe asthma. In: Reinberg, A, and Halberg, F (eds), *Chronopharmacology*. Oxford: Pergamon, pp. 213–221.

Hetzel, MR, and Clark, TJH (1980) Comparison of normal and asthmatic circadian rhythms in peak expiratory flow rate. Thorax 35:732–738.

Hetzel, MR, Clark, TJH, and Branthwaite, MA (1977a) Asthma: analysis of sudden deaths and ventilatory arrests in hospital. Br Med J 1:808–811.

Hetzel, MR, Clark, TJH, and Houston, K (1977b) Physiological patterns in early morning asthma. Thorax 32:418–423.

Hewitt, D (1962) A study of temporal variations in the risk of fetal malformation and death. Am J Public Health 52:1676–1688.

Hildebrandt, G (1962) Biologische Rhythmen und ihre Bedeutung fur die Bäder- und Klimaheilkunde. In: Amelung, W, and Evers, A (eds), *Handbuch der Bäder- und Klimaheilkunde*. Stuttgart: Schattauer-Verlag, pp. 730–785.

Hildebrandt, G, Rohmert, W, and Rutenfranz, J (1973) Über Jahresrhythmische Häufigkeitsschwankungen der Inanspruchnahme von Sicherheitseinrichtungen durch die Triebfbfahrzeugführer der Deutschen Bundesbahn. Int Arch Arbeitsmed 31:73–80.

Hopkins, H (1933) The time of appearance of epileptic seizures in relation to age, duration and type of the syndrome. J Nerv Ment Dis 77:153–162.

Hoseason, AS (1938) Vasomotor rhinorrhoea with asthma, associated with menstruation. Br Med J 2:703–704.

Hrdlicka, J, Krutova, K, and Malek, J (1950) Frequency of premature deliveries according to weight and length of fetuses and their seasonal rhythm. Cs Gynec 29:26–34.

Hughes, E (1931) *Seasonal Variation in Man.* London: Lewis.

Hunt, JR (1917) Progressive atrophy of the globus pallidus (primary atrophy of the pallidal system). Brain 40:58–148.

Huntington, E (1938) *Season of Birth; Its Relation to Human Abilities.* New York: Wiley.

Hutchison, R, and Moynihan, BGA (1909) Hunger pain and duodenal ulcer. Br Med J 1:926–927.

Illingworth, CFW, Scott, LDW, and Jamieson, RA (1944a) Acute perforated peptic ulcer. Frequency and incidence in the west of Scotland. Br Med J 2:655–658.

Illingworth, CFW, Scott LDW, and Jamieson, RA (1944b) Acute perforated peptic ulcer. Frequency and incidence in the west of Scotland. Br Med J 2:617–620.

Ilmarinen, J, Rutenfranz, J, Kylian, H, and Klimt, F (1975) Untersuchungen zur Tagesperiodik verschiedener Kreislauf- und Atemgrößen bei submaximalen und maximalen Leistungen am Fahrradergometer. Europ J Appl Physiol 34:255–267.

Islam, MS (1981) Seasonal rhythm of airway resistance and intrathoracic gas volume in healthy females and males. Respiration 42:193–199.

Job, C, Reinberg, A, and Delbarre, F (1981) Chronoeffectiveness of indomethacin in four patients suffering from an evolutive coxarthrosis or gonarthrosis. Int J Chronobiol 7:65.

Johnasson, BW (1972) Myocardial infarction in Malmö—1960–1968. Acta Med Scand 191:505–515.

Johnson, LC, Tepas, DI, Colquhoun, WP, and Colligan, MJ (1981) *Biological Rhythms, Sleep and Shift Work.* New York: SP Medical and Scientific Books.

Jongbloet, PH (1970) Chromosomal aberrations and month of birth. Lancet 2:1317–1318.

Jongbloet, PH (1971) Month of birth and gametopathy. An investigation into patients with Down's, Klinefelter's and Turner's syndrome. Clin Genet 2:315–330.

Jares, A, and Frees, J (1937) Die Tageschwankungen der Schmerzempfindung. Dtsch Med Worchenschr 63:962–963.

Kales, A, Beall, GN, Bajor, GF, Jacobson, A, and Kales, JD (1968) Sleep studies in asthmatic adults: relationship of attacks to sleep stage and time of night. J Allergy 41:164–173.

Kalter, H (1959) Seasonal variation in frequency of cortisone-induced cleft palate in mice. Genetics 44:518–519.

Kamraj-Mazurkiewicz, K (1971) Significance of the diurnal pattern in epileptic seizures in children. Neurol Neurochir Pol 5:197–204.

Kashiwagi, T, McClure, JN Jr, and Wetzel, RD (1972) The menstrual cycle and headache type. Headache 12:103–104.

Katavisto, M (1965) The diurnal variations of ocular tension in glaucoma. Acta Ophthalmol (Suppl) 78:1–131.

Katz, G (1953) Seasonal variation in incidence of premature births. Nord Med 50:1637–1638.

Kaufmann, MW, Gottlieb, G, Kahaner, K, Peselow, E, Stanley, M, Casadonte, P, and Deutsch, S (1981) Circadian rhythm and myocardial infarct: a preliminary study. IRCS Med Sci (Biochem) 9:557.

Kendell, RE, and Marshall, J (1963) Role of hypotension in the genesis of transient focal cerebral ischaemic attacks. Br Med J 2:344–348.

Klein, KE, Brüner, H, Voigt, ED, and Wegmann, HM (1966) Comparative studies on physiological indices of fitness in man under exercise, low pressure and acceleration. In: Yoshimura, H, and Weiner, JS (eds), *Human Adaptability and Its Methodology.* Tokyo: Jpn. Soc. Promot. Sci., pp. 234–247.

Klein, KE, and Wegmann, HM (1980) Significance of circadian rhythms in aerospace operations. In: *Sleep, Wakefulness and Circadian Rhythms.* NATO, AGARD Lecture Series 105, pp 2-1–2-17.

Kleitman, N, and Ramsaroop, A (1946) Body temperature and cutaneous sensitivity to tingling and pain. Fed Proc 5:56.

Kluger, MJ (1979) *Fever: Its Biology, Evolution and Function.* Princeton: Princeton University Press.

Kovar, WR, and Taylor, RJ (1960) Is spontaneous abortion a seasonal problem? Obstet Gynecol 16:350–353.

Kowanko, IC, Knapp, MS, Pownall, R, and Swannell, AJ (1982a) Domiciliary self-measurement in rheumatoid arthritis and the demonstration of circadian rhythmicity. Ann Rheum Dis 41:453–455.

Kowanko, IC, Pownall, R, Knapp, MS, Swannell, AJ, and Mahoney, PGC (1982b) The time of day of prednisolone administration in rheumatoid arthritis. Ann Rheum Dis 41:447–452.

Kowanko, IC, Pownall, R, Knapp, MS, Swannell, AJ, and Mahoney, PGC (1981) Circadian variations in the signs and symptoms of rheumatoid arthritis and in the therapeutic effectiveness of flurbiprofen at different times of the day. Br J Clin Pharmacol 11:477–484.

Krieger, DT (ed) (1979) *Endocrine Rhythms*. New York: Raven Press.

Kripke, DF, Mullaney, DJ, Atkinson, M, and Wolf, S (1978) Circadian rhythm disorders in manic-depressives. Biol. Psychiatry 13:335–351.

Kripke, DF (1981) Phase advance theories for affective illnesses. In: Goodwin, F, and Wehr, T (eds), *Circadian Rhythms in Psychiatry: Basic and Clinical Studies*. California: Boxwood Press.

Kronauer, RE, Czeisler, CA, Pilato, SF, Moore-Ede, MC, and Weitzman, ED (1982) Mathematical model of the human circadian system with two interacting oscillators. Am J Physiol 242:R3–R17.

Kunkle, EC (1964) Time patterns in headache; their diagnostic and therapeutic significance. J Maine Med Assoc 55:77–82.

Kunkle, EC, Pfeiffer, JB Jr, Wilhoit, WM, and Hamrick, LW Jr (1952) Recurrent brief headache in "cluster" pattern. Trans Am Neurol Assoc 77:240–243.

Kuroiwa, A (1978) Symptomatology of variant angina. Jpn Circ J 42:459–476.

Lagoguey, M, and Reinberg, A (1981) Circadian and circannual changes of pituitary and other hormones in healthy human males: their relationship with gonadal activity. In: Van Cauter, E, and Copinschi, G (eds), *Human Pituitary Hormones*. The Hague: Martinus Nijhoff, pp. 261–278.

Laidlaw, J (1956) Catamenial epilepsy. Lancet 2:1235–1237.

Langdon-Down, M, and Brain, WR (1929) Time of day in relation to convulsions in epilepsy. Lancet 1:1029–1032.

Langley, D, and Swanljung, H (1951) Ocular tension in glaucoma simplex. Br J Ophthalmol 35:445–458.

Lee, RE, Smolensky, MH, Leach, CS, and McGovern, JP (1977) Circadian rhythms in the cutaneous reactivity to histamine and selected antigens, including phase relationship to urinary cortisol excretion. Ann Allergy 38:231–236.

Leech, SH, and Kumar, P (1981) Cyclic urticaria. Ann Allergy 46:201–203.

Leffingwell, A (1982) *Illegitimacy and the Influence of Seasons upon Conduct; Two Studies in Demography*. London: Sonnenschein and Co.

Levine, H, Halberg, F, Hillman, DC, Fanning, R, Cornelissen, G, and DePrins, J (1979) Alteration of circadian core temperature rhythm characteristics and values outside habitual idiochronodesm as a result of laryngitis and transmeridian flight. Chronobiologia 6:127–128.

Li, TA (1936) Seasonal variation of the birth weight of the newborn. J Pediatr 8:459–469.

Lu, MC, Smolensky, MH, Hsi, B, and McGovern, JP (1980a) Seasonal changes in immunoglobulin and complement levels in atopic and non-atopic persons. In: Smolensky, MH, Reinberg, A, and McGovern, JP (eds), *Recent Advances in the Chronobiology of Allergy and Immunology*. Oxford: Pergamon Press, pp. 261–273.

Lu, MC, Smolensky, MH, Hsi, B, and McGovern, JP (1980b) Seasonal variation in total and specific IgE. In: Smolensky, MH, Reinberg, A, and McGovern, JP (eds), *Recent Advances in the Chronobiology of Allergy and Immunology*. Oxford: Pergamon Press, pp. 275–285.

MacFarland, A (1978) Variations in number of births and perinatal mortality by day of week in England and Wales. Br Med J 2:1670–1673.

Magnussen, G (1936) 18 cases of epilepsy with fits in relation to sleep. Acta Psychiatr Neurol 11:289–321.

Manery, JF (1979) Ions and body temperature. In: Lomax, P, and Schönbaum, E (eds), *Body Temperature. Regulation, Drug Effects, and Therapeutic Implications*. New York: Marcel Dekker, pp. 119–150.

Mansfield, CM, Carabasi, RA, Wells, W, and Borman, K (1973) Circadian rhythm in the skin temperature of normal and cancerous breasts. Int J Chronobiol 1:235–243.

Mansfield, CM, Wallace, JD, Curley, RF, Kramer, S, Southard, ME, and Driscoll, D (1970) A comparison of the temperature curves recorded over normal and abnormal breasts. Radiology 94:697–698.

Marshall, J (1977) Diurnal variation in occurrence of strokes. Stroke 8:230–231.

Martin, EG, Bigelow, GH, and Wilbur, GB (1914) Variations in the sensory threshold for faradic stimulation in normal human subjects. II. The nocturnal variation. Am J Physiol 33:415–422.

Master, AM (1960) The role of effort and occupation (including physicians) in coronary occlusion. JAMA 174:942–948.

Master, AM, Dack, S, and Jaffe, HL (1937) Factors and events associated with onset of coronary artery thrombosus. JAMA 109:546–549.

Master, AM, and Jaffee, HL (1952) Factors in the onset of coronary occlusion and coronary insufficiency. JAMA 148:794–798.

McGovern, JP, Smolensky, MH, and Reinberg, A (1977a) Circadian and circamensual rhythmicity in cutaneous reactivity to histamine and allergenic extracts. In: McGovern, JP, Smolensky, MH, and Reinberg, A (eds), *Chronobiology in Allergy and Immunology.* Springfield: Thomas, pp. 79–116.

McGovern, JP, Smolensky, MH, and Reinberg, A (1977b) *Chronobiology in Allergy and Immunology.* Springfield: Thomas.

McKeown, T, and Record, RG (1951) Seasonal incidence of congenital malformations of the central nervous system. Lancet 1:192–196.

Meyers, A, and Dewar, HA (1975) Circumstances attending 100 sudden deaths from coronary artery disease with coroners' necropsies. Br Heart J 37:1133–1143.

Miettiner, OS, Reiner, ML, and Nadas, AS (1970) Seasonal incidence of coarctation of the aorta. Br Heart J 32:103–107.

Milne, J, and Gandevia, B (1969) Occupational asthma and rhinitis due to Western (Canadian) red cedar (*Thuja plicata*). Med J Aust 2:741–744.

Mitchell, C (1970) Occupational asthma due to Western or Canadian red cedar (*Thuja plicata*). Med J Aust 2:233–235.

Moore, JG, and Englert, E Jr (1970) Circadian rhythm of gastric acid secretions in man. Nature 226:1261–1262.

Moore-Ede, MC, Sulzman, FM, and Fuller, CA (1982) *The Clocks that Time Us.* Cambridge: Harvard University Press.

Moynihan, BGA (1910a) *Duodenal Ulcer.* Philadelphia: Saunders, pp. 101–121.

Moynihan, BGA (1910b) Some remarks on dyspepsia. Dublin J Med Sci 130(no. 463, 3rd series):1–15.

Moynihan, BGA, and Childe, CP (1909) Hunger pain and duodenal ulcer. Br Med J 1036–1037.

Murray, AB, Ferguson, AC, and Morrison, B (1980) The seasonal variation of allergic respiratory symptoms induced by house dust mites. Ann Allergy 45:347–350.

Nasu, H, Aoyama, T, and Morisada, A (1958) Four cases of juvenile paralysis agitans in a family. Psychiatr Neurol Jpn 60:178–183.

Neffen, H, Oehling, A, and Sanz, M-L (1980) Variations of the circadian rhythm in cAMP in bronchial asthma after administration of fenoterol. Allerg Immunopathol 8:545–552.

Newell, FW, and Krill, AE (1965) Diurnal tonography in normal and glaucomatous eyes. Am J Ophthalmol 59:840–853.

Newmark, ME, and Penry, JK (1980) Catamenial epilepsy: a review. Epilepsia 21:281–300.

Nicholson, PA, and Bogie, W (1973) Diurnal variation in the symptoms of hay fever: implications for pharmaceutical development. Curr Med Res Opin 1:395–400.

Nielsen, J, and Friedrich, U (1969) Seasonal variation in non-disjunction of sex chromosomes. Humangenetik 8:258–260.

Nielson, J, Peterson, GB, and Therkelsen, AJ (1973) Seasonal-variation in birth of children with aneuploid chromosome abnormalities—Report from Danish Cytogenetic Central Register. Hum Genet 19:67–74.

Nowlin, JB, Troyer, WG, Collins, WS, Silverman, G, Nichols, CR, McIntosh, HD, Estes, EH, and Bogdonoff, MD (1965) The association of nocturnal angina pectoris with dreaming. Ann Intern Med 63:1040–1046.

O'Brien, IM, Harries, MG, Burge, PS, and Pepys, J (1979) Toluene diisocyanate induced asthma. 1. Reactions to TDI, MDI, HDI and histamine. Clin Allergy 9:1–6.

Orie, NGM, Sluitter, HF, Tammeling, GJ, DeVries, K, and Wal, AMVD (1964). Fight against bronchitis. In: Orie, HGM, and Sluiter, NJ (eds), *Bronchitis: 2nd International Bronchitis Symposium.* Springfield IL: Thomas, pp. 352–369.

Ortavant, R, and Reinberg, A (1980) *Rythmes et Reproduction.* Paris: Masson.

Osterman, PO, Lovstrand, KG, Lundberg, PO, Lundquist, S, and Muhr, C (1981) Weekly headache periodicity and the effect of weather changes on headache. Int J Biometeorol 25:39–45.

Osterman, PO, Lundberg, PO, Lundquist, S, Lovstrand, KG, and Muhr, C (1980) Weekly periodicity of headache and the effect of changes in weather on headache. Ups J Med Sci (Suppl) 31:23–26.

Ostfeld, AM (1963) The natural history and epidemiology of migraine and muscle contraction headache. Neurology 13:11–15.

Otto, W (1960) Jahreszeitliche Verteilung von

Lebendgeborenen, Frühgeborenen, Totgeborenen und Gestorborenen. Artzl Forsch 14:404–411.

Ouvrier, RA (1978) Progressive dystonia with marked diurnal fluctuation. Ann Neurol 4:412–417.

Ozkaragoz, K, and Cakin, F (1970) The effect of menstruation on immediate skin reactions in patients with respiratory allergy. J Asthma Res 7:171–175.

Paloheimo, J (1961) Seasonal variations of serum lipids in healthy men. Ann Med Exp Biol. Fenn 39(Suppl 8) pp. 1–88.

Parkes, AS (1968) Seasonal variation in human sexual activity. In: Thoday, JM and Parkes, AS (eds) *Genetic and environmental influences on behavior;* Eugenics Soc Symposium 4:128–145.

Patry, FL (1931) The relation of time of day, sleep and other factors to the incidence of epileptic seizures. Am J Psychiatr 87:789–813.

Pell, S, and D'Alonzo, CA (1963) Acute myocardial infarction in a large industrial population. JAMA 185:831–838.

Pengelley, ET (ed) (1974) *Circannual Clocks: Annual Biological Rhythms.* New York: Academic Press.

Pepys, J (1977) Clinical and therapeutic significance of patterns of allergic reactions of the lungs to extrinsic agents. Am Rev Resp Dis 116:573–587.

Pepys, J, and Davies, RJ (1978) Occupational asthma. In: Middleton, E, Reed, CE, and Ellis EF (eds), *Allergy, Principles and Practice.* New York: Mosby, p. 812–842.

Pepys, J, and Hutchcroft, BJ (1975) Bronchial provocation tests in etiologic diagnosis and analysis of asthma. Am Rev Resp Dis 112:829–859.

Piazzini, M, Guaxxelli, R, Montali, E, Conti, C, and Bigozzi, U (1981) On the epidemiology of certain auxopathological conditions caused by numerical chromosomal aberrations: an investigation into the possibility of seasonal variations. Acta Med Auxol 13:185–192.

Pickering, G (1972) Hypertension: definitions, natural histories and consequences. Am J Med 52:570–583.

Pickering, TG, Harshfield, GA, Kleinert, HD, Blank, S, and Laragh, JH (1982) Blood pressure during normal daily activities, sleep and exercise. JAMA 247:992–996.

Pinatel, MC, Czyba, JC, and Souchier C (1982)

Seasonal-changes in sexual hormones secretion, sexual-behavior and sperm production in man. Int J Andr Suppl 5:183–190.

Pinatel, MC, Souchier, C, Croze, JP, and Czyba, JC (1981) Seasonal variation of necrospermia in man. J Interdiscipl Cycle Res 12:225–235.

Pittendrigh, CS (1960) Circadian rhythms and the circadian organization of living systems. Cold Spring Harbor Symp Quant Biol 25:159–184.

Polani, PE, and Campbell, M (1960) Factors in the causation of persistent ductus arteriosus. Ann Hum Genet 24:343–357.

Pöllmann, L (1982) Uber tagesrhythmische Unterschiede der Wirkungsdauer eines Lokalanästhetikums. Dtsch Zahnärztl Z 37:388–390.

Pöllmann, L, and Harris, PHP (1978) Rhythmic changes in pain sensitivity in teeth. Int J Chronobiol 5:459–464.

Pöllmann, L, and Hildebrandt, G (1979) Circadian variations of potency of placebos on pain threshold in healthy teeth. Chronobiologia 6:145.

Pounder, RE, Hunt, RH, Vincent, SH, Milton-Thompson, GJ, and Misiewicz, JJ (1977) 24-hour intragastric acidity and nocturnal acid secretion in patients with duodenal ulcer during oral administration of cimetidine and atropine. Gut 18:85–90.

Prevost, RJ, Smolensky, MH, Reinberg, A, Raymer, WJ, and McGovern, JP (1980) Circadian rhythm of respiratory distress in asthmatic, bronchitic and emphysemic patients. In: Smolensky, MH, Reinberg, A, and McGovern, JP (eds), *Recent Advances in the Chronobiology of Allergy and Immunology.* Oxford: Pergamon Press, pp. 237–250.

Prinzmetal, M, Kennamer, R, Merliss, R, Wada, T, and Bor, N (1959) Angina pectoris. I. A variant form of angina pectoris. Am J Med 27:375–388.

Proccacci, P, Buzzelli, G, Passeri, I, Sassi, R, Voegelin, MR, and Zoppi, M (1972) Studies on the cutaneous pricking pain threshold in man. Circadian and circatrigintan changes. Res Clin Stud Headache 3:260–276.

Proccacci, P, Corte MD, Zoppi, M, and Maresca, M (1974) Rhythmic changes of the cutaneous pain threshold in man. A general review. Chronobiologia 1:77–96.

Puchelle, E, Da Costa De Moraes, R, and Zahm,

JM (1975) Variations diurnes da la visco-elasticite des secretions bronchiques chez le bronchitique chronique. Biorheology 12:67–71.

Puscass, I, Turi, Z, and Chiu, A (1979) Critical consideration on the diagnostic value of nocturnal gastric secretion in duodenal ulcer patients. Rev Med Intern 31:445–446.

Quetelet, MA (1842) A treatise on man and the development of his faculties (R Knox, translator.) In: Chambers, W, and Chambers, R (eds), *Chamber's Information for the People*. Edinburgh: W and R Chambers.

Ramirez-Lassepas, M, Haus, E, and Lakatua, DJ (1978) Seasonal and circadian periodicity of spontaneous intracerebral hemorrhage. *Proc. American Heart Association,* 3rd International Joint Meeting on Stroke and Cerebral Circulation, Feb. 16–18, New Orleans, Louisiana.

Ramirez-Lassepas, M, Haus, E, Lakatua, DJ, Sackett, L, and Swoyer, J (1980) Seasonal (circannual) periodicity of spontaneous intracerebral hemorrhage in Minnesota. Ann Neurol 8:539–541.

Record, RG (1961) Anencephalus in Scotland. Br J Prev Soc Med 15:93–105.

Reinberg, A (1968) The hours of changing responsiveness or susceptibility. Perspect Biol Med 11:111–128.

Reinberg, A (1973) Biological rhythms and human biometeorology. Int J Biometeorol (Suppl) 16:97–112.

Reinberg, A (1979a) Circadian and circannual rhythms in healthy adults: sleep, wakefulness and circadian rhythm. In: *Sleep, Wakefulness and Circadian Rhythms.* NATO AGARD Lecture Series. 105 pp. 1-1–1-27.

Reinberg, A (1979b) *Chronobiological field studies of oil refinery shift workers.* Chronobiologia 6 (Suppl 1):1–119.

Reinberg, A (1980) La chronobiologie humaine (buts et definitions). In: Ortavant, R, and Reinberg, A (eds), *Rhythmes et Reproduction.* Paris: Masson, pp. 1–14.

Reinberg, A (1982) Human chronobiology and adaptation. In: Hildebrandt, G, and Hensel, H (eds), *Biological Adaptation.* Stuttgart: Thieme Verlag, pp. 64–67.

Reinberg, A, Gervais, P, Halberg, F, Gaultier, M, Roynette, N, Abulker, C, and Dupont, J (1973) Mortalité des adultes: rythmes circadiens et circannuels dans un hôpital parisien et en France. Nouv Presse Med 2:289–294.

Reinberg, A, Gervais, P, Morin, M, and Abulker, C (1971a) Rhythme circadian humain du seuil de la réponse bronchique a l'acétylcholine. CR Acad Sci 272:1879–1881.

Reinberg, A, Ghata, J, and Sidi, E (1963) Nocturnal asthma attacks: their relationship to the circadian adrenal cycle. J Allergy 34:323–330.

Reinberg, A, Guillet, P, Gervais, P, Ghata, J, Vignaud, D, and Abulker, C (1977) One month chronocorticotherapy (Dutimelan, 8–15 mite). Control of the asthmatic condition without adrenal suppression and circadian rhythm alteration. Chronobiologia 4:295–312.

Reinberg, A, and Lagoguey, M (1978a) Annual endocrine rhythms in healthy young adult men: their implication in human biology and medicine. In: Assenmacher, I, and Farner, DS (eds), *Environmental Endocrinology.* Berlin: Springer-Verlag, pp. 113–121.

Reinberg, A, and Lagoguey, M (1978b) Circadian and circannual rhythms in sexual activity and plasma hormones (FSH, LH, testosterone) of five human males. Arch Sex Behav 7:13–30.

Reinberg, A, Lagoguey, M, Chauffournier, JM, and Cesselin, F (1975) Circannual and circadian rhythms in plasma testosterone in five healthy young Parisian males. Acta Endocrinol (Kbh) 80:732–743.

Reinberg, A, Schuller, E, Clench, J, and Smolensky, MH (1980) Circadian and circannual rhythms of leukocytes, proteins, and immunoglobulins. In: Smolensky, MH, Reinberg, A, and McGovern, JP (eds), *Recent Advances in the Chronobiology of Allergy and Immunology.* Oxford: Pergamon Press, pp. 251–259.

Reinberg, A, Schuller, E, Dlasnerie, N, Clench, J, and Helary, M (1971b) Rhythmes circadiens et circannuels des leucocytes, protéines totales, IgA, IgM, IgG d'adultes et sains. Nouv Presse Med 6:3819–3823.

Reinberg, A, and Smolensky, MH (1974) Circatrigintan secondary rhythms related to hormonal changes in the menstrual cycle. General considerations. In: Ferin, M, Halberg, F, Richart, RM, and Vande Wiele, RL (eds), *Biorhythms and Human Reproduction.* New York: Wiley, pp. 241–258.

Reinberg, A, Smolensky, MH, Ghata, J, Gervais, A, and Gervais, P (1974) Approche chronobiologique des rhythmes mensuels des femms saines spontanément réglées. Ann Endocrinol 35:309–310.

Reinberg, A, Vieux, N, and Andlauer, P (eds) (1981) *Night and Shift Work: Biological and Social Aspects*. Oxford: Pergamon Press.

Rippey, RM (1981) Overview: seasonal variations in cholesterol. Prev Med 10:655–659.

Rogers, EJ, and Vilkin, B (1978) Diurnal variation in sensory and pain thresholds correlated with mood states. J Clin Psychiatry 39:431–438.

Rosenberg, LA, and Heinonen, OP (1974) Seasonal occurrence of ventricular septal defect. Lancet 2:903–904.

Rosenblatt, LS, Shifrine, M, Hetherington, NW, Paglieroni, T, and MacKenzie, MR (1982) A circannual rhythm in rubella antibody titers. J Interdiscipl Cycle Res 13:81–88.

Rossolini, A, and Chieffi, O (1964) On relationships between asthma and sex hormones in the woman. Atti Accad Fisiocrit Siena Medicofis 13:231–247.

Rothman, KJ, and Fyler, DC (1974) Seasonal occurrence of complex ventricular septal defect. Lancet 2:193–197.

Rothman, KJ, and Fyler, DC (1976) Association of congenital heart defects with season and population density. Teratology 13:29–34.

Rowland, JM, Potter, DE, and Reiter, RJ (1981) Circadian rhythm in intraocular pressure: a rabbit model. Curr Eye Res 1:169–173.

Rutstein, DD, Nickerson, RJ, and Heald, FP (1952) Seasonal incidence of patent ductus arteriosus and maternal rubella. Am J Dis Child 84:199–213.

Salber, EJ, and Bradshaw, ES (1952) Birth weights of South African babies. III. Seasonal variation in birth weight. Br J Soc Med 6:190–191.

Sandahl, B (1974) A study of seasonal and secular trends in incidence of stillbirths and spontaneous abortions in Sweden. Acta Obstet Gynecol Scand 53:251–257.

Sandahl, B (1977) Seasonal incidence of some congenital malformations in the central nervous system in Sweden, 1965–1972. Acta Paediatr Scand 66:65–72.

Sargent, F (1967) Introduction to human biometeorology: Its concepts and problems. In: *Seminar on Human Biometeorology*. Environmental health Series: Air Pollution.

U.S.D.H.E.W., Public Health Service Publication No. 999-AP-25, pp. 1–23.

Sauerbier, I (1979) Circadian aspects of the teratogenicity of cytostatic drugs. Chronobiologia 6:152.

Sauerbier, I (1980) Recent findings relative to teratology and chronobiology. In: Scheving, LE, and Halberg, F (eds), *Chronobiology: Principles and Applications to Shifts in Schedules*. Alphen aan den Rijn, The Netherlands: Sijthoff and Noordhoff, pp. 535–540.

Saundby, R, Moynihan, BGA, Maylard, AE, and Herschell, G (1909) Diagnosis in stomach surgery/The diagnostic value of hunger pain. Br Med J 1:814–815.

Schenck, E, and Kruschke, U (1975) Familial progressive dystonia with diurnal fluctuation. Klin Wochenschr 53:779–780.

Scott, JT (1960) Morning stiffness in rheumatoid arthritis. Ann Rheum Dis 19:361–368.

Segawa, M, Hosaka, A, Miyagawa, F, Nomura, Y and Imai, H (1976) Hereditary progressive dystonia with marked diurnal fluctuation. Adv Neurol 14:215–233.

Sensi, S, Manzoli, U, Capani, F, Domenichelli, B, Lucente, M, Schiavoni, G, and Coppola, E (1980) Circadian rhythm of ventricular ectopy. Chest 77:580.

Shackelford, PG, and Feigin, RD (1973) Periodicity of susceptibility to pneumococcal infection: influence of light and adrenocortical secretions. Science 182:285–287.

Shelley, WB, Preucel, RW, and Spoont, SS (1964) Autoimmune progesterone dermatitis. JAMA 190:35–38.

Shifrine, M, Garsd, A, and Rosenblatt, LA (1982) Seasonal variation in immunity of humans. J Interdiscipl Cycle Res 13:157–165.

Shifrine, M, Rosenblatt, LS, Taylor, N, Hetherington, NW, Matthews, VJ, and Wilson, FD (1980a) Seasonal variations in lectin-induced lymphocyte transformation in beagle dogs. J Interdiscipl Cycle Res 11: 219–226.

Shifrine, M, Taylor, NJ, Rosenblatt, LS, and Wilson, FD (1980b) Seasonal variation in cell-mediated immunity of clinically normal dogs. Exp Hematol 8:318–326.

Siehr, P (1899) Zwei Fälle von Paralysis agitans im jugendlichen Alter. Dissertation: Königsberg.

Simpson, HW (1977) Aspects of cancer chronotherapy: mammary chronothermography and its perspective for treatment of breast carcinoma. In: *14th Therapeutic International Congress,* Montpellier, France. Paris: Expansion Scientifique, pp. 197–210.

Siracusa, A, Curradi, F, and Abbritti, G (1978) Recurrent nocturnal asthma due to toluene di-isocyanate: a case report. Clin Allergy 8:195–201.

Slater, BCS, Watson, GI, and McDonald, JC (1964) Seasonal variation in congenital abnormalities. Preliminary report of a survey conducted by the research committee of council of the college of general practitioners. Br J Prev Soc Med 18:1–7.

Slatis, HM, and DeCloux, RJ (1967) Seasonal variation in stillbirth frequencies. Hum Biol 39:284–294.

Smals, AGH, Kloppenborg, PWC, and Benraad, TJ (1976) Circannual cycle in plasma testosterone levels in man. J Clin Endocrinol Metab 42:979–982.

Smolensky, MH (1973) Chronobiology applied to therapy of human breast cancer. In: *Time: The Fourth Dimension of Medicine,* Vol. 2. New Orleans, La.: Upjohn Symposium, November 3–4, 1973, pp. 6–7.

Smolensky, MH (1975) Chronobiologic aspects of cutaneous reactivity, an example of endogenous rhythmicity and implications upon the evaluation of environmental quality. In: Gervais, P. (ed), *Asthme, Allergie Respiratoire et Environnement Socio-Écologique.* Le Mont-Dore, pp. 41–60.

Smolensky, MH (1980) Chronobiologic aspects of the epidemiology of human reproduction and fertility. In: Ortavant, R, and Reinberg, A (eds), *Rythmes et Reproduction.* Paris: Masson, pp. 219–242.

Smolensky, MH (1981) Chronobiologic factors related to the epidemiology of human reproduction. In: Cortés-Prieto, J, Campos da Paz, A, and Nevese-Castro, M (eds), *Research on Fertility and Sterility.* Lancaster: MTP Press, pp. 157–181.

Smolensky, MH, Bicakova-Rocher, A, Reinberg, A, and Sanford, J (1981a) Chronoepidemiological search for circannual changes in the sexual activity of human males. Chronobiologia 8:217–230.

Smolensky, MH, and Halberg, F (1977) Circadian rhythms in airway patency and lung volumes. In: McGovern, JP, Smolensky, MH, and Reinberg, A (eds), *Chronobiology in Allergy and Immunology.* Springfield, IL: Thomas, pp. 117–138.

Smolensky, MH, Halberg, F, Reinberg, A, and Stupfel, M (1974) CO_2 respiratory regulation and chronobiology. In: Nahas, G, and Schafer, KE (eds), *Carbon Dioxide.* New York: Springer-Verlag, pp. 118–124.

Smolensky, MH, Halberg, F, and Sargent, F (1972) Chronobiology of the life sequence. In: Itoh, S, Ogata, K, and Yoshimura, H (eds), *Advances in Climatic Physiology.* Tokyo: Igaku Shoin, pp. 281–318.

Smolensky, MH, Reinberg, A, Lee, RE, and McGovern, JP (1973) Secondary rhythms related to hormonal changes in the menstrual cycle: Special reference to allergology. In: Ferin, M, Halberg, F, Richart, RM, and Vande Wiele, RL (eds), *Biorhythms and Human Reproduction.* New York: Wiley, pp. 287–306.

Smolensky, MH, Reinberg, A, Prevost, RJ, McGovern, JP, and Gervais, P (1980) The application of chronobiologic findings and methods to the epidemiological investigation of the health effects of air pollutants on sentinel patients. In: Smolensky, MH, Reinberg, A, and McGovern, JP (eds), *Recent Advances in the Chronobiology of Allergy and Immunology.* Oxford: Pergamon Press, pp. 211–236.

Smolensky, MH, Reinberg, A, and Queng, J (1981b) The chronobiology and chronopharmacology of allergy. Ann Allergy 47(4):234–252.

Smolensky, MH, Tatar, SE, Bergman, SA, Losman, JG, Barnard, CN, Dacso, CC, and Kraft, IA (1976) Circadian rhythmic aspects of human cardiovascular function: a review by chronobiologic statistical methods. Chronobiologia 3:337–371.

Soutar, CA, Carruthers, M, and Pickering, CA (1977) Nocturnal asthma and urinary adrenaline and noradrenaline excretion. Thorax 32:677–683.

Soutar, CA, Costello, J, Ijaduola, O, and Turner-Warwick, M (1975) Nocturnal and morning asthma. Relationship to plasma corticosteroids and response to cortisol infusion. Thorax 30:436–440.

Steinbach, K, Eder, A, Glogar, D, Joskowicz, G, and Weber, H (1978) Circadian variations in the frequency of arrhythmia and quantitative analysis of rhythm disturbances. Acta Med Aust 5:132–134.

Stempel, DA, Davis, VL, Moussey, LJ, and Helms, RW (1981) Seasonal variations of serum IgE levels in normal children. Ann Allergy 47:14–16.

Stephens, S, Smolensky, MH, Kennelly, BM (in preparation) Temporal factors in cardiac morbidity.

Stoller, A and Collmann, RD (1965) Incidence of infective hepatitis followed by Down's syndrome nine months later. Lancet 2:1221–1223.

Strempel, H (1977) Circadian cycles of epicritic and protopathic pain threshold. J Interdiscipl Cycle Res 8:276–280.

Suda, M, Hayaishi, O, and Nakagawa, H (eds) (1979) *Biological Rhythms and Their Central Mechanism: A NATO Foundation Symposium.* Amsterdam: Elsevier/North Holland Biomedical Press.

Symonds, C (1956) A particular variety of headache. Brain 79:217–232.

Tähti, E (1956) Studies of the effect of X-radiation on 24-hour variations in the mitotic activity in human malignant tumours. Acta Pathol Microbiol Scand (Suppl) 117:1–61.

Tammeling, GJ, DeVries, K, and Kruyt, EW (1977) Circadian pattern of bronchial reactivity to histamine in healthy subjects and in patients with obstructive lung-disease. In: McGovern, JP, Smolensky, MH, and Reinberg, A (eds), *Chronobiology in Allergy and Immunology.* Springfield, IL: Thomas, pp. 139–149.

Tarquini, B (1978) Nouve vedute sull'ulcera peptica. Recent Prog Med 64:24–44.

Tarquini, B, Brocchi, A, Buricchi, L, Cappelli, G, Costa, A, Neri, B, and Cagnoni, M (1977) Circadian study on serum gastrin in patients with duodenal ulcers and in a control group. Chronobiologia 4:49–55.

Tarquini, B, Rosati, I, Serantoni, C, Orzales, R, Ciani, P, Cagnoni, M, and Rosene, G (1976) Circadian studies on gastric mitotic index in patients with duodenal ulcer and in a control group. Chir Gastroenterol 11:369–371.

Taylor, AN, Davies, RJ, Hendrick, DJ, and Pepys, J (1979) Recurrent nocturnal asthmatic reactions to bronchial provocation tests. Clin Allergy 213–219.

Taylor, AN, Longbottom, JL, and Pepys, J (1977) Respiratory allergy to urine proteins of rats and mice. Lancet 2(8043): 847–849.

Thiry, A, Heusghem, C, and Legentil, P (1954) Study of the urinary excretion of estrogens, 17-ketosteroids and reducing steroids in epilepsy, particularly the so-called catamenial epilepsy. Rev Med Liege 9:238–246.

Thomas, CB, Holljes, HWD, and Eisenberg, FF (1961) Observation on seasonal variation in total serum cholesterol level among healthy young prisoners. Ann Intern Med 54:413–430.

Tjoa, WK, Smolensky, MH, Hsi, BP, Steinberger, E, and Smith, KD (1982) Circannual rhythm in human sperm count revealed by serially independent sampling. J Fertil Infertil 38:454–459.

Todisco, T, Grassi, V, Dorbini, CA, Sottorini, M, de Benedictis, FM, Costellucci, G, and Romano, S (1980) Circadian rhythms of respiratory functions in asthmatics. Respiration 40:128–135.

Tonnesen, MG, Jubiz, W, Moore, JG, and Frailey, J (1974) Circadian variation of prostaglandin E(PGE) production in human gastric juice. Am J Dig Dis 19:644–648.

Toole, JF (1968) Nocturnal strokes and arterial hypotension. Ann Intern Med 68:1132–1133.

Townsend, RE, Prinz, PN, and Obrist, WD (1973) Human cerebral blood flow during sleep and waking. J Appl Physiol 35:620–625.

Tromovitch, TA, and Heggli, WF (1967) Autoimmune progesterone urticaria. Calif Med 106:211–212.

Tromp, SW (1963) *Medical Biometeorology: Weather, Climate and the Living Organism.* New York: American Elsevier.

Trousseau, A (1865) *Clinique Médicale de l'Hôtel Dieu de Paris,* Vol. 2. *Asthme.* Paris: Baillière, p. 373.

Udry, JR, and Morris, NM (1967) Seasonality of coitus and seasonality of birth. Demography 4:673–680.

Van Cauter, E (1973) *Problémes dans l'analyse des séries chronologiques courtes.* Mémoire, de licence en Sciences actuarielles. Faculté des Sciences, Université Libre de Bruxelles.

Voigt, ED, Engle, P, and Klein, H (1967) Daily fluctuations of the performance-pulse index. Germ Med Mon 12:394–395.

Voutilainen, A (1953) Ueber die 24-Stunden-Rhythmik der Mitosenfrequenz in malignen Tumoren. Acta Pathol Microbiol Scand (Suppl) 99:1–104.

Watanabe, G, and Aoki, S (1956) Climatic effect on the serum cholesterol levels. Jpn J Med Prog 43:301–306.

Waters, WE, and O'Connor, PJ (1971) Epidemiology of headache and migraine in women. J Neurol Neurosurg Psychiat 34:148–153.

Weitzman, ED (1981) Sleep and its disorders. Ann Rev Neurosci 4:381–417.

Weitzman, ED, Czeisler, CA, Coleman, RM, Spielman, AJ, Zimmerman, JC, Dement, W, Richardson, G, and Pollak, CP (1981) Delayed sleep phase syndrome. A chronobiological disorder with sleep-onset insomnia. Arch Gen Psychiat 38:737–46.

Weitzman, ED, Czeisler, CA, Zimmerman, JC, Ronda, JM, and Knauer, RS (1982) Chronobiologic disorders: analytic and therapeutic techniques. In: Guilleminault C (ed) *Sleeping and Waking Disorders*. Calif.: Addison Wesley pp. 167–188.

Wertheimer, L, Hassen, AZ, and Delman, AJ (1972) The 24-hour (circadian) rhythm of the cardiovascular system. Clin Res 20:404.

Wesche, DL, and Frederickson, RCA (1981) The role of the pituitary in the diurnal variation in tolerance to painful stimuli and brain enkephalin levels. Life Sci 29:2199.

Wolff, HG (1963) *Headache and Other Head Pain*. New York: Oxford University Press.

Wongwiwat, M, Sukapanit, S, Triyanond, C, and Sawyer, WD (1972) Circadian rhythm of the resistance of mice to acute pneumococcal infection. Infect Immunol 5:442–448.

Wright, RA, and Judson, FN (1978) Relative and seasonal incidences of the sexually transmitted diseases—2-year statistical review. J Vener Dis 54:433–440.

Wulfsohn, NL, and Politzer, WM (1964) Bronchial asthma during menses and pregnancy. S Afr Med J 38:173.

Yamamura, Y, Sobue, I, Ando, K, Iida, M, Yanagi, T, and Kono, C (1973) Paralysis agitans of early onset with marked diurnal fluctuation of symptoms. Neurology 23:239–244.

Yasue, H, Omote, S, Takizawa, A, Nagao, M, Miwa, K, Kato, H, Tanaka, S, and Akiyama, F (1978) Pathogenesis and treatment of angina pectoris at rest as seen from its response to various drugs. Jpn Circ J 42:1–10.

Yasue, H, Omote, S, Takizawa, A., Nagao, M, Miwa, K, and Tanaka, S (1979) Circadian variation of exercise capacity in patients with Prinzmetal's variant angina: role of exercise-induced coronary arterial spasm. Circulation 59:938–948.

Zondech, B, and Bromberg, YM (1947) Endocrine allergy: clinical reaction of allergy to endogenous hormones and their treatment. J Obstet Gynecol Br Comm 54:1–19.

Zuckerman, S (1957) The human breeding season. New Scientist 1:12–20.

6

Clinical Chronopharmacology
An Experimental Basis for Chronotherapy

Alain Reinberg

The practical significance of biological temporal structure is well illustrated by chronobiologic findings pertaining to the administration of medicines. Metabolic pathways are neither open with the same level of efficiency nor oriented continuously in the same direction (Reinberg 1974b, 1976a,b). The sensitivity of target systems to chemical substances varies rhythmically, too. New experimental methods and concepts have been developed to research, comprehend, and describe bioperiodic changes in drug effectiveness and tolerance. The major aim of clinical chronopharmacology is the optimization of therapeutic interventions. By manipulating therapeutic administrations as a function of the organism's biological time structure, it is possible to enhance the desired and reduce the undesired effects of several types of medications.

Introduction

With reference to medical tradition, but not necessarily to scientific rationale, medicines are prescribed for specified clock hours. The timing of therapeutic measures today is related more frequently to psycho-social considerations, less frequently to empirical observations. Sometimes the homeostatic hypothesis is offered as the basis for a treatment schedule. Only occasionally, before the 1960's, was an experiment designed to evaluate objectively, for a given agent, the advantage of a well-defined chronotherapy. In light of many new findings, it is now pertinent to reexamine the present-day rationale for administering treatments at particular times of the day and/or night.

The scheduling of treatments is based primarily upon prevailing scientific hypotheses as well as achieving patient compliance. With regard to the latter, involving *psychosocial considerations,* patients are instructed to ingest or inject prescribed medications at meal times with the hope that a high level of compliance will be attained. With regard to the former concern, the *homeostatic hypothesis* implies that the pharmacologic, therapeutic, and toxicologic effects of chemical substances should be the same, independent of the timing of treatment. Both desired and undesired effects of medications are expected to be identical no matter the hour, day, or month of administration. This hypothesis has been demonstrated to be invalid each time it has been tested in chronopharmacologic and chronotoxicologic experiments (see the following review papers: Ceresa and Angeli 1977; Halberg 1960, 1962, 1963, 1967, 1969, 1974, 1975; Halberg and Reinberg 1967; Halberg et al. 1967, 1969a,b, 1977a,b; Haus et al. 1974; Menzel 1955; Montalbetti 1974; Moore-Ede 1973; Reinberg 1965, 1967, 1971, 1973, 1974b,c, 1975, 1976a,b, 1977a,b; Reinberg and Ghata 1977; Reinberg and Halberg 1971; Reinberg and Smolensky 1982; Scheving et al. 1974; Smolensky et al. 1979, 1980; Walker 1974). Based on currently available data, the homeostatic philosophy of therapeutic management has to be viewed as obsolete and in some cases inappropriate or even dangerous. A chronobiologic approach often is indispensable for solving a set of therapeutic problems, including the reduction of undesired effects.

The belief that chronotherapeutics has important and practical application in medicine is not a recent one. In 1814 Julien Joseph Virey wrote that Thomas Sydenham, who based his judgment on empirical observations, recommended the narcotic opium (laudanum) be given in the late evening rather than in the morning to achieve best therapeutic effect. It was not until more than 150 years later that chronopharmacologic investigations of anesthetics, barbiturates, and narcotics on rats by Scheving et al. (1974), Nair (1974), and Bruguerolle et al. (1979) and on men by Fukami et al. (1970), Nicholson and Stone (1977), and Simpson et al. (1973) confirmed this empirical observation. Recognition must be given to Jöres (1938), Möllerström (1953), and Menzel (1955); their pioneer work constitutes the foundation of today's chronopharmacologic and chronotherapeutic studies. These investigators recognized 40 years ago that the bioperiodicities of human beings must be taken into account and, if need be, restructured when treating disease. Specific chronobiologic methods are now available to achieve these goals (Aschoff et al. 1975; Halberg 1960, 1969, 1975; Halberg

et al. 1967, 1972; Haus et al. 1974; Philippens 1974; Reinberg 1971, 1974b, 1976a; Reinberg and Halberg 1971; Scheving et al. 1974; Sturtevant 1976; Reinberg and Smolensky 1982).

Development of Clinical Chronopharmacology

Modern chronopharmacology involves both the investigation of drug effects as a function of biological timing and the investigation of the effects of drugs on the characteristics of biological rhythms: period, τ; acrophase, ϕ; amplitude, A; and the rhythm-adjusted mean or mesor, M. Regular and thus predictable changes in biological susceptibility and response to a large variety of physical as well as chemical agents (including foods and drugs) are now viewed as rather common phenomena. This is true for both plants and animals (Haus et al. 1974; Reinberg 1974b; Reinberg and Halberg 1971; Scheving et al. 1974), including man. Experimental evidence of circadian ($\sim$24 hr), circamensual ($\sim$30 day), and circannual ($\sim$1 year) changes in human biological responses to various chemical and physical agents has been presented elsewhere in review papers (Halberg 1962, 1969; Halberg and Reinberg 1967; Halberg et al. 1967, 1969, 1972; Reinberg 1965, 1967, 1971, 1974a–c; Reinberg and Halberg 1971).

The findings of earlier chronobiologic studies led to concepts such as the hours of changing responsiveness (Halberg 1960, 1962, 1963; Reinberg 1965, 1967), chronopharmacology (Reinberg and Halberg 1971), chronosusceptibility (Reinberg 1967), chronotolerance (Halberg et al. 1977), as well as chronesthesy, chronopharmacokinetics, and chronergy (Reinberg 1976a; Reinberg et al. 1975) as depicted in Fig. 1. Recognizing that review papers have been published recently on this and related topics, the aim of this chapter is to provide illustrative examples of human circadian chronopharmacology and chronotherapy.

The objective demonstration of chronopharmacologic phenomena demands

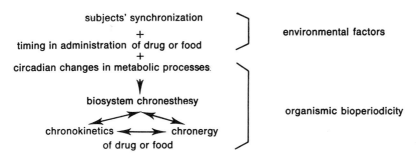

Fig. 1. The *chronesthesy* of a biosystem refers to rhythmic changes in the biosystem's susceptibility; it includes both molecular and membrane phenomena and related metabolic processes. The chronesthesy involves cells, tissues, organs, and organ systems of the host as well as the susceptibility of parasites, bacteria, tumors, etc. The *chronopharmacokinetics* of an agent denotes rhythmic changes in either its bioavailability, pharmacokinetics, and/or excretion in the urine, feces, sweat, saliva, etc. Statistically significant rhythms have been demonstrated in the parameters used to characterize the pharmacokinetics of several agents. The *chronergy* of a chemical (or a physical) agent refers to rhythmic changes in any of its effect(s), either desired ("chronoeffectiveness") or undesired. The chronergy of a chemical agent involves its chronopharmacokinetics as well as the chronesthesy of a set of biosystems. The acrophase of the chronergy need not coincide in time with the acrophase of its blood level. (From Reinberg 1976a.)

the use of appropriate methodology. Chronobiologic investigations must follow a set of elementary rules regarding (1) the synchronization of subjects (the timing and regularity of the socioecologic synchronizer, i.e., clock hours of light-on and light-off, meal timing) (Apfelbaum et al. 1972; Reinberg 1974c); (2) the collection of time series on each of the physiological and/or pathological variables monitored [with consideration for the accuracy of measurements or determinations, span of time for data gathering—at least 24-hr sampling durations with the interval (Δt) between tests or measurements being 4 hr, etc.]; and (3) the statistical analyses of time series thus obtained by Cosinor and/or related methods (Halberg et al. 1967, 1977, 1972). These were discussed in detail in Chap. 2. It should be pointed out that circadian rhythms can be modulated and modified by coexisting rhythms of about 1 year and about 30 days (the latter mainly, but not exclusively, found in women). Therefore, the month of the year and/or the day of the menstrual cycle in women must be given when presenting findings of chronopharmacologic research (Reinberg and Lagoguey

1978; von Mayersbach et al. 1977; Procacci et al. 1974; Reinberg 1974a; Smolensky et al. 1974).

Reports of changes in the effects of chemical substances according to circadian stage in human beings are numerous. Relevant information is available, for example, for histamine (Lee et al. 1977; Reinberg 1965; Reinberg et al. 1965, 1967, 1974; Smolensky et al. 1974; De Vries et al. 1962), sodium salicylate (Reinberg et al. 1967, 1974), acetylcholine (Reinberg et al. 1971, 1974), halothane (Fukami et al. 1970), prostaglandin F-2α (Smith et al. 1973), lidocaine (Reinberg and Reinberg 1977), clofibrate (Andersen and Hellström 1982), digoxin (Avlisi et al. 1978; Del Ponte et al. 1979), hydrochlorothiazide (Mills et al. 1975), oxymetholone (Moore-Ede and Burr 1973), insulin (Serio et al. 1971), theophylline (Smolensky et al. 1982), and many others. Table 1 summarizes the findings of chronopharmacologic studies on asthmatic patients treated with synthetic corticosteroids, while Tables 2 and 3 summarize the effects of various chemical agents as a function of the rat's (Table 2) and man's (Table 3) circadian-system-stage

214   Alain Reinberg

Table 1. *Chronopharmacologic Studies on Synthetic Corticosteroids.*

Group studied	Corticosteroid[a] tested	Explored circadian rhythms	Ref.
Asthmatic children	Prednisone (c) (per os)	PEF Urinary K$^+$	Reindl et al. (1969)
Asthmatic adults	Dutimelan[b] (c) (per os)	PEF Plasma cortisol	Serafini et al. (1976)
Asthmatic adults	Dutimelan[b] (c) (per os)	Plasma ACTH, cortisol, insulin, gastrin, urinary 17-OHCS, bronchial patency	Crepaldi et al. (1974)
Symptom-free asthmatic children	Methylprednisolone (a) (s.c. injection)	PEF	Reinberg et al. (1974d)
Asthmatic adults	Dutimelan mite[b] (c) (per os)	PEF, oral temperature, grip strength, self-rating of dyspnea, urinary 17-OHCS, K$^+$, Ca^{++}, Na$^+$	Reinberg et al. (1977)

[a] Corticosteroid fixed dose, multiple test times; (c) = chronic; (a) = acute medication.

[b] Dutimelan 8/15 mite. Dragée A ingested at 0800 contains prednisolone acetate (4 mg) and prednisolone alcohol, 2 mg; dragée B ingested at 1500 contains prednisolone alcohol (2 mg) and cortisone acetate (8 mg). Dutimelan 8/15 mite contains only one-half the amount of corticoid dose as Dutimelan 8/15.

Note: Studies demonstrate no or slight adrenal inhibition and no or slight alteration of subject's temporal structure (e.g., acrophase shift and/or changes in mean level) occurs when the corticosteroid is given once or twice a day not far from the expected acrophase of the plasma cortisol circadian rhythm (i.e., around 0800 for allergic subjects synchronized with diurnal activity from 0700 to 2300 alternating with nocturnal rest). In addition, a relatively large dose of corticosteroids given at 2000 not only induces undesired effects but also is ineffective on both bronchial patency and dyspnea in allergic patients (Reinberg et al., 1983).

with respect to induced sleep, general anesthesia, and related phenomena.

Circadian rhythm dependencies of drugs are relatively easy to demonstrate and describe. Another type of effect, drug-induced alteration of human circadian rhythms due to timed administrations of medications, requires elaborate experimental protocols. For example, determination of circadian rhythm characteristics for a set of biologically meaningful variables is necessary prior to, during, and after drug administration to evaluate the effect of timing with regard to clock hour apart from other conventional pharmaceutical considerations such as route, dose, and form. This is necessary since findings substantiate the alteration of biological time structure, for example, following the administration of reserpine (Halberg 1962); cyproheptadine (Reinberg and Sidi 1966); insulin (Serio et al. 1971; Gibson et al. 1974); hypoglycemic agents (Sensi et al. 1975; Mirouze and Selam 1977); glucagon (Melani et al. 1975); oxymetholone (Moore-Ede and Burr 1973);

metyrapone (Angeli et al. 1975; Touitou et al. 1976); lithium and other antidepressant agents used in psychiatry (Wirz-Justice et al. 1980; Wirz-Justice and Wehr 1983); and ACTH, cortisol, and other corticosteroids (see Table 1). For example, acrophases may be phase-shifted (phase-advanced or phase-delayed relative to pretreatment control values) as well as mesors lowered or enhanced as a result of the timed administration of either corticosteroid or ACTH as shown for the urinary excretion of 17-OHCS and electrolytes, grip strength, peak expiratory flow (PEF), blood eosinophils, etc.

A set of most interesting findings deals with the fact that some drugs possess the property of lengthening the period of certain circadian (and ultradian) rhythms, specifically when studies are performed under conditions allowing rhythms to free-run. Most of these drugs—lithium, imipramine (a tricyclic agent), and clorgyline (a second generation mono-amine oxidase inhibitor)—are effectively used in psychiatry to

Table 2. *Effects of Drugs as a Function of the Rat's Circadian-System-Stage on Induced Sleep, General Anesthesia, and Related Phenomena.*

Strain, age, sex	Chemical agent (fixed dose and multiple test times)	Variable investigated	Synchronization[a]	Chronopharmacologically induced changes	Refs.
Sprague-Dawley, adult	Pentobarbital sodium	Duration of anesthesia	L: 0600 to 1800 / D: 1800 to 0600 / And continuous L or D	Longest duration (peak time at ~1900) / Persisting rhythm in continuous L and/or D	Scheving et al. (1968)
Sprague-Dawley, adult	Pentobarbital sodium	Duration of anesthesia	L: 0800 to 2000 / D: 2000 to 0800	Longest duration of anesthesia at ~1700 coinciding with trough time of brain amines	Walker (1974)
Wistar, adult	Pentobarbital sodium	Induction time and duration of anesthesia	L: 0800 to 2000 / D: 2000 to 0800	Induction time and duration of anesthesia have their peak time at ~2000	Simmons et al. (1974)
Wistar, old	Hexobarbital sodium	Duration of anesthesia; hexobarbital oxidation in liver	L: 0700 to 1900 / D: 1900 to 0700	Longest duration of anesthesia and lowest oxidation at ~1800	Müller (1974)
Sprague-Dawley, adult	Hexobarbital sodium	Duration of anesthesia; hexobarbital oxidation in liver	L: 0600 to 1800 / D: 1800 to 0600	Longest duration of anesthesia and lowest enzyme activity at ~1400	Nair (1974)
Wistar, adult	Pentobarbital sodium	Induction time of anesthesia	L: 0600 to 1800 / D: 1800 to 0600	Peak time at ~1100 (January–May)	Bruguerolle et al. (1979);
Wistar, adult	Althesin	Induction time of anesthesia	L: 0600 to 1800 / D: 1800 to 0600	Peak time at ~1600 in October / Peak time at ~1000 in March	Bouyard et al. (1974)
Wistar, adult	Curarizing agents, e.g., pancuronium bromide	Neuromuscular activation	L: 0600 to 1800 / D: 1800 to 0600	Peak of the curarizing effect at 0800 in March and October	

[a] L = light; D = dark.

Table 3. *Effects of Various Agents, as a Function of Man's Circadian-System-Stage, on Induced Sleep, General Anesthesia, and Related Phenomena.*

Chemical agent (multiple test times)	Variable investigated	Synchronization	Chronopharmacologically induced changes	Ref.
Laudanum	Efficiency as narcotic	Presumably diurnally active subjects	Most efficient at night when going to sleep	Virey (1814)
Halothane	Lowest amount needed for anesthesia	Presumably diurnally active subjects	Best efficiency between midnight and 0600	Fukami et al. (1970)
Ethanol, 0.67 g/kg body weight	Iterative self-rating of ebriety; speed of random number additions	Sleep–rest (midnight to 0700); activity (0700 to midnight)	Maximum of ebriety and poorer performance follow ethanol at 1900 and 2300	Reinberg et al. (1975)
Dipotassic clorazepate, 50 mg p.o.	Circadian changes in plasma bioavailability	Diurnally active subjects	Greatest plasma peak height and shortest half-life when taken at 0700 (versus 1900)	Aymard and Soulairac (1979)
Diazepam and its hydroxylated metabolites, fixed doses	Sleep recording and self-evaluation of sleep	Diurnally active subjects	Activity of metabolites of diazepam may exhibit a circadian rhythm	Nicholson and Stone (1979)
(3-Alkyl pyrazolyl) piperazine (tranquilizer), 10 mg p.o.	Self-evaluation of sleep, etc.	Simulated abrupt 8-hr time zone shift	Better "quality" of sleep, less broken sleep, less tired on retiring than control (placebo)	Simpson et al. (1973)
Clemastine (antihistamine), 3 mg p.o.	Iterative self-rating of sleepiness	Sleep–rest (midnight to 0700); activity (0700 to midnight)	Increase of sleepiness by > 25% versus control (placebo)	Reinberg et al. (1978)
Terfenadine (antihistamine), 60 mg p.o.	Iterative self-rating of sleepiness	Sleep–rest (midnight to 0700); activity (0700 to midnight)	Decrease of sleepiness by < 25% versus control more often for R_x at 1900 than at 0700	Reinberg et al. (1978)

control unipolar depression and manic-depressive illness (Wirz-Justice and Wehr, 1983). The example of lithium effectiveness in changing the free-running circadian period is well documented. According to Wirz-Justice and Wehr (1982), lithium-induced lengthenings of free-running τ's have been exhibited by various types of functions in several different species: in Kalanchoe, a tropical plant—petal opening in constant green light (Engelman 1973); in cockroach—rest–activity cycle in constant dim light (Hofmann et al. 1978); in aplysia—action potentials of the isolated eye of this marine invertebrate in DD (Strumwas-ser and Viele, 1981); in desert rat—rest–activity cycle in constant dim light (Engelman 1973); in rat—rest–activity cycle in DD (Kripke and Wyborney 1980); in man—rest–activity cycle and temperature rhythm of healthy subjects in LL during the Arctic summer (Johnsson et al. 1979, 1980).

Changes in the circadian τ's resulting from the administration of lithium and also other antidepressant agents help to explain, at least in part, their effectiveness in the treatment of depression. If mental depression is related to an internal desynchronization [e.g., either changes in the phase relationship between circadian oscillators or changes in the period length of one or more oscillators, or both (Kripke 1982; Wehr et al. 1979, 1982)], antidepressant agents provide a chronopharmacologic tool for helping to control or minimize the pathological alteration of rhythms.

Understanding that chronopharmacology may entail two types of effects, i.e., different levels of effectiveness or toxicity as a function of the timed administration or effects upon temporal structure, is important from both a theoretical and practical point of view. Any drug, whether it be ethanol (Reinberg et al. 1975; Rutenfranz and Singer 1967) or a corticosteroid (Reinberg and Smolensky 1982), is capable of producing different effects depending on its biological timing. This capability is revealed by quantitative changes in rhythm characteristics—mainly the ϕ's and M's—of certain circadian variables. For example, corticosteroids quite often induce contingent alteration of pituitary–adrenal activities, including their circadian rhythms. The latter has repercussions on a wide range of functions because so many metabolic rhythms at the cellular level are synchronized by the circadian pattern of adrenocortical secretion, which plays the role of a pacemaker (Halberg 1967; Reinberg et al. 1971b).

Although most of our knowledge about chronopharmacology comes from studies involving circadian rhythms, the field of chronopharmacology is not restricted only to rhythms of 24 hr; chronopharmacologic applications involving periods of approximately 1 hr, 30 days, and 1 year (Knobil 1980; Reinberg and Lagoguey 1978; von Mayersbach et al. 1977; Reinberg 1974a; Smolensky et al. 1974) have been demonstrated. For example, a circamensual chronopharmacology in women has been explored in terms of the days of changing responsiveness to (1) chemical agents such as histamine (Smolensky et al. 1974), ethanol (Jones and Jones 1975), and synthetic estradiol (Yen and Tsai 1972) as well as to physical agents such as radiant heat and (2) drug-induced menstrual-rhythm alterations (Procacci et al. 1974; Reinberg 1974b; Smo-

lensky et al. 1974). However, only the circadian chronopharmacology is presently well documented.

New Concepts in Clinical Chronopharmacology
Chronopharmacokinetics (Chronokinetics)

Chronopharmacokinetics refers to rhythmic changes in either the bioavailability, disposition, pharmacokinetics, and/or excretion of a medicine via the urine, feces, sweat, saliva, or other route. When the administration time is manipulated, for example, when a medication is given as a single daily dose so that four fixed times of treatment are studied with respect to the 24-hr scale and with each time point of administration explored at weekly intervals, statistically significant circadian rhythms are usually demonstrable in the pharmacokinetics, that is "peak height," "span of time to peak," "half-life," "disappearance rate," and "area under the time-concentration curve (AUC)," etc.

For example, at the time of this writing, chronopharmacokinetic dependencies have been substantiated for certain analgesic and non-steroid antiinflammatory agents (Table 4) such as sodium salicylate (Reinberg et al. 1967; Reinberg et al. 1975), aspirin (Markewicz and Semenowicz 1979b), indomethacin (Clench et al. 1981), acetominophen and phenacetin (Shively and Vesell 1975), and aminopyrine (Shively et al. 1981). Chronopharmacokinetic changes have been detected also for theophylline and digitalis (Table 5), i.e., regular theophylline (Kyle et al. 1980a,b) and sustained-release theophylline (Scott et al. 1981; Smolensky et al. 1981, 1982), and digitalis (Carosella et al. 1979). This is the case for many drugs used in neurology and psychiatry (Table 6), including dipotassic clorazepate (Aymard and Soulairac 1979), hexobarbital (Altmayer et al. 1979), lithium carbonate (Lambinet et al. 1981), diphenylhydantoin (Garrettson and Jusko 1975), and nortripty-

Table 4. Clinical Chronokinetics of Analgesic and Nonsteroid-Antiinflammatory Agents.

Drug (dose/24 hr)[a]	Clock hours of R_x	Number and type subjects	Variables investigated	Major circadian changes of pharmacokinetic parameters	Refs.
Sodium salicylate (1 g) (a) per os	0700 1100 1900 2300	6 healthy adults, 3M, 3F	Urinary salicylate excretion	Duration of excretion longest with R_x at 0700 (22 ± 1.36 h). Urinary excretion 4 hr post-R_x greatest with R_x at 2300, smallest with R_x at 0700	Reinberg et al. (1967); Reinberg et al. (1975b)
Aspirin (1500 mg) (a) per os	0600 1000 1800 2200	6 healthy males, 20–21 yr	Plasma levels	Peak height (C_{max}) and largest area under the curve (AUC) both greatest with R_x at 0600, smallest C_{max} and AUC with R_x at 2300	Markiewicz and Semenowicz (1979b)
Indomethacin (100 mg) (a) per os	0700 1100 1500 1900 2300	9 healthy young adults, 7M, 2F	Plasma levels	Peak height greatest at 0700 and 1100, shortest t_{max} ~0700. No circadian change in AUC	Clench et al. (1977, 1981)
Acetaminophen (1 g) (a) per os	Before sleep and at 0830	4 healthy adult males	Acetaminophen urinary excretion	The rate of urinary drug excretion when R_x taken before sleep less than when taken at 0830	Mattok and McGilveray (1973)
Acetaminophen (975 mg/70 kg) per os	0600 1400	8 healthy adults	Plasma half-life	Half-life: 131.1 ± 8.0 min at 0600; 111.4 ± 9.8 min at 1400 (equaling a decrease of 15%; $P < 0.025$)	Shively and Vesell (1975)
Phenacetin (1.5 mg/70 kg) (a) per os	0600 1400	10 healthy adult males	Plasma half-life	Half-life: 57.3 ± 10.9 min at 0600; 48.1 ± 7.4 min at 1400	Shively and Vesell (1975)
Aminopyrine (2 mg/kg) (a) per os	0800 2000	12 healthy adults	Plasma and saliva	Circadian rhythms in aminopyrine half-life obliterated by fast. Reversal of eating times, reverses the diurnal variation. No effect of sleep deprivation	Shively et al. (1981)

[a] (a) = acute; (c) = chronic.

Note: Subjects synchronized with diurnal activity and nocturnal rest.

Table 5. *Clinical Chronokinetics of Theophylline, Digitalis, and Propranolol.*

Drug[a] (dose/24 hr)	Clock hours of R_x	Number and type subjects	Variables investigated	Major circadian changes of pharmacokinetic parameters	Refs.
Theophylline as Theolair (4 mg/kg) (c) 8 days per os	0100 0700 1300 1900	12 healthy adults, 8M, 4F	Plasma and salivary levels	AUC largest with R_x at 1900; longest time to peak with R_x at 1900. Peak height greatest with R_x at 0700. Elimination rate fastest with R_x at 0100	Kyle et al. (1980a,b)
Sustained-release theophylline as TheoDur (18.8 mg/kg/24 hr) (c) per os	0800 2000	13 asthmatic children (6–13 yr)	Plasma level	During the 4-hr span post-R_x when theophylline taken at 0800, drug levels higher ($\sim$7 μg/ml) (than those following the R_x at 2000 ($P < 0.001$)	Scott et al. (1981)
Theophylline (4.4 mg/kg/24 hr) (a) per os	0100 0700 1300 1900	1 healthy adult male	Plasma levels	Time to peak shortest with R_x at 0100 (longest with R_x at 1900). Peak height greatest with R_x at 0700 (least with R_x at 1900)	Kyle et al. (1979)
Theophylline (6.9 to 18.2 mg/kg) (c) 6 days per os	0800 2000	14 healthy adults, 7M, 7F	Serum levels	Serum concentration greater following R_x at 0700 vs 1300 with a nonalcohol aminophylline solution) and greater for a controlled-release capsule given at 0800 vs 2000	Lesko et al. (1980)
Digitalis (1 mg) (a) per os and i.v.	6 time points/24 hr	36 healthy adult males	Serum and urinary levels	With R_x at 1200 and 1600 plasma curves show a late second concentration peak. With R_x at 0800 no second peak but exponential disappearance rate	Carosella et al. (1979)
Propranolol (80 mg) (a) per os	0200 0800 1400 2000	8 healthy adult males	Plasma propranolol	Peak concentration of drug lower after R_x at 1400 than after R_x at 0800, 2000, and 0200 ($P = 0.1$, $P = 0.02$, respectively). AUC after R_x at 1400 lower than after R_x at 0800, 2000, and 0200 ($P < 0.005$, $P < 0.05$, $P < 0.005$, respectively)	Markiewicz et al. (1980)

[a] (a) = acute; (c) = chronic.

Note: Subjects synchronized with diurnal activity and nocturnal rest.

Table 6. *Clinical Chronokinetics of Drugs Used in Neurology and Psychiatry.*

Drug[a] (dose/24 hr)	Clock hours of R_x	Number and type subjects	Variables investigated	Major circadian changes of pharmacokinetic parameters	Ref.
Dipotassic clorazepate (50 mg) (a) per os	0700 1900	5 healthy adults	Plasma levels of N-desmethyl diazepam	At 0700 time to peak (1 hr) and half-life (3 hr) shortest, at 1900 time to peak (4 hr) and half-life (30 hr) longest	Aymard and Soulairac (1979)
Hexobarbital (500 mg) (a) per os	0200 1000 1800	6 healthy adults, 4M, 2F	Plasma levels	Terminal elimination slower at 1800 than at 0200; at 0200 $T_{max} = 1.8$ hr, $C_{max} = 7.5$ µg/l; at 1800 $T_{max} = 3.1$ hr, $C_{max} = 4.6$ µg/ml	Altmeyer et al. (1979)
Lithium carbonate (0.75–1 g) (c) per os	3 types of schedules	5 manic depressive adults	Urinary Li^+, creatinine, and urea	1/3 of the daily dose at 1200 and 2/3 at 2000 reduces both drug nephrotoxicity and large circadian changes in urinary Li^+ compared to 3 equal doses daily or a large dose only in the morning	Lambinet et al. (1981)
Diphenylhydantoin (overdose: 5 to 18 mg/kg) (c) per os	Unknown DPH plasma levels 44–76 mg/l	4 children, 2M, 2F (6–11 yr)	Plasma DPH, urinary HPPH	Urinary 5-(p-hydroxyphenyl)-5-phenylhydantoin (HPPH) excretion larger during the day (up to 75%/24 hr) than the night	Garrettson and Jusko (1975)
Nortriptyline (100 mg/dose) (a) per os	0900 2100	Healthy adults 10 M	Plasma nortriptyline, 10-hydroxy-nortriptyline	x̄ plasma nortriptyline level higher 2 and 3 hr post R_x at 0900 than at 2100 ($P < 0.05$); x̄ plasma 10-hydroxynortriptyline (10-HP) higher 1, 2, 3 and 4 hr post R_x at 0900 than at 2100; T_{max} for 10-HP faster after R_x at 0900 than 2100 ($P < 0.05$)	Nakano and Hollister (1978)

[a] (a) = acute; (c) = chronic.

Note: Subjects synchronized with diurnal activity and nocturnal rest.

Table 7. *Clinical Chronokinetics of Antibacterial, Anticancerous, and Other Agents.*

Drug[a] (dose/24 hr)	Clock hours of R_x	Number and type subjects	Variables investigated	Major circadian changes of pharmacokinetic parameters	Ref.
Erythromycin (250 mg × 4) (c) per os every 6 hr/3 days	0200 0800 1400 2000	24 healthy male adults	Plasma erythromycin	Peak height greatest at ~1130; time to peak shortest at ~2000; AUC largest at ~1200	Di Santo et al. (1975)
Ampicillin (500 mg) (a) per os	6 time points/ 24 hr	6 healthy male adults	Plasma ampicillin	Greatest plasma level 1 hr postadministration occurred ~1100	Sharma et al. (1979)
Sulfasymazine, sulfanilamide (1.5–3.0 g) (c) per os	0700 1900	14 adult patients, various diseases	Plasma levels and urinary excretions	Sulfasymazine: disappearance rate from plasma faster for R_x between 0700 to 1900 (half-life 2.6 times shorter) than between 1900 to 0700. Sulfanilamide: same trend but no statistically significant differences	Dettli and Spring (1966)
Cis-diammine-dichloroplatinum (60 mg m²) (a) i.v.	0600 1800	11 cancer patients	Urinary cis-DDP and creatinine	cis-DDP urinary concentration: peak height and largest AUC with R_x at 0600. Minimum nephrotoxicity (gauged by creatinine clearance) with R_x at 1800	Hrushesky et al. (1980)
D-Xylose (10 g) (a) per os	6 time points/ 24 hr	11 healthy young adults	Plasma and urine levels	Plasma peak height greatest at ~1100; plasma AUC largest at ~1130. Largest urinary excretion 2 hr post-absorption at ~1200	Markiewicz and Semenowicz (1979a)
Ferrous sulfate (100 mg) (a) per os	0700 1000 1900 2200	8 healthy adults, 4M, 4F	Plasma iron	Sideremia greater at 1900 (64.4 + 13.1 μg/100 ml) than at 0700 (28.0 ± 9.8)	Tarquini et al. (1979)
Potassium chloride (37 mEq) (a) i.v.	1200 0000	healthy adults, 5M	Plasma potassium	Plasma potassium increased by 40% more ($P < 0.01$) for R_x at 0000 than at 1200	Moore-Ede et al. (1978)

[a] (a) = acute; (c) = chronic.

Note: Subjects synchronized with diurnal activity and nocturnal rest.

line (Nakano and Hollister 1978). Table 7 indicates chronopharmacokinetic phenomena have been detected for antibacterial, anticancerous, and other medicines including erythromycin (Di Santo et al. 1975), ampicillin (Sharma et al. 1979), sulfasymazine, sulfanilamide (Dettli and Spring 1966), cis-diamminedichloroplatinum (cis-DDP) (Hrushesky et al. 1981), D-xylose (Markewicz and Semenowicz 1979a), ferrous sulfate (Tarquini et al. 1979), and potassium chloride (Moore-Ede et al. 1978). The chronokinetics of ethanol and corticosteroids have been studied as well and will be discussed subsequently in later sections of this chapter.

From a methodological point of view it should be mentioned that the data summarized in Tables 3–7 were obtained from subjects synchronized with diurnal activity and nocturnal rest. Information about the dose/24 hr (or range of plasma levels), acute and/or chronic administrations, and route (mainly per os or IV) is provided for each investigation. The number of timed administrations used, each one corresponding to a different test for the chronopharmacokinetic studies both with acute and chronic dosings of the investigated drug, is also indicated. In some experiments (erythromycin and diphenylhydantoin), administration is iterative (e.g., 250 mg erythromycin every 6 hr for 3 days) or as an overdose (diphenylhydantoin) leading to temporally varying, but persisting, high plasma levels. For the most part, chronopharmacokinetic studies were performed on healthy volunteers when common drugs (e.g., ethanol, aspirin, etc.) were investigated. Chronopharmacokinetic studies of drugs involving a toxic risk (e.g., lithium, cis-DPP, etc.) were investigated in patients requiring specific treatment.

In general, it appears that several (if not all) of the parameters characterizing the disposition of a drug vary predictably ac-

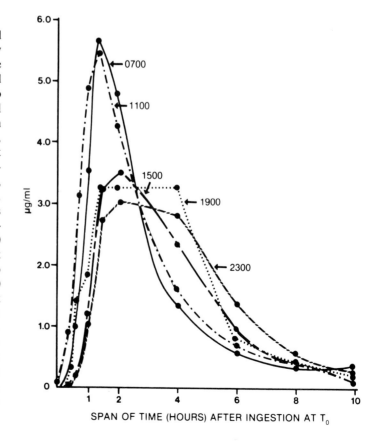

Fig. 2. In random order and at weekly intervals, 9 healthy subjects, 19–29 years of age (two females), synchronized with activity from 0700 to 0000, received a single oral dose (100 mg) of indomethacin at fixed hours: 0700, 1100, 1500, 1900, and 2300 (not at 1100 for two participants). Venous blood (sampled at 0, 0.33, 0.67, 1.0, 1.5, 2.0, 4.0, 6.0, 8.0, and 10.0 hr postingestion) was obtained for plasma drug determinations. Ingestion at 1900 and/or 2300 led to the smallest peak height and longest time to peak, while ingestion at 0700 and/or 1100 led to the largest peak height, shortest time to peak, greatest AUC, and fastest disappearance rate. A circadian rhythm of both peak height and time to peak was detected. (From Clench et al. 1981, reproduced with permission.)

SPAN OF TIME (HOURS) AFTER INGESTION AT T_0

cording to the time (clock hour) when treatment is given. In most cases, the amplitude (or the magnitude) of the circadian changes is not trivial. This fact can be deduced from inspecting Figs. 2 and 3 for indomethacin and Figs. 4 and 5 for theophylline. The data presented in the tables and figures provide further evidence that the metabolic fate of a pharmacologic agent should not be expected to be the same when administered at different times, and clearly prove that rhythms strongly influence the metabolism of medications. As discussed in the subsequent sections, it is likely that metabolic pathways are neither open permanently, nor open with the same patency throughout the 24-hr span.

Ethanol Chronopharmacokinetics. Over the years, there have been many studies of the chronokinetics of ethanol. Critical evaluation of the earlier conducted investigations was published by F. M. Sturtevant and colleagues (1975, 1976). The aim of these review papers was to substantiate the circadian rhythmicity of this well-investigated drug using both pharmacokinetic methods and models. F. Sturtevant concluded that the disappearance of ethanol from the blood follows the simplest of kinetic models. Special attention was given to the quantity β, Widmark's slope, of the ethanolemia linear decay curve. In addition, theoretical considerations were presented for chronovariation of the elimination constants for hypothetical drugs following exponential and zero-order models. F. Sturtevant concluded that: "1) rhythmicity within elimination curves can only be determined by repetition of the experiment at different times of the dial [24-hr] period and 2) the expectation that a rate constant estimated at one time of the day may be valid for another part of the day carries with it an unknown risk." The discussion that F. Sturtevant and this author commenced in 1975 still continues. For chronopharmocokinetic investigations, Sturtevant advocates the use of pharmacokinetic models based on sophisticated mathematical formulations, while the au-

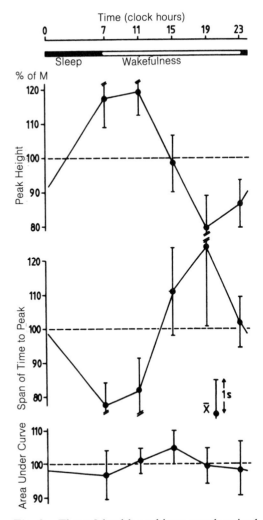

Fig. 3. These 9 healthy subjects synchronized with diurnal activity (0700–0000) and nocturnal rest were studied as described in the caption of Fig. 2. The results for the 3 parameters used to characterize the indomethacin bioavailability are expressed as a percentage of the group 24-hr mean, M, or circadian mesor for each considered variable. M (± 1 SE) is equal to (1) 5.09 $\pm$ 1.43 μg/ml for the peak height, (2) 2.17 $\pm$ 0.73 hr for the time to peak, and (3) 16.18 $\pm$ 0.56 μg/hr/ml for the AUC. Statistically significant peak–trough differences, amounting to more than 40% M, was observed for peak height (t = 3.9; P < 0.0025) and time to peak (t = 2.2; P < 0.0025), but not for the AUC. The greatest plasma concentration (peak height) occurred for an ingestion time (IT) between 0700–1100; the lowest corresponded to an IT of 1900. The shortest time to peak occurred for an IT between 0700–1100 and the longest for an IT of 1900. (From Clench et al. 1981, reproduced with permission.)

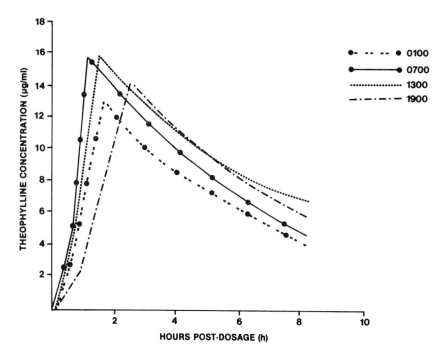

Fig. 4. Model time-concentration curves constructed with data from 13 diurnally active persons adhering to a 6-hr theophylline dosing schedule for 8 consecutive days. The model curves for the eighth day of dosing indicate theophylline when taken at 0700 or at 1300 was more quickly absorbed and produced higher immediate blood levels than when taken at 1900, when theophylline was eliminated most rapidly. (From Kyle et al. 1980a, reproduced with permission.)

thor of this chapter emphasizes the importance of more conventional methods and models (e.g., quantification of circadian changes based on the indices of peak height, time to peak, and AUC).

For example, orally induced ethanolemia was studied by Reinberg et al. (1975). Data were gathered from six healthy young adult males studied at fixed clock hours (0700, 1100, 1900, and 2300) with an interval of 1 week between consecutive tests and a 12-hr fast before the commencement of each. The order of the tests was randomized. Venous blood for ethanol determination was sampled immediately before and 15, 30, 60, 90, 120, 240, and 480 min after the ingestion of the fixed ethanol test dose, 0.67 g ethanol/kg body weight, under standardized conditions. Circadian rhythms were reported for the peak height (greatest peak for ethanol ingestion, R_x, at 0700), time to peak (short-

est time for R_x at 0700), AUC (largest AUC for R_x at 1900), and ethanolemia 140 min post-R_x (lowest for R_x at 0700). The calculated disappearance rate was greatest when ethanol was consumed at 0700. Similar results were obtained by Swoyer et al. (1975).

F. Sturtevant felt the conclusions of Reinberg and co-workers were not "wholly warranted" because T_{max} and C_{max} are affected by absorption and dosage in addition to ethanol elimination. With regard to the chronokinetic aspect, we agree with F. Sturtevant that, in 1975, the findings of many experiments had to be regarded as preliminary. However, new findings from experiments on both man and rat have added more information about the chronokinetics of ethanol. Minors and Waterhouse (1979) demonstrated a statistically significant circadian rhythm in the rate of ethanol

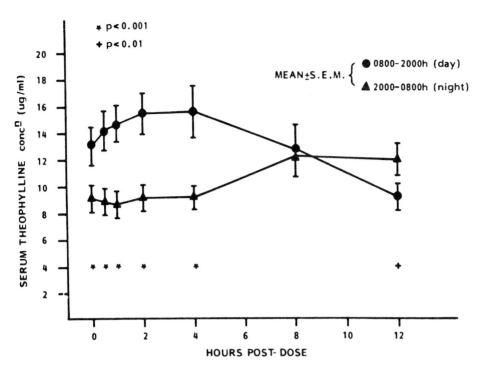

Fig. 5.   Differences in the blood levels of theophylline in 13 diurnally active young asthmatic patients given sustained-release theophylline (SRT) doses at 0800 and 2000. So-called "steady state" levels were achieved prior to samplings for theophylline. Blood levels of the SRT for the 4-hr span after the 0800 treatment in comparison to the 4-hr span after the 2000 treatment were statistically significantly greater. The SRT when given at 0800 immediately resulted in theophylline levels within the therapeutic range of 10–20 μg/ml; this was not the case for the 2000 SRT. (From Scott et al. 1981, reproduced with permission.)

removal in eight subjects (three males and five females). They ingested 0.8 g ethanol/ kg body weight once weekly; data on blood and urinary ethanol levels were obtained at regular intervals for the following administration times: 0100, 0500, 0900, 1300, 1700, and 2100. The rate of disappearance (β) of ethanol from the body was estimated from a least-squares regression of ethanol concentration in the series of 5 urine samples collected during the span from 120 min until 300 min post-ingestion. The acrophase of β, representative of the administration time resulting in fastest elimination, was 0757 for the male and 0244 for the female groups.

Investigations performed on mature male Charles River rats by R. P. Sturtevant (1978) and R. P. Sturtevant and Garber (1979) also demonstrated a circadian rhythm in the pharmacokinetics of ethanol. Animals were synchronized with 12 hr of light (L) alternating with 12 hr of darkness (D). Ethanol (1.5 g/kg body weight) was injected intraperitoneally at 6 different test times, equally distributed over the 24-hr scale. The ethanol disappearance rate was characterized by a large-amplitude circadian rhythm with the maximum occurring around the change from D to L (beginning of the inactivity phase) and a minimum 12 hr later. The LD cycle was an efficient synchronizer; when the LD cycle was advanced or delayed by 4, 8, or 12 hr, the acrophase of the circadian rhythm was similarly shifted in time. This circadian rhythm in β hypothetically is related to 24-hr rhythms in liver enzyme processes related to the oxidation of ethanol, e.g., into acetaldehyde. In fact R. P. Sturtevant and Graber (1981) demonstrated a circadian rhythm in liver alcohol dehydrogenase (ADH), a cytosolic enzyme using NAD^+ as coenzyme. The acrophase of this rhythm fits well with the hypothesis that this enzyme plays a role in the chronokinetics of ethanol, at least in acute administrations. According to R. P. Sturtevant (personal communication, 1981), circadian rhythmicity of microsomal ethanol-oxidizing enzymes utilizing $NADP^+$, rather than NAD^+, as coenzyme could be involved in the chronokinetics of rats chronically treated with ethanol.

With regard to the chronergy of ethanol in man, emphasis must be given to the fact that circadian changes in the effects of the drug have been demonstrated in rats (Walker and Soliman 1975) and man. The acrophase of self-rated ethanol-induced ebriety coincides with ethanol ingestion at 2300; on the other hand, the largest ethanol-induced decrease of oral temperature (24-hr mean) is associated with an ingestion at 0700 (Reinberg et al. 1975) (see Fig. 11).

Corticosteroid   Chronopharmacokinetics. Many experiments on rats and man have demonstrated that the occurrence or magnitude of side effects including adrenal suppression and desired effects such as increased grip strength and bronchial patency of various drugs, for example, corticosteroids, depends upon the circadian timing (Ceresa et al. 1975; Grant et al. 1965; Montalbetti 1974; Reinberg 1975; Reinberg et al. 1971; Reinberg et al. 1977; Reinberg and Halberg 1974; Segre 1966; Smolensky 1974; Smolensky et al. 1980). An important question still awaiting an answer is whether changes in effectiveness are related either to the chronokinetics of corticosteroids or to the chronesthesy of the target organs for these active agents, or to both. McAllister et al. (1981) studied the disposition of plasma prednisolone in six healthy male subjects (acute administration; 20 mg/24 hr; R_x at 0800 and 2000 on different experimental days scheduled at least 1 week apart) and in five chronic stable asthmatics who

had been treated previously with prednisolone daily for at least 6 months. No significant differences were found between the nighttime and daytime studies for any of the pharmacokinetic data (half-life, C_{max}, T_{max}, AUC, etc.) in either the asthmatic or healthy participants. On the contrary, Morselli et al. (1970) demonstrated chronopharmacokinetic changes for exogenously administered cortisol in man, mainly in the plasma disappearance rate. Their data showed the half-life of cortisol to be shorter when given at 1600 than 0800. In experiments on adult male Norwegian rats by English and Marks (1981), a circadian rhythm in the plasma disposition of methylprednisolone was demonstrated. Separate studies during which methylprednisolone (1 mg/kg body weight) was injected into the femoral vein were conducted at 0000, 0600, 1200, and 1800. The maximum half life (32.5 ± 1.5 min) of this corticoid occurred when it was injected at 1800, while the minimum (10.8 ± 0.9 min) occurred when it was injected at 1200.

It could well be that synthetic derivatives of corticosteroid hormones and cortisol have different chronopharmacokinetics, including an absence of circadian rhythmicity; however, with respect to the latter, the evidence is not convincing. Angeli et al. (1978, 1981) have shown that prednisolone as well as natural adrenocortical hormones exhibit a circadian rhythm in transcortin (the blood carrier protein for corticosteroid) binding. The lowest binding capacity occurs during the night around 0400; the highest capacity occurs around 1600. This means that higher free, and thus effective, plasma corticosteroid (both hormones and hormonoids) levels are reached during the morning and early afternoon. In addition, Angeli et al. (1981) have shown patients suffering from alcohol-induced chronic liver disease exhibit an altered circadian rhythm of plasma corticosteroid binding protein.

These illustrative examples demonstrate that (1) the quantification of the chronopharmacokinetics of an agent (especially in the case of corticosteroids) can be rather complex and (2) the chronergy of an agent (with regard to both desired and undesired effects) depends upon both its chronopharmacokinetics and the chronesthesy of the target biosystem(s).

Changes in Aspects of the Pharmacokinetic Curve of Certain Medications with Regard to the Timing of their Administration.   The pharmacokinetics of a given substance can be characterized by a curve of simple or complex shape. For the sake of both precision and standardization in quantification, mathematical pharmacokinetic models have been developed. The chronopharmacologic approach shows that, depending on the timing of some medications, not one, but two (or more) pharmacokinetic models are necessary. The pharmacokinetic model for most substances investigated thus far (see Tables 4–7) is roughly that of an open one-compartment type. This means that independent of the time (clock hours) of drug administration the curve used to describe the pharmacokinetics has only one peak. In such cases, chronopharmacokinetic changes concern parameters such as T_{max}, C_{max}, AUC, half-life, disappearance rate, etc. However, for some medications the pharmacokinetic curve may exhibit one peak when administered at one time of day, yet exhibit two peaks when administered at another. Two examples illustrate this point.

The first example deals with digoxin (Carosella et al. 1979). A single oral dose of 1 mg beta-methyl-digoxin (BMD) was given to 6 healthy diurnally active subjects at each of 6 different test times (0800, 1200, 1600, 2000, 0000, and 0400), each scheduled at weekly intervals. The administration of BMD at 2000 and 0000 was followed by a first order kinetics (one-compartment model) as evidenced by plasma concentrations. When given at each of the other times, the model was different. A second peak, characteristic of a two-compartment model, was exhibited when BMD was given at 0400, 0800, and 1200. The second peak of the time-concentration curve following

treatment at 1200 was found to be statistically significant using a computer program designed for quantifying pharmacokinetic phenomena. BMD given as a single dose (0.8 mg) intravenously at 1400 also exhibited a two-compartment model (Carosella et al. 1979). Moreover, a second peak was detected in the kinetics of BMD when given by injection at 1400. No matter how administered at 1400, there was roughly a 12-hr difference between the occurrence of the two peaks in the time-concentration curve.

The second example deals with mequitazine (Primalan), an antihistaminic medication derived from phenothiazine (with a quinuclidinyl group located on the nitrogen of position 10). The chronopharmacokinetics of this medication was studied by collecting urine samples from 6 healthy subjects treated at 0700 or 1900 (A. Reinberg, J. B. Fourtillant, F. Lévi, C. Peiffer, and A. Bicacova-Rocher, unpublished data 1983). A single 5-mg dose of mequitazine was given orally at 0700 and 1900, with the 2 time-point studies done at 7-day intervals. Urinary determination of the metabolites of mequitazine requires the combination of both gas-liquid-chromatography and mass spectrometry (so-called mass-fragmentography) for high precision, specificity, and reproducibility. The administration of the antihistamine at 0700 was associated with a time-concentration curve with 2 peaks, while its administration at 1900 was associated with an open one-compartment kinetics (Fig. 6). These time-related differences were depicted by all the subjects for both total mequitazine and conjugated mequitazine. At the present time, there is no explanation for the time-dependent nature of the pharmacokinetic models for either BMD or mequitazine. It could well be that circadian changes in the enterohepatic circulation play an important role, but this has not been demonstrated as yet.

Biomechanisms Presumably Involved in Chronopharmacokinetic Changes.   All the pathways affected by a chemical following entry into an organism may exhibit circa-

228   Alain Reinberg

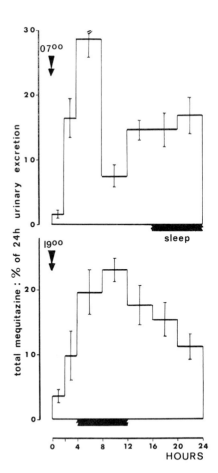

Fig. 6. Circadian time-dependency of pharmacokinetic models. A 5-mg dose of mequitazine (an antihistaminic agent) was given orally to 6 healthy subjects at 0700 and 1900, 1 week apart. They were synchronized with diurnal activity from ~0700 to ~2300, alternating with nocturnal rest. Determinations of mequitazine were made by mass-fragmentography techniques in total urine voidings collected at first every 2 hr (twice) and thereafter at 4 hr intervals during 24 hr. The results are graphed as the total mequitazine excreted per urinary collection interval, expressed relative to the entire 24-hr excretion, following each time-specified treatment, at 0700 or 1900. The kinetics were characterized by 2 peaks (a two-compartment model) when the antihistamine was ingested at 0700, and by 1 peak (a one-compartment model) only when given at 1900. (A. Reinberg, J. B. Fourtillan, F. Lévi, C. Peiffer, and A. Bicakova-Rocher 1983, unpublished data.)

dian rhythmicity. Thus, depending on the biological time, a particular metabolic pathway for a given drug may be open or closed. Moreover, the capacity to metabolize the drug may differ between pathways at different circadian stages. Some of these possibilities were considered above when discussing the chronopharmacokinetics of ethanol and corticosteroids. Obviously any biomechanisms thought to have a role in the pharmacokinetics of a drug must be explored from a chronopharmacokinetic point of view. However, relatively few medicines have been studied in this manner thus far, mainly in laboratory animal experiments.

Liver Metabolic Pathways. Radzialowski and Bousquet (1968) studied the circadian rhythmic activities of certain hepatic drug-metabolizing enzymes, such as aminopyrine N-demethylase, 4-di-

methyl-aminobenzene reductase, *p*-nitroanisole, and O-demethylase in male and female Holtzman rats and in male Swiss-Webster mice synchronized with light from 0630 to 2000 alternating with darkness. Livers were removed from groups of animals at 2-hour intervals over 24 hr. The activity of each of the enzyme systems exhibited a circadian rhythm with a peak around 0200 (second half of the activity span) and a trough around 1400 (second half of the rest span). Some of these circadian rhythms appear to be dependent upon adrenal activity, since they are altered by adrenalectomy and thereafter are restored by the administration of corticosteroids. Alteration of circadian rhythmicity also has been observed in rats pretreated for 4 days with phenobarbital, although the circadian rhythm of plasma corticosterone was not affected.

Nair (1974) found circadian variations in

both the hexobarbital effect (induced-sleep duration) and the hepatic hexobarbital oxidase activity (Fig. 7). Male Sprague–Dawley rats synchronized with 12 hr light (0600–1800) alternating with 12 hr darkness were given 150 mg/kg hexobarbital sodium intraperitoneally. The longest duration of induced sleep coincided in time (R_x at 1400—during the second half of the rest span) with the lowest enzyme (hexobarbital) activity and presumably the highest plasma disposition of the drug. These findings agree well with human data for induced-sleep duration (Reinberg 1981) and hexobarbital chronopharmacokinetics (Altmayer et al. 1979).

Pertinent to this discussion is the report of a circadian rhythm in the liver enzyme activity of tyrosine transaminase by Axelrod in 1968. In rats synchronized with light from 0500 to 1900 alternating with darkness, the acrophase of hepatic tyrosine transaminase activity occurs around 2300. When the lighting regimen is reversed (light from 1900 to 0500 and darkness from 0500 to 1900), the acrophase shifts; the ϕ occurs around 1200. Finally, when animals are maintained in constant darkness, the circadian rhythm of enzyme activity continues.

Kidney Metabolic Pathways. The excretion of some drugs is affected by the urinary pH. This is presumably the case, at least in part, for sodium salicylate, aspirin, and sulfasymazine. Dettli and Spring (1966) postulated the circadian chronopharmacokinetics of sulfasymazine is related to the circadian rhythm of urinary pH. Their data support this hypothesis (see Table 7). These authors suggest the kidneys may be regarded as a major oscillator when drug excretion is dependent on urinary pH. This is not the case with sulfanilamide, a drug for which these authors failed to find a statistically significant difference between disposition at 0700 and 1900.

A second example is provided by *cis*-DDP—an antitumor agent (Hrushesky 1981; Lévi 1982). Circadian rhythms in its urinary excretion, nephrotoxicity, and antitumor effectiveness have been detected. The *cis*-DDP urinary concentration shows

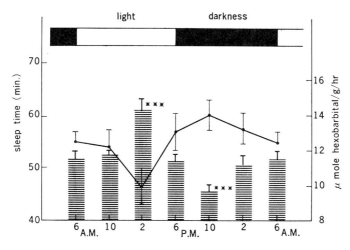

Fig. 7. Circadian variation in the duration of hexobarbital-induced sleep (*vertical bars*) compared to the circadian changes in hepatic hexobarbital oxidase activity (*solid line*). The duration of induced sleep at each clock hour of study represents the average of 6–10 animals. Hexobarbital sodium (150 mg/kg) was given intraperitoneally. The enzyme activity is expressed as μmoles of hexobarbital metabolized per gram tissue per hour; each datum represents the mean of 6–8 animals. The shorter *vertical lines* represent the standard errors; *** = $P < 0.001$. The timing of highest and lowest hexobarbital oxidase activity at 2200 and 1400 coincides with shortest and longest hexobarbital-induced sleep. (From Nair 1974, reproduced with permission.)

both greatest peak height and largest AUC when given at 0600. The lowest nephrotoxicity (gauged by creatinine clearance) occurs when it is given at 1800, a time when the *cis*-DDP urinary concentration reaches both lowest peak height and smallest AUC. A circadian rhythm of a tubular brush border lysozymal enzyme (n-acetyl glucose aminidase) seems to be involved in the circadian differences in the drug-related nephrotoxicity of *cis*-DDP. Chronopharmacologically, the best tolerance to *cis*-DPP corresponds in time to its highest effective antitumor activity.

A third example is provided by Lambinet et al. (1981) who manipulated the timed administration schedules of lithium carbonate for patients suffering from depression. In comparison to other schedules investigated, namely, equal doses at 0800, 1200, and 2000 or two-thirds of the daily dose at 0800 and the remaining one-third at 1200, lithium carbonate provided as one-third of the daily dose (750 to 1000 mg) at 1200 and the remaining two-thirds at 2000 reduced both the drug-associated nephrotoxicity (gauged by both creatinine and urea clearance) and the large-amplitude circadian rhythm of urinary Li^+ excretion.

Effects of Meal Timing. There is no doubt that the ingestion of food may affect the pharmacokinetics of an ingested drug. In addition, from a chronobiologic point of view, meal timing in man (e.g., single daily meal as a big breakfast versus a big dinner) is able to phase shift the acrophase of certain variables, such as plasma insulin, glucagon, and iron (Goetz et al. 1976) (see Chap. 7). For the most part, in human beings the acrophase of a great many circadian rhythms, such as plasma hormones, body temperature, blood cells, and psychological performance, remains unchanged or exhibits only minor alteration. These latter findings infer meal timing is not a powerful synchronizer in man, even if some rhythms show a temporal dissociation (Reinberg and Smolensky 1982). In comparison to human beings, meal timing in rodents (upon which

much chronopharmacologic research is conducted) can be a more important synchronizer for certain rhythms. Nonetheless, even in rodents meal timing is not a strong synchronizer for circadian systems, such as mitosis in some tissues (Pauly et al. 1975; Scheving et al. 1974; Philippens et al. 1977). Based on findings revealing meal timing to be a weak synchronizer at best in human beings, it is surprising, therefore, to read that the circadian rhythm in the half-life of aminopyrine is obliterated by fasting and the reversal of eating times inverts the "diurnal" variation (Shively et al. 1981). This might be true; however, before forming this conclusion the data from this experiment must be complemented with those from additional administration-time studies, since only two time points (0800 and 2000) have thus far been used.

The importance of this methodological aspect, i.e., the provision in experimental protocols of a sufficient number and distribution of time-point studies over 24 hr, must not be understated, especially when the conclusion is either alteration or absence of a drug's chronopharmacokinetics. With respect to this, the validity of McAllister's (1981) conclusion regarding the absence of chronopharmacokinetics for plasma prednisolone must be questioned since only two time points (0800 and 2000) were investigated. Again, it is possible that prednisolone fails to exhibit chronokinetics, but to be certain additional times of study, selected for pertinence with regard to both the synchronization schedule and biological temporal structure, are necessary.

Chronopharmacokinetic Changes with Regard to Some Physicochemical Properties of Drugs. Bélanger et al. (1981) demonstrated that chronokinetic differences between medications depend, at least in part, upon their physicochemical and dispositional properties. In their research, drugs were administered to male Sprague–Dawley rats. Data were analyzed using the open one-compartment model to calculate pharmacokinetic parameters. No circadian variation in the *absorption of drugs* was found if they were readily hydrosoluble, i.e., antipyrine, acetaminophen, and hydrochlorothiazine. On the other hand, significant circadian variation in the absorption rate constant was detected for the poorly soluble drugs, such as furosemide, indomethacin, and phenylbutazone. Temporal variations also were found for the *hepatic clearance of drugs* with high extraction ratios, like acetaminophen and antipyrine, but not for those with low extraction ratios, such as indomethacin and phenylbutazone. The *rate of elimination* of hydrochlorothiazide, a drug mainly excreted via tubular secretion, displayed circadian rhythmicity. Such changes have to be taken into account when explaining circadian differences in the effects of hydrochlorothiazide on the urinary excretion of potassium and sodium in man (Mills et al. 1975).

Circadian Changes in Plasma Proteins. Following absorption, some drugs become bound to plasma proteins; thus it is important to recognize the fact that plasma proteins undergo a circadian rhythm (Touitou et al. 1979). The discussion of transcortin in an earlier section of this chapter, based on the findings of Angeli et al. (1978, 1981), constitutes one example. In general, healthy young adults display a small-amplitude circadian rhythm in plasma proteins with a peak at 1600 and a trough at 0400. In elderly persons, the peak is slightly different, occuring around 0800; the trough still is at 0400. Due to this temporal pattern, a rapid change of about 20% may be found in the plasma protein levels of elderly persons between those clock hours corresponding to midsleep and awakening. This latter finding has been confirmed by Haus (personal communication, 1982).

Practical Implications of Chronopharmacokinetic Changes. Circadian rhythms in drug disposition must be taken into account for achieving, in comparison to non-time-qualified pharmacokinetic trials, both a better precision and a better understanding of the metabolic fate of medicines. Several examples serve to illustrate this.

Better Precision. In attempting to minimize the occurrence of undesired side-effects from theophylline (a bronchodilator used to treat asthma), it is recommended that the plasma concentration be occasionally monitored for up to several hours after an administration to ensure proper dosage. The aim of such clinical studies is to control the variability of plasma levels within narrow limits ($\sim$10–20 μg/ml), to ensure therapeutic goals, and to prevent side effects. When considering the results depicted in Figure 4, one can see that it is possible for the plasma theophylline levels to vary dramatically, from 3 to 15 μg/ml 1 or 2 hr after an oral administration of a nonsustained release form, depending upon the timing of the drug. Such temporal variation occurs with both acute and chronic administration schedules (Kyle et al. 1980; Smolensky et al. 1981). The interpretation of plasma theophylline determinations is meaningful only when the physician is provided with the particulars related to (1) the patient's synchronization schedule (particularly the timing of lights-on and lights-off), (2) the timing of the theophylline, (3) the timing of the blood sampling relative to the last administration time, and (4) other conventional information, such as dose, form, route, sex, age, and weight.

Better Understanding. Theophylline serves once again to illustrate this point. It is believed (and advertised) that sustained-release preparations ensure a relatively stable (constant) plasma level since the pharmacokinetics (presumably based on studies conducted during the daytime when the drug is given at 0800) exhibit a trapezoid-shaped curve with a plateau of the blood theophylline level within the therapeutic range. The latter does in fact occur, but with the possibility of dramatic differences between administration times as shown in

Figs. 4 and 5 (Scott et al. 1981; Smolensky et al. 1981, 1982; Kyle et al. 1980).

Based on new findings, it appears that the administration of a sustained-release or depot form of theophylline does not necessarily lead to a constant disposition. This point is very important not only for theophylline, but for other medicines as well. Even if a galenic preparation or a molecule has a rather long half-life, even if a drug is given iteratively as a constant dose and at short intervals, its pharmacokinetics (Di Santo et al. 1975; Lambinet et al. 1981) as well as its effectiveness (Touitou et al. 1976) with high probability will exhibit a circadian rhythm.

The metabolic fate of a pharmacological agent and nutrient (Apfelbaum et al. 1972; Gibson et al. 1974; Hardeland et al. 1973; Melani et al. 1975; Mirouze and Selam 1977; Reinberg 1974; Furuya and Yugari 1974) should not be expected to be the same for administrations during the day versus those during the night, since their metabolism will vary as a function of the (circadian) timing. Rhythms strongly influence the metabolism of medications and nutrients (Apfelbaum et al. 1972; Melani et al. 1975; Reinberg 1974b,c; Reinberg and Halberg 1971; Sensi et al. 1975). Metabolic pathways are neither continuously open; nor are they open with a constant patency over 24-hr or other bioperiodic domains. Furthermore, any rhythmic change in the pharmacokinetics of a medicine or in its effects presupposes rhythmic change in the susceptibility of the affected biosystem(s).

Chronesthesy of a Biosystem

Chronesthesy, defined as temporal changes in a biosystem's susceptibility to medications, takes into account rhythms of both molecular and membrane phenomena (see Chap. 3). The chronesthesy results from chronobiologic processes occurring in receptors, cells, tissues, organs, and systems of organs and gives rise to temporal susceptibilities observed in human beings, parasites, bacteria, and tumors. The organismic temporal structure accounts for the observation that biosystems can be completely unresponsive to a medication when given at one time in the 24-hr scale and yet be highly receptive (to the same dose) when given at another.

The chronesthesy can be expressed and quantified in terms of bioperiodic changes of receptors (Hughes et al. 1976; Spelsberg et al. 1979; Wirz-Justice et al. 1980, 1981; Wirz-Justice and Wehr 1983). For example, circadian rhythms of several rat brain neurotransmitter receptors have been reported by Wirz-Justice and Wehr (1983) and Wirz-Justice et al. (1981). Particular attention was given to the binding of ^{3}H-WB4101 to the α_1-adrenergic receptor, ^{3}H-dihydroalpronolol to the β-adrenergic receptor, ^{3}H-quinuclidinylbenzylate to the muscarinic receptor, ^{3}H-nalaxone to the opiate receptor, and ^{3}H-diazepam to the benzodiazepine receptor in forebrain homogenates. Both the α and β adrenergic as well as the opiate receptors were found to be most abundant during the dark (activity) span; the number of benzodiazepine receptors decreased to a minimum around the end of the light span. These findings were reproduced in studies during October and December–January. On the other hand, the cholinergic receptors exhibited a circadian periodicity only in December–January (peak at the beginning of the dark span). In October a 12-hr ultradian rhythm was exhibited with one peak during the mid-dark and another during the mid-light spans, respectively. Lithium, clorgylin, as well as fluphenazine may influence both the mesor and acrophase of some of the circadian rhythms of brain receptors (Wirz-Justice and Wehr 1983; Kafka et al. 1982). Circannual changes of receptors also have been detected. This is the case of the estrogen receptors of the uterus in ovariectomized female pigs (Hugues et al. 1976) as well as the progesterone receptors and nuclear acceptors of the chick oviduct (Spelsberg et al. 1979).

The chronesthesy of medications and other agents has been investigated more or less directly in human beings. Directly means here that the investigated agent reaches the target organ (e.g., bronchi, skin, perineural space, etc.) without being distributed by the blood and which does not involve chronokinetic changes. For example (Fig. 8), one measures the bronchial reactivity to inhaled aerosols such as histamine (De Vries et al. 1962; Tammeling et al. 1977), acetylcholine (Reinberg et al. 1971, 1974), orciprenaline—a β-receptor stimulating agent (Gaultier et al. 1975, 1977), iapropium bromide (SCH 1000)—a vagolytic agent (Gaultier et al. 1975, 1977), and

house dust extract in sensitized patients (Gervais et al. 1977). The chronesthesy of other types of agents is known also, for example the cutaneous reaction to intradermally injected histamine (Lee et al. 1977; Reinberg et al. 1965, 1969; Scheving et al. 1978, 1980; Smolensky et al. 1974), and to a histamine liberator (Reinberg et al. 1965) as well as the anesthetic response to betoxicaine, lidocaine, or mepivacaine (Reinberg and Reinberg 1977; Pöllmann 1980). Aspects of the chronesthesy of the latter are shown in Fig. 9.

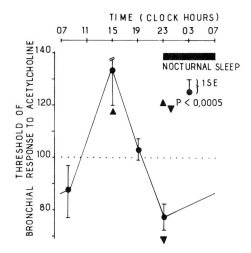

Fig. 8. These 8 healthy adults—smokers or exsmokers (4 women: 28–47 years of age and 4 men: 24–48 years of age)—were synchronized with L(0700–2300) and D(2300–0700). Serial determinations of the bronchial response to acetylcholine (ACh) were made at fixed hours (0800, 1500, 1900, and 2300) as one test per day on 5 different days, each separated by an interval of about 1 week. The order of the tests was randomized among the subjects. The ACh test at 1500 or at 0800 was done twice. Each measurement session began with 3 determinations of 1-sec forced expiratory volume ($FEV_{1.0}$). By successive assays the smallest quantity of ACh via aerosol inhalation (particle size $\sim 1~\mu$mm) was determined which provoked a 15–20% decrease of the $FEV_{1.0}$ recorded at the beginning of each session. The lowest threshold occurred at 2300 and the highest at 1500. (The variation between test times is shown as relative values from the group mean for all tests.) (From Reinberg et al. 1971a.)

Chronergy of Chemical and Physical Substances

Chronergy, defined as rhythmic variations in the effect(s) of any substance, whether desired (as a chronoeffectiveness) or undesired (as an iatrogenically induced chronotoxicity or even chronopathology), involves both chronopharmacokinetics and chronesthesies. It is not often that the chronesthesy of a medication coincides closely in time with the occurrence of the greatest blood level. Phase differences in rhythms of 24 hr, for example, in metabolic pathways and processes at various hierarchical levels of biological organization underlie the possible noncoincidence in timing of the acrophases of chronergies and serum drug levels, as exemplified by ethanol (Reinberg et al. 1974a, 1975a). For the purpose of simplicity and clarity, the information presented in Fig. 10 deals only with chronergies rather than chronokinetics. The data in this figure reveal that the antihistamimic effects of terfenadine in doses of either 20 mg or 60 mg differ in intensity and duration, as gauged by the inhibition of the cutaneous responsiveness, i.e., the erythema and wheal to intradermally injected histamine depending upon its administration time.

The chronergy of a medicine is not always easily demonstrable by usual methodological procedures. Pöllman (1980a), concerned with evaluating the effects of an analgesic, noramidopyrine (Novalgine),

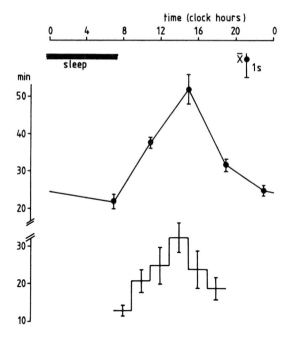

Fig. 9. Circadian changes in the duration (min) of local anesthesia produced by lidocaine. **Top curve:** In 6 apparently healthy adults synchronized with diurnal activity from 0700–0000 and nocturnal rest, 0.1 ml of a 2% lidocaine solution was injected intradermally every 4 hr during 24 hr, at specified clock hours. The flexor surface of both forearms was used exclusively. The duration of anesthesia was determined by measuring the time in minutes from injection to the recovery of cutaneous sensitivity. The duration was only about 20 min at 0700; it was 52 min at 1500 and about 25 min at 2300. Differences between the longest and shortest durations are statistically significant (P < 0.0005). **Bottom curve:** For rigorous standardization the study was restricted to selected patients suffering from decay (dentin caries) in a living, single-rooted upper front tooth. Lidocaine (2 ml 2% solution) was injected in the para-apical region. A stop watch was started at the end of the injection. Thereafter, the tooth was drilled to remove decay, but the cavity was left unfilled until the return of sensitivity as determined by a set of tests. A group of 35 subjects (apparently healthy apart from their tooth decay) was investigated. Each patient was treated only once. The timing of treatment was randomized between 0700 and 1900. There were 6 subgroups of 5–7 patients studied at 2-hr intervals. All subjects had diurnal activity and nocturnal rest. The duration of local anesthesia was about 12 min for the test interval from 0701 to 0900, about 32 min for that of 1301–1400 (P < 0.005), and about 19 min for that of 1701–1900 (P < 0.025). For both of these experiments illustrating the chronesthesy of a biosystem, differences between the longest and shortest effect are statistically significant. (From Reinberg and Reinberg 1977.)

used in addition a placebo. At several time points the effectiveness of the placebo and medication was tested against the application of a pain-inducing cold stimulus to the front teeth. Pöllman not only discovered circadian rhythmicity in the effectiveness of noramidopyrine, but found as well the same for the placebo. The chronergy of both the placebo and the analgesic did not

differ in peak (morning) and trough (night) times, although variance in the amplitude values between the rhythms of the analgesic and placebo effect was detected. At the peak time (1500), the analgesic was more effective than the placebo, while at the trough time, the difference between the effects of the two were small.

Many medications possess circadian

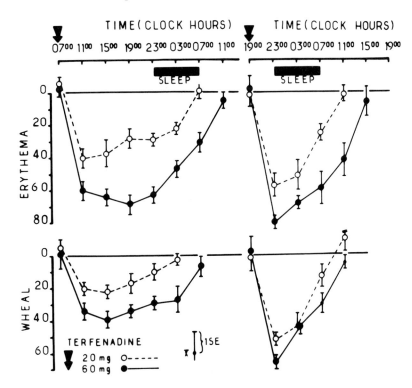

Fig. 10. Changes as a function of time (0700 vs. 1900) in the inhibitory effect of an antihistaminic agent (terfenadine) on skin reactions to histamine. There were 12 healthy human subjects (21–30 years of age) synchronized with diurnal activity from 0700 to 2300 and nocturnal rest. Ingestion of the antihistamine occurred at different times, i.e., 0700 or 1900, at weekly intervals. A double-blind and randomized (Latin square) procedure was used to test the effects of placebo and terfenadine (Merrell, Toraude), 20 and 60 mg, respectively. Intradermal (ID) injections of histamine (2 μg/0.1 ml saline solution) were made on the flexor surfaces of both forearms at 4-hr intervals and specified times during 28- to 43-hr study spans. Exact areas of both wheal and erythema were measured 10 min after the ID injections. The observed change for each variable—agent, dose, time point, subject—was expressed as a percentage of the corresponding value on the control curve (placebo). With reference to the histamine-induced erythema and wheal: (1) the duration of the antihistaminic effect was longer when terfenadine was ingested at 0700; (2) the maximum effect also was greater when it was ingested at 1900; (3) the time to reach maximum effect was longer when it was given at 0700; (4) the antihistaminic effects (extent and duration) of terfenadine were greater with 60 than with 20 mg, both at 0700 and 1900. (From Reinberg et al. 1978.)

chronergies manifested by effects upon processes related to sleep and anesthesia (Reinberg 1981) (see Tables 2 and 3). Circadian rhythms have been demonstrated in the effects of drugs used to anesthetize rodents and man. A circannual rhythm also has been detected (Bruguerolle et al. 1979). Chronopharmacologically induced changes of this nature over 24 hr presumably are causally related to circadian rhythms of brain amines (Walker 1974), liver enzymes (Müller 1974; Nair 1974), neuromuscular excitability (Bouyard et al. 1974; Bruguerolle et al. 1979), and certain toxic effects (Scheving et al. 1968, 1974). It is probable that any chronopharmacologic effect on sleep or anesthesia involves many circadian systems, so-called component rhythms, at various hierarchical levels of biological organization.

In man, circadian rhythms in performance and the subjective feelings of sleepiness can be objectively demonstrated and quantified. Subjects can be given forms to record iteratively every 4 hr at fixed clock hours self-assessments of eye–hand and random number addition skills as well as subjective ratings of fatigue and sleepiness. At each of several time points in the 24-hr span subjects indicate by a pencil stroke in the space of a horizontal rectangle (5 × 22 mm) a quantitive index of sleepiness. "Not sleepy at all" corresponds to making a mark at the far left side of the rectangle. The more the pencil mark is positioned to the right, the greater the sleepiness. Such autorhythmometric methods are useful for detecting and quantifying chronopharmacologic changes resulting from drugs which influence vigor, sleepiness, and vigilance.

Using these methods, Reinberg with Clench and others (1975) demonstrated circadian rhythmicity in the level of ebriety from ethanol ingestion in a dosage of 0.67 g/ kg body weight. The peak level of ebriety, self-rated 60 min after each ethanol ingestion, occurred after consumption of the dosage at 2300; least ebriety corresponded to ethanol ingestions at 0700 or 1100. The lowest decrement of performance in the random number addition test occurred after ethanol ingestion at 0700 and 1100. The best performance, without alcohol consumption, occurred around 1500, as is usually the case.

The circadian rhythm of ebriety differed in phase from those rhythms describing the ethanol chronokinetics. In diurnally active healthy subjects, the greatest peak height, shortest span of time to reach this peak, and shortest disappearance rate corresponded to an early morning, 0700, ingestion of ethanol. In comparison, ingestion at night, 1900 or 2300, was associated with the lowest peak of ethanolemia, the longest span of time to reach this peak, and longest disappearance rate. In consideration of the chronokinectics of ethanol, it is evident that the highest plasma level of a drug (i.e., ethanol) need not necessarily correspond to the maximum of its given effect—(i.e., for ethanol, ebriety and performance decrement).

Chronergic effects of ethanol on the oral temperature circadian rhythm have been detected in man by Reinberg et al. (1974, 1975). No matter when ethanol was ingested, no statistically significant induced change in the circadian A or ϕ of the oral temperature rhythm resulted. On the contrary, important changes were observed in the 24-hr mesor of this rhythm when it was ingested at 0700. The control M value (without ethanol) was 36.42° ± 0.06°C (1 SE). When the drug was ingested at 0700, a statistically significant decrease of M to 36.27° ± 0.06°C was observed. At other test times, ethanol failed to induce statistically significant changes in comparison with the control value (Fig. 11). For example, the M corresponding to the ethanol ingestion at 1900 was 36.45° ± 0.05°C. Figure 11 also illustrates the ethanol-induced change in the 24-hr mean (mesor) urinary excretion of adrenalin and noradrenalin. When ethanol was ingested at 1900, a statistically significant raise (as shown by the M value) in catecholamine excretion, relative to the control and the 0700 ethanol ingestion, occurred.

Hypothermia is reported to be associated with acute ethanol intoxication (Fournier and Gaultier 1955; Gervais 1966). In the chronopharmacologic investigation by Reinberg et al. (1974, 1974), no overt toxic effect was produced since the amount of ethanol administered was small. Nonetheless, the decrease of body temperature occurring after the 0700 test could represent a potential risk of a toxic effect. Following the 0700 administration, no change in the catecholamine M occurred. On the contrary, after the 1900 test an increased level of urinary (and presumably blood) catecholamines resulted without change in the body temperature M. Based on these findings, complementary mechanisms are proposed. According to Bruinvels (1979) noradrenaline can act centrally at the level of the hypothalamus to induce a temperature

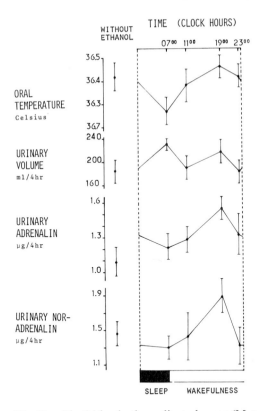

TIME (CLOCK HOURS)

WITHOUT
ETHANOL

07⁰⁰ 11⁰⁰   19⁰⁰ 23⁰⁰

ORAL
TEMPERATURE
Celsius

URINARY
VOLUME
ml/4hr

URINARY
ADRENALIN
μg/4hr

URINARY NOR-
ADRENALIN
μg/4hr

SLEEP   WAKEFULNESS

Fig. 11. The 24-hr rhythm-adjusted mean (M ± 1 SE) of 4 physiological variables after the ingestion of ethanol (0.67 g/kg body weight) at different test times (0700, 1100, 1900, and 2300). Control data were collected without ethanol. Tests were performed at least 1 week apart in random order. Subjects were 6 healthy young adult males synchronized with activities from about 0700 to 0000 and nocturnal rest. Subjects were fasting about 7 hr before and 7 hr after each ethanol ingestion. Measurements and integrated urine samples were gathered at 4-hr intervals. Relative to the respective control values, ethanol ingested at 0700 induced a decrease of temperature M but no change in catecholamine Ms; ethanol ingested at 1900 induced a rise of catecholamine Ms but no change of temperature M. The temperature decrease due to ethanol at 0700 is presumably related to drug-induced peripheral vasodilation not being counteracted at this time by a change in catecholamines. On the contrary, ethanol ingestion at 1900 being followed by higher levels of catecholamines presumably resulted in peripheral vasoconstriction compensating for the ethanol-induced vasodilation with no change of body temperature. (From Reinberg et al. 1975.)

rise. Gillespie (1967) and Wilkin (1981) found that ethanol has a peripheral vasodilatory effect on the cutaneous blood vessels which presumably results in heat loss. On the contrary, catecholamines have a vasoconstrictive effect. It could well be that temperature decrease occurring after the ethanol test at 0700 is associated with an ethanol-induced vasodilatory effect uncompensated by catecholamine stimulation when ingestion takes place at this time of day.

With regard to the chronopharmacokinetics of ethanol, the phasing of the circadian rhythm in a given effect need not coincide in time with the phasing of the rhythms in the peak height of ethanolemia or in disappearance rate. [According to Sturtevant (1976), change in the disappearance rate of ethanol from the blood is a better pharmacokinetic index than is peak height. Nevertheless, the circadian rhythms of these two parameters occur in phase with one another.] In the chronopharmacokinetic study by Reinberg (1974), the major body temperature decrease coincided with an ethanol ingestion at 0700. At this ingestion time, both the largest peak height and the fastest disappearance rate of this drug from the blood took place. However, the strongest stimulation of catecholamine excretion occurred when it was ingested at 1900, when both the peak height and the disappearance rate were relatively low. This finding, among others, was precisely the reason why the concepts of chronesthesy and chronergy were proposed in addition to (and in connection with) that of chronopharmacokinetics (Reinberg 1976a,b; Reinberg et al. 1975a,b).

Chronergic studies of ethanol also have a practical interest (Reinberg 1976b). Since a decreased body temperature is a symptom of a potentially harmful effect of ethanol, a higher chronotoxicity may be expected after its ingestion around 0700 than after other times, since this is the only time when a hypothermic effect, although slight, was noted with the dosage selected for research. Circadian changes in the acute chronotoxicity of ethanol have been examined in mice by Haus and Halberg (1959). Different groups of genetically similar animals standardized for rhythm study and then treated by a one-time-only injection of a fixed dose of ethanol responded differently depending on the circadian time of testing. Ethanol-induced mortality was highest when injections were given around the beginning of the animals' nocturnal activity phase; it was lowest in those animals injected with ethanol just before the beginning of their diurnal rest phase. Thus, results of experiments on mice and men are in good agreement; the harmful effects of ethanol are greatest when it is consumed at the start of the activity span. In keeping with the fact that ethanol is a toxic agent, its consumption in the morning has to be considered very dangerous for diurnally active man, especially if exposure to low environmental temperature occurs at this time of day.

Circadian changes in both the chronopharmacokinetics and chronergy of indomethacin, a nonsteroid antiinflammatory medication, for healthy persons were reported by Clench et al. (1975, 1977, 1981) as well as for the rat by Labrecque et al. (1979). In addition, the chronotherapeutics of this agent were studied by Job et al. (1981) in rheumatoid patients.

To investigate the indomethacin chronergy in human beings, several physiological variables were investigated at 2-hr intervals on control (without drug) as well as on test days using an open randomized, five-way crossover pilot study. A statistically significant oral temperature circadian rhythm was detected ($p < 0.05$) on control days and also on test days when indomethacin was given at 0700, 1900, and 2300, but not when given at 1100 or 1500. Moreover, a drug-induced rhythm alteration of both the A and ϕ occurred when 100 mg of indomethacin were administered at 1100 and 1500. There was no detectable difference between the temperature 24-hr mean (mesor) of the control and any of the test day values.

The rhythm alterations mentioned above appear to be related to transient changes occurring "n" minutes postabsorption. These transient changes expressed, for example, as the ratio of the *temperature 240 min postabsorption/temperature control day measured at the same clock hour* (T_{240}/T_c) also displayed circadian rhythmicity. A statistically significant transient decrease of oral temperature occurred when indomethacin was ingested at 1100 ($T_{240}/T_c = 0.98 \pm 0.001$), while an increase occurred when indomethacin was ingested at 2300 ($T_{240}/T_c = 1.019 \pm 0.001$). It can be concluded that the acute administration of 100 mg indomethacin at 1100 in diurnally active healthy subjects induced a transient decrease of the oral temperature which was responsible for the alteration of this circadian rhythm. Such transient effects on oral temperature did not result when indomethacin was administered at 0700, 1900, or 2300.

Job et al. (1981) studied the chronoeffectiveness of indomethacin in 4 nonhospitalized volunteer patients suffering from osteoarthritis during a 4-week, double-blind crossover, placebo-controlled and randomized chronotherapeutic study. Tablets were ingested at the fixed clock hours of 0800, 1200, and 2000. During 1 week, a placebo was given as a control. During the other weeks, only 1 of the 3 daily timed administrations contained the active 50 mg dose of indomethacin. Patients were given thermometers and forms to measure and record their oral temperature and to self-rate their pain and stiffness at 0700, 1100, 1500, 1900, and 2300 daily during the entire span of the study. Patients were socially synchronized with diurnal activity from about 0700 to about 2300 and nocturnal rest.

The acrophase of each detected circadian rhythm was not altered by changes in the timing of the drug's administration. Relative to the control span and the other times of treatment, indomethacin ingested at 1200 (50 mg/24 hr/7 days) appeared to have the most effect on the self-rated variables—a decrease of 60% in the 24-hr adjusted mean (mesor, M) of pain ($P < 0.0005$), a decrease of 54% in the M of stiffness ($P < 0.0005$), as well as a decrease of the oral temperature M. However, interindividual differences in the effectiveness of indomethacin given at either 0800 or 2000 were observed. Relative to the control span, three of the four patients exhibited a statistically significant (P < 0.025 to P < 0.0025) decrease of the oral temperature M when indomethacin was ingested at noon. The decrease of the temperature M for the fourth subject when given indomethacin at 1200 was not statistically significant. A decrease in the M also was noted in two patients treated at 0800 but in only one when treated at 2000. These findings again support the existence of a chronopharmacologic effect of indomethacin on the body temperature rhythm.

Time series of self-measurements and self-ratings have been used to study changes also in drowsiness induced by antihistaminic agents. For example, in a double-blind placebo, crossover study performed by Reinberg et al. (1978), clemastine (3 mg) was found to enhance sleepiness at all the time points of measurements, every 4-hr after taking the medication either at 0700 in one trial or at 1900 in another. On the contrary, terfenadine (60 mg) did not induce sleepiness in comparison with the placebo. When ingested at 1900, the antihistamine induced a decrease, rather than an increase, in sleepiness. These results agree well with those of Nicholson and Stone (1979), who used a different methodology to study the induced sleep resulting from several agents. Most antihistamines, such as clemastine, induce sleepiness, while terfenadine appears to do the opposite; it enhances vigilance.

The chronopharmacokinetics of a benzodiazepine have been investigated by Aymard and Soulairac (1979). Ingestion of 50 mg dipotassic clorazepate at 0700 was associated with the highest peak in plasma, the shortest time to reach this peak (1 hr), and the shortest half-life (3 hr) with reference to results obtained when the drug was taken at 1900. At this latter time, the span to reach the peak blood level was 4 hr and the half-life was as long as 30 hr.

Simpson and his coworkers in 1973 evaluated the potential of a tranquilizer: (3-alkyl pyrazolyl) piperazine or Quiadon as a chronobiotic—a drug which specifically affects aspects of the biological time structure. In this study, a double blind (Quiadon versus placebo) protocol was used. Twelve healthy males were submitted to a simulated 8-hr time zone change. Starting on the day of the "shift," each subject took his dose, approximately 10 mg daily at 2230. The "quality" of sleep was significantly better with Quiadon; subjects of this group felt less tired when retiring to sleep, had fewer total awakenings while at rest, and did not feel the need for a full 8-hr allocation of recumbency. By contrast, on the average, control subjects tended to have more disturbed sleep. Although feeling upon awakening "as rested as usual," they were "more tired than usual" on retiring.

Experimental results obtained thus far on man (Table 3) are in agreement with the empirical observations of Sydenham and Virey: if narcosis, general anesthesia, and drug-induced sleep are desired, medication promoting such effects should be administered not long in time before the anticipated beginning of spontaneous sleep. Both laboratory and field research document the existence of a "best (biological) time to sleep" (Akerstedt et al. 1981; Reinberg et al. 1973; Weitzman et al. 1970). However, the coincidence between the Sydenham–Virey phenomenon and the best time to sleep requires further investigation to gain a better comprehension of the involved mechanisms.

Pertinent to the chronergy of drugs which influence sleep states is the practical problem of sleep disturbances in shift-workers. Shift- and night-workers, being involved in nocturnal activities, must obtain sleep during the daytime. Chronobiologic and other types of studies have been devoted to adjustments of such employees to (1) "new" timings of activity and rest after each shift, i.e., resynchronization, (2) tolerance for shift work, and (3) interindividual differences in both resynchronization and tolerance (Colquhoun 1971; Rutenfranz 1978; Reinberg 1979; Reinberg et al. 1980).

Some employees seem to tolerate shift-work without difficulty and without health impairment for as long as 25 years or more. As a rule, tolerant subjects do not suffer sleep disturbances. In comparison those who are incapable of tolerating shift work exhibit sleep disturbances immediately, usually within 8 months or less, or at a much later age when reaching their forties or fifties, even after as many as 15 to 20 years of shift-work experience. Symptoms of intolerance are persisting fatigue (physiological fatigue disappears after a regular rest), gastrointestinal troubles, emotional irritability, mood alteration, and sleep disturbance—poor subjective quality of sleep, difficulty falling asleep, and disrupted sleep with frequent awakening. Clinical symptoms observed in workers intolerant of shift-work are in almost all cases associated with the use of sleeping pills—barbiturates, tranquilizers, antihistaminics, and other medications derived from plant alkaloids. In occupational medicine, regular reported use of sleeping pills is considered a clinical sign of intolerance to shiftwork (Andlauer et al. 1978; Scherrer 1980). Even if sleeping pills are useful under certain circumstances for short spans of time, such as a week or so, their regular use is of no aid in solving problems of intolerance to shiftwork or transmeridian flight (e.g., desynchronization related to jet lag).

Clinical Chronopharmacology and Drug Optimization

Although present chronobiologic research involves the examination of several different types of medications in preparation for clinical trials of specific drugs, chronopharmacologic findings have already made significant impact in the clinic with regard to the scheduling of long-term synthetic corticosteroid therapy. A higher degree of benefit and safety, in comparison to conventional (nonchronobiologic) administration schedules, has been achieved with various types of synthetic corticosteroids through consideration of the existing chronergies manifested at different hierarchical levels. Taking into account both time-dependent benefits and risks has resulted in a so-called chronoptimization for these types of medications. Adverse and undesired effects of conventionally timed (homeostatically scheduled) corticosteroid administration both during and following treatment are related at least in part to the critical drop of the endogenous glucocorticoid production following corticosteroid-induced ACTH inhibition. This often results in low cortisol secretion following drug withdrawal; sometimes the result is an iatrogenically induced adrenal insufficiency. Both conditions are undesired and dangerous side effects of corticotherapy. Another type of adverse effect, disturbance of the circadian temporal structure, results from conventionally scheduled corticosteroid treatment. This is exhibited not only by the pituitary–adrenal axis but also by certain other circadian functions, such as those underlying airway patency, muscular strength and activity, urinary and plasma 17-OHCS, as well as potassium and sodium metabolism (D'Agata et el. 1968; Martin and Hellman 1964; Martin and Mintz 1965; Montelbetti 1974; Nichols et al. 1965; Reinberg et al. 1971, 1974c,d, 1978; Reindl et al. 1969; Segre and Klaiber 1966; Serafini and Bonini 1974; Smolensky 1974; Smolensky et al. 1980).

Traditional attempts to reduce the major, undesired side effects of synthetic corticosteroids most often have involved changes in their molecular structure, their vehicle, or route of administration. These interventions, which are conventional ones, are based upon homeostatic conceptualizations of pharmacologic processes. The level of success achieved by the conventional approach has not been very encouraging; the chronopharmacologic approach, on the other hand, has contributed significantly (see Table 1). The chronotherapy of corticoids consists of treatment at fixed hours in the 24-hr scale so as not to inhibit the endogenous secretion of cortisol. For subjects with diurnal activities and nocturnal rest from about 2300 to 0700, the plasma cortisol acrophase is expected in the morning, around 0800. When a synthetic (or natural) corticosteroid preparation is given at a time differing greatly from the cortisol acrophase, for example, 10–12 hr later or earlier, as a single daily dose (Ceresa and Angeli 1977; Ceresa et al. 1969; Martin and Hellman 1964; Segre and Klaiber 1966; Reinberg et al. 1971b, 1974c; Reindl et al. 1969) or when the total daily amount is given in equally divided doses with different timings (Grant et al. 1965; Nichols et al. 1965; Reinberg et al. 1971b, 1974c; Smolensky and Reinberg 1976), endogenous cortisol secretion is inhibited and reduced and/or a set of physiological circadian rhythms is altered.

A significant step forward toward a practical chronocorticotherapy was achieved by Ceresa et al. (1969), Montalbetti (1974), and Reinberg et al. (1978). Utilizing a particular

combination of corticoids, each one having different characteristics of absorption and metabolism, and scheduling administrations to specified clock hours (0800 and 1500 with consideration of the synchronizer, i.e., sleep–wakefulness pattern in the 24-hr scale) to minimize inhibition of endogenous ACTH production, a way was found to preserve the temporal structure without sacrificing clinical and pharmacologic objectives obtainable by the conventional administration of larger doses of corticoids but which have been associated with undesired side effects (Montalbetti 1974). The favorable results achieved by this so-called plurichronocorticoid (the preparation consists of more than one type and form of synthetic corticoids which are administered at specific clock hours coinciding with designated circadian stages) represent a practical and new application of corticoid chronopharmacokinetics and pituitary–adrenal chronesthesies. Table 8, summarizing Cosinor findings, shows that for one pluricorticoid, Dutimelan 8–15, the

Table 8. *Circadian Rhythm in 17-OHCS Urinary Excretion of Nine Asthmatic Adults Before (no R_x) and During (R_x) 1-Month Chronotherapy: Dutimelan 8–15 mite.*

Experimental situation	Rhythm detection (P)	Rhythm adjusted mean (M ± 1 SE)	Amplitude A (95% CL)	Acrophase ϕ in hr and min ϕ ref: 0000 (95% CL)
Before Dutimelan day −2 and −1	<0.005	0.93 ± 0.13	0.45(0.29–0.62)	1333(1207–1458)
During Dutimelan				
R_x days no. 10–11	<0.005	1.11 ± 0.23	0.59(0.33–0.84)	1235(1048–1419)
R_x days no. 20–21	<0.005	1.38 ± 0.25	0.53(0.21–0.86)	1410(1141–1639)
R_x days no. 30–31	<0.005	1.16 ± 0.21	0.41(0.18–0.64)	1130(0908–1346)

Units for M and A = mg/4 hr.

M values correspond to 4-hr excretion; M × 6 = 24 hr excretion.

Urinary 17-hydroxycorticoids. Single Cosinor summary.

The aim of the study was to test (during a 1-month chronic administration) the optimization of corticoid medication resulting from a standardized time-treatment. Subjects: 9 adults (5 females: 18–55 years; 4 males: 41–60 years) suffering from allergic asthma with a previous history of steroid dependency. Synchronization: diurnal activity from ~0700 to ~2300 and nocturnal rest; spontaneous diet. Corticoids: Dutimelan 8–15 mite (DTMm) with dragée A (prednisolone acetate: 4 mg; prednisolone alcohol: 2 mg) at 0800; dragée B (prednisolone alcohol: 1.5 mg; cortisone acetate: 7.5 mg) at 1500. Total urine voidings were collected every 4 hr at specified times during a 48-hr span on control days and on days 10–11, 20–21 and 30–31 thereafter. 17-hydroxycorticosteroids (17-OHCS, Porter Silber) were determined in each sample. Statistically significant circadian rhythms were validated in the studied variables both before and during the sustained chronocorticotherapy. More specifically, this latter had no effect either on the acrophase (peak time) or on the mesor M (24-hr mean) of the urinary 17-OHCS circadian rhythm.

Source: Reinberg et al. (1977).

level of urinary 17-OHCS (indicative of adrenocortical function) did not decrease over several weeks' administration during which the successful management of asthma was achieved. It also reveals that the ϕ of the urinary 17-OHCS rhythm during treatment did not vary relative to the control span. This indicates at least for this variable, nondisturbance of temporal structure.

However, as far as drug chronoptimization is concerned, an important question was not completely answered. With regard to allergic asthma, do corticosteroid administrations at 0800 and 1500 [e.g., Dutimelan 8–15 (referred to as DTM 8–15)] differ in effect in comparison to when they are administered later, such as at 1500 and 2000? To answer this question a double-blind, cross-over randomized, and placebo-controlled chronotherapeutic study was designed by Reinberg et al. (1983). During an 8-day span, 8 patients suffering from corticosteroid-dependent allergic asthma were given DTM 8–15 plus a placebo at 2000. (At 0800 the administration contained 7 mg prednisolone acetate plus 4 mg prednisolone alcohol; at 1500 it contained 15 mg cortisone acetate plus 3 mg prednisolone alcohol.) During another 8-day span, patients were given placebo at 0800, while at 1500 they were given an administration containing 15 mg cortisone acetate plus 3 mg prednisolone alcohol and at 2000 they were given 7 mg prednisolone acetate plus 4 mg prednisolone alcohol. This latter administration schedule is referred to as R_x 15–20. During wakefulness between 0700 and 2300, every 2 hr at fixed clock hours, peak expiratory flow (PEF) and dyspnea were self-measured and self-rated. For each of the 8 patients the PEF 24-hr mean was lower, and the nocturnal dip was greater (P < 0.05 to P < 0.0005) with R_x 15–20 than with DTM 8–15. Moreover, the nocturnal dyspnea was greater with R_x 15–20 than with DTM 8–15. Chronic administration of the DTM 8–15 was more effective in controlling asthma and improving PEF than was the R_x 15–20. Considering both the side

effect of adrenal inhibition and the beneficial effect of improved airway function, it appears that the chronocorticotherapy with DTM 8–15 as opposed to R_x 15–20 resulted in the more successful optimization.

Steroid-responsive disorders may be managed by adrenocorticotrophic hormone (ACTH) and/or synthetic corticosteroids. Investigation of circadian chronergies of the adrenal cortex reveals both *quantitative* as well as *qualitative* time-dependencies of ACTH. In a recent study, both the clinical and metabolic attributes of a new synthetic peptide with 17 amino acids, ACTH 1–17 (Synchrodyn), were evaluated using a chronopharmacologic methodology (Reinberg et al. 1980b, 1981a,b). Eight healthy adult males between 18 and 30 years of age volunteered for the study. All were synchronized with diurnal activity from 0700 to 0000 and nocturnal rest. Investigations extended over 6 consecutive weeks (19 January to 25 February 1980) with individual time-point trials at weekly intervals during a series of 3-day tests starting on a Saturday and lasting until the subsequent Monday. On separate Sundays, a control or ACTH test was conducted at 0700, 1400, and 2100 during which either saline or 100 μg ACTH 1–17 was injected IM.

During each 3-day test of 72 hr duration a number of variables were evaluated every 4 hr, at fixed clock hours: self-rating of fatigue, oral temperature, heart rate, grip strength, peak expiratory flow (for estimation of bronchial patency), and urinary excretion of 17-OHCS, K^+, Na^+, Ca^{2+}, and Mg^{2+}. On Sundays, venous blood was sampled prior to control or ACTH injections at one of the study times, i.e., 0700, 1400, or 2100, as well as 20, 40, 60, 90, 120, 150, and 180 min thereafter. Plasma cortisol, testosterone, and aldosterone were radioimmunoassayed.

With regard to the 24-hr mean of the considered physical variables, injection of ACTH 1–17 at 0700 was followed, relative to control data, by the largest diminution of fatigue and the largest gain in both grip strength and PEF. The 24-hr mean of both oral temperature and heart rate was not altered. In comparison to the control data, ACTH injection at 1400 resulted in a small, but statistically significant, rise of both the PEF and oral temperature 24-hr means. Relative to control data, ACTH at 2100 was followed by a reduction in fatigue and an improved grip strength. With respect to effects upon human circadian time structure, as gauged by acrophase shifts and/or rhythm detections, no alterations due to ACTH injection at 0700 resulted. In comparison, the circadian rhythms of fatigue, oral temperature, heart rate, grip strength, and PEF were altered by ACTH injection at 1400, as were the circadian rhythms of fatigue and heart rate when ACTH was injected at 2100.

A strong and statistically significant rise of plasma cortisol was induced after every one of the timed ACTH injections. The obtained mean response curves were similar in form and parallel. Greatest plasma cortisol response followed the 0700 injection; the smallest one followed treatment at 2100 (Figs. 12 and 13). The plasma cortisol response to ACTH 1–17 at 1400 was intermediate. Cosinor analysis of the time series data indicates that the largest cortisol response to ACTH 1–17 is in phase with the crest time (ϕ) of the circadian rhythm of plasma cortisol as found by control studies. Both saline (nonstimulated) and ACTH-stimulated plasma cortisol levels had a ϕ of 0900.

Circadian rhythms of ACTH-induced

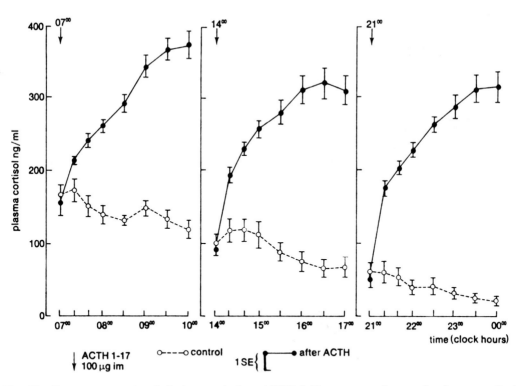

Fig. 12. Response curves of plasma cortisol to ACTH 1-17 represent changes in plasma cortisol levels (ng/ml) from before saline or ACTH injections at, respectively, 0700, 1400, and 2100 and at 20, 40, 60, 90, 120, 150, and 180 min after each timed injection. Control values varied according to the expected circadian rhythm of the healthy subjects. A strong response to the 100 μg ACTH injection was obtained regardless of the time of day. However, over all time points the highest levels followed the ACTH injection at 0700; the lowest ones followed ACTH at 2100. (From Reinberg et al. 1980b.)

244   Alain Reinberg

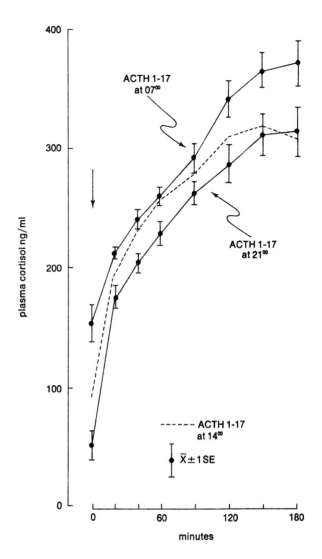

Fig. 13. Comparison of response curves of plasma cortisol with reference to the selected clock hours of ACTH injection. The 3 curves exhibit the same trend but at different overall levels. The highest response curve corresponds to ACTH 1-17 injected at 0700; the lowest corresponds to ACTH 1-17 injected at 2100. (From Reinberg et al. 1980b.)

changes in urinary 17-OHCS are displayed in Figure 14. Greatest elevation followed the injection of ACTH 1–17 at 0700, while the smallest elevation followed that given at 2100. Such changes can be seen also by examining the total urinary excretion of 17-OHCS over each 24-hr span subsequent to each time point of ACTH injection. Reference values are given by the 24-hr urinary excretion of 17-OHCS on control days when saline was injected. Differences between control and ACTH treatments were statistically significant. Statistically significant differences were noted also between the time points of ACTH treatment. ACTH

injected at 0700 induced a 24-hr urinary excretion of 17-OHCS approximately 4 times greater than control values [ACTH = 17.00 ± 1.70 mg/24 hr ($\bar{x}$ ± 1 SE); control = 4.51 ± 0.39 mg/hr]. Injections at 1400 or 2100 led to an output of 17-OHCS which was approximately 3 times and 2 times the control values, respectively (at 1400 ACTH = 11.60 ± 1.20 mg/24 hr, control = 4.47 ± 0.45 mg/24 hr; and at 2100 ACTH = 8.49 ± 0.80 mg/24 hr, control = 4.25 ± 0.42 mg/24 hr).

With regard to the circadian acrophase of the urinary 17-OHCS rhythm, only a small shift occurred after ACTH injection

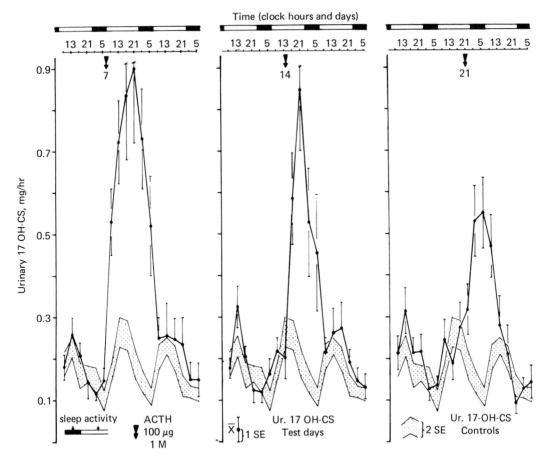

Fig. 14. Changes in the 4-hr urinary excretion of 17-OHCS due to ACTH 1-17 (100 μg). There were 8 healthy young subjects studied. For both control and ACTH-related changes, urinary 17-OHCS are expressed in mg/hr; the represented time point corresponds to the middle of the 4-hr span of each total urine voiding (e.g., time point at 0500 corresponds to the amount of 17-OHCS in the urinary sample collected from 0300 to 0700). *Shaded area:* reference circadian rhythm substantiated 3 times during a 72-hr span. Shaded area extends from −1 to +1 SE before (R_x day −1 day) and after (R_x day and R_x day +1 day) each of the ACTH injections (test days). The greatest change in 17-OHCS excretion (both amount and duration) occurred after the ACTH injection at 0700; while the smallest change occurred after the ACTH injection at 2100. There was no alteration in the peak time of the urinary 17-OHCS rhythm after the injection of ACTH at 0700. The peak time was delayed, with regard to the saline control, when ACTH was injected at 1400 or at 2100. (From Reinberg et al. 1980b.)

at 0700; while a large shift occurred after the injection at 2100 (Fig. 14). These acrophase shifts (Δφ) were quantified by Cosinor analyses. With reference to the acrophase of the circadian rhythm of urinary 17-OHCS which was found to be 1453 during the control span, the Δφ was approximately 4, 6, and 14 hr due to ACTH at 0700, 1400, and 2100, respectively.

As stated before, experiments with ACTH were performed in January-February 1980. In order to investigate the hypothesis that the effectiveness of ACTH is not only related to its administration with regard to the time of day but also to the time of year, a second experiment was conducted during June-July 1981. Both experiments were conducted under almost identical conditions and with the same subjects. Figure 15 presents the 24-hr adjusted means for the urinary concentration of 17-OHCS. Drastic differences in the ACTH-induced changes are evident for both the time of day and the time of year. In winter the stimulation was greatest when ACTH was injected at 0700; it was least when it was injected at 2100 ($P < 0.0005$). In summer the circadian time of greatest effect was different; during this time of the year ACTH produced its greatest effect when given at 1400 ($P < 0.05$

to $P < 0.02$). There was no statistically significant seasonal difference between the ACTH-induced response at 0700 or 2100. In addition, the adrenocortical responsiveness was greater in summer than in winter, particularly when ACTH was injected at 1400 or 2100 ($P < 0.0005$); the 17-OHCS Ms were twice as high in summer as in winter. The difference in the Ms at 0700 was not statistically significant. Control values were higher in winter than in summer.

It must be remembered that any change thus expressed as a 24-hr excretion in fact corresponds to the area under a time-concentration curve. This is one index which can be used to analyze the ACTH-induced response; others include the peak height (C_{max}) and the span of time to reach the peak (T_{max}). Peak height as well as the span of time to reach it from individual time series and experimental circumstances were measured precisely. Peak heights were expressed in μmol/hr and thereafter averaged as shown in Fig. 16. It is clear that the peak height was greatest for ACTH stimulation at 0700 and least at 2100, both in winter ($P < 0.0025$) and summer ($P < 0.05$). In addition, the peak heights were greater in summer than in winter for both ACTH when administered at 1400 ($P < 0.01$) and at 2100 ($P < 0.0025$); the peak height also was greater in summer than in winter for ACTH administered at 0700 ($P < 0.05$). Since the urine voidings were collected every 3 to 4 hr after treatment, this parameter could be rather accurately estimated. Overall, it appears that the strongest ACTH-induced stimulation occurred after the ACTH injection at 0700, both in winter and summer. This was the case for each of the subjects as well as the group average.

Time to peak (T_{max}) with regard to sampling intervals was measured (in hours and decimal fractions) from the injection time to the middle of the sampling interval during which the 17-OHCS peak occurred. There was no statistically significant difference in the time to peak related to either the time of the day or the time of the year. T_{max} corresponding to the injection of ACTH at 0700

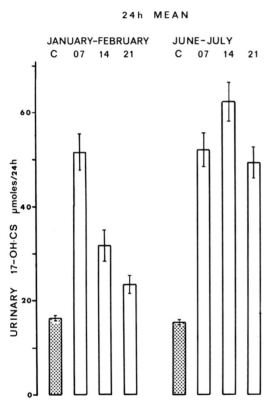

Fig. 15. Change in the 24-hr excretion of urinary 17-OHCS resulting from ACTH 1-17 injections (100 μg IM) at 3 different clock hours (0700, 1400, and 2100) both in winter (January-February) and summer (June-July). Placebo control: *shaded areas*. Means are given in μmol/ 24 hr ± 1 SE. Maximal stimulation occurred for ACTH at 0700 in winter ($P < 0.0005$) and at 1400 in summer ($P < 0.05$ to $P < 0.025$) in comparison to the other time points of ACTH injection studied.

PEAK   HEIGHT

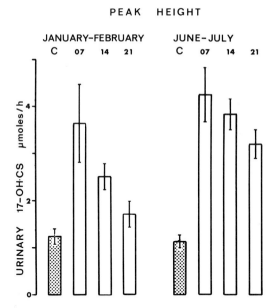

Fig. 16. Changes in the peak height (C_{max}) of urinary 17-OHCS following an IM injection of 100 μg ACTH 1-17 in January-February and June-July at each of 3 separate clock hour studies (0700, 1400, and 2100). Means are given in μmol/hr $\pm$ 1 SE. Maximal stimulation always occurred after ACTH injection at 0700; least stimulation followed that at 2100 ($P < 0.0025$ in winter and $P < 0.05$ in summer).

was 10.6 $\pm$ 1.4 hr ($\pm$ SE) in winter and 10.8 $\pm$ 1.8 hr in summer; T_{max} corresponding to the injection of ACTH at 1400 was 8.3 $\pm$ 0.9 hr in winter and 9.4 $\pm$ 1.4 hr in summer. Unlike the C_{max}, the T_{max} of the adrenal response to ACTH apparently depends on neither the time of the day nor the time of the year. It is of interest to note that both in the winter and in the summer, ACTH (100 μg IM) injected at 0700 reduced fatigue and enhanced both grip strength and bronchial patency of the healthy young diurnally active adults without alteration of the circadian time structure of these rhythms.

In summary, ACTH (100 μg IM) injected at *0700* reduced fatigue and enhanced both the grip strength and bronchial patency of healthy young diurnally active adults without alteration of the circadian time structure of these rhythms. These desirable ef-

fects are presumably related in part to the fact that the greatest effect of ACTH upon the adrenal cortex, that is, cortisol stimulation, occurred when given in the morning at 0700. This is when cortisol levels ordinarily are most elevated in comparison to 1400 and/or 2100 when lowest levels are expected. In addition, however, desirable ACTH 1-17-induced effects may be related to non-corticoadrenal-mediated events (Reinberg et al. 1980b, 1981a,b).

Based on these examples of synthetic corticosteroids and ACTH, the importance of rhythmically modulated therapy should not be underestimated. This is exemplified also by the treatment of adrenal insufficiency whether due to Addison's disease or hypophysectomy. Substitution steroid therapy for patients suffering from adrenal insufficiency achieves best therapeutic efficiency when a chronopharmacologic approach is used (Reinberg et al. 1971b, 1974c, 1979). Unequally timed doses of cortisol, such as two-thirds or three-fourths of the daily dosage in the morning around 0700 and the remaining fraction later around 2300, produces better results than does the homeostatic one consisting of three equal doses daily—one before or after each meal.

The specific effectiveness of both synthetic corticosteroids and ACTH with regard to the large organ chronesthesy and the persistence of the temporal structure indicates that these two hormonal substances possess statistically and clinically significant circadian chronopharmacologies. Yet it appears that hormonal effects may exhibit not only a circadian chronopharmacology, but also a circannual one, as suggested by studies of human chorionic gonadotropin (HCG) as well as ACTH. Lagoguey et al. (1980) and Lagoguey and Reinberg (1981) studied both time of day and time of year (May–June and October–November) differences in the testicular response to HCG of 4 healthy young adult male volunteers. Each subject was studied twice yearly for responses to a set of 6 different tests. The effect on plasma testosterone of 2500 IU/0.5 ml HCG (Organon) or saline given as intramuscular injections was evaluated at 3 different time points. Studies were done at weekly intervals. The weeks and order of the fixed clock-hour treatments of the 6 tests (3 control and 3 HCG) were randomized. Venous blood was sampled immediately before and 30, 60, 90, 150, and 240 min after each injection of saline or HCG. Changes occurring after the IM administration of HCG in each individual, both with respect to the time of day and the time of year, were referenced to the plasma testosterone control values of the corresponding time of day and year.

Plasma testosterone changes were evident in several ways. The mean plasma testosterone level *without HCG stimulation* was higher in the morning as compared to the evening. It was higher in autumn than in spring. For all subjects and times of year, HCG given at 0700 failed to increase the testosterone level relative to the control values. On the contrary, a statistically significant rise of testosterone (P < 0.01 to < 0.0005) relative to the control levels followed the 2000 HCG injection. HCG stimulation at 1400 resulted in an intermediate effect compared to responses at other times of administration (Fig. 17).

The area under the plasma testosterone concentration-time curve also varied with treatment time. The area (in arbitrary units, for example, cm^2) was expressed individually for each subject in each situation—time of day, time of year, control, and after HCG stimulation—and averaged thereafter. Control values ($\bar{x} \pm 1$ SE) were taken as reference. The response to HCG was strongest at 2000 and weakest at 0700 (Fig. 18). The response was stronger during May and June than during October and November, for example at 2000.

Although several examples of hormonal chronopharmacologies have been put forth, the fact is a wide variety of chemical substances exhibit highly significant circadian rhythms in effects. Such chronopharmacologies constitute the basis for the chronoptimization of therapeutic agents, including carcinostatic ones. Even though Chapter 4

reviews the chronergy of carcinostatic medications, the topic is relevant here as well. Findings from several large-scale investigations on rodents conducted by Halberg (1974), Halberg et al. (1977b), and Haus et al. (1972, 1974) substantiate circadian susceptibility–resistance cycles to cyclophosphamide and arabinofuranosylcytosine (ara-C), two widely used antitumor medications, in mice experimentally given L-1210 acute lymphatic leukemia. A conventional treatment schedule, consisting of 8 equal doses given at equal intervals, of ara-C over the 24-hr span was compared with eight sinusoidally varying dose schedules, each schedule differing from one another in phasing with respect to the acrophase and bathyphase (trough) over the 24-hr span. Both survival time and cure' rate, when compared to the conventional equal-interval dosing schedule (homeostatic approach), were statistically significantly improved by the chronochemotherapy (Halberg et al. 1977b; Haus et al. 1974). These findings as well as others (Levine and Halberg 1972; Simpson 1977; Taviada et al. 1975) (see also Chap. 4) suggest the importance of a chronotherapeutic approach for administering highly potent treatments associated with undesired side effects or toxicity.

Attempts already have been made to chronoptimize the use of powerful anticancerous agents such as *cis*-diamminedichloroplatinum (*cis*-DDP). This agent has proved to be efficient for cancer therapy but harmful to the kidney. Recently, Hrushesky et al. (1980), Lévi et al. (1980), and Lévi (1982) demonstrated the advantage of chronotherapy for *cis*-DDP. Nephrotoxicity can be reduced relative to that produced by conventional *cis*-DDP schedules, even with the administration of high doses to achieve desired effects. Preliminary results obtained from a limited number of patients have shown that adriamycin given at 0600 with *cis*-DDP given at 1800 is better tolerated and apparently more effective (with regard to a set of conventional indices) than when the same drugs in the

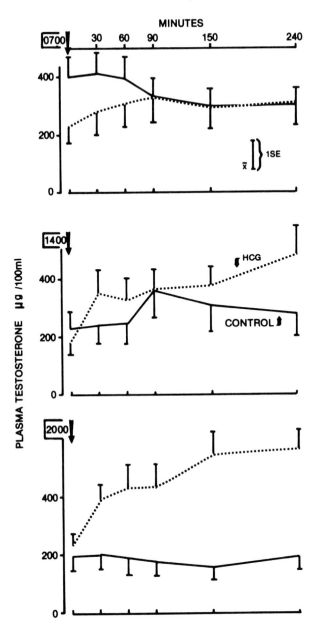

MINUTES

Fig. 17. Circadian rhythm in the responsiveness of the gonads as the rise in the level of plasma testosterone of 4 healthy young males given HCG (2500 IU HCG organon IM). At weekly intervals, HCG or saline (control) was injected at a fixed clock hour (0700, 1400, and 2000). The 6 (3 control and 3 HCG) tests were randomized. Venous blood was sampled immediately before and 30, 60, 90, 150, and 240 min after each injection of saline or HCG. Tests were performed twice in May–June (trough of plasma testosterone circannual rhythm) and in October–November (peak of plasma testosterone circannual rhythm). Raw data were pooled (May–June and October–November) and averaged for each time point determination ($\bar{x} \pm 1$ SE) to visualize the response curve for HCG. A statistically significant stimulation occurred only when HCG was injected at 2000. (From Lagoguey and Reinberg 1980, reproduced with permission.)

same doses are timed in a reverse manner (e.g., *cis*-DDP at 0600 and adriamycin at 1800).

The findings discussed in this section make clear the error of the homeostatic approach for chemotherapy, that is the belief that repeated constant doses in the 24-hr scale lead to consistent and constant effects. As shown by Scheving et al. (1974) and Haus et al. (1972, 1974) in mice, the ef-

fect of equal, time-invariant doses results, as a rule, in unequal responses. Similar findings have been demonstrated in man for medications other than cytostatic agents including time-invariant doses of ethanol (Wilson et al. 1966), erythromycin (Di Santo et al. 1975; Halberg 1974); lithium (Lambinet et al. 1981), and metyrapone (Touitou et al. 1976). Administration of these agents at different circadian stages

TEST TIME OF BOTH DAY AND YEAR

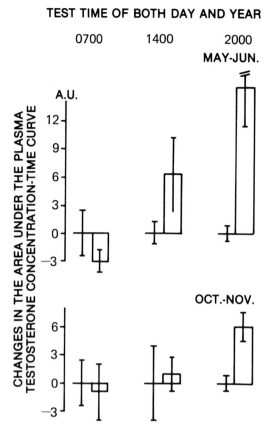

Fig. 18. Circannual rhythm in the responsiveness of the testes of 7 healthy young human males to 2500 IU HCG, IM. See caption for Fig. 17 for the experimental design of the study. Relative changes in the area under the plasma testosterone concentration-time curve are presented in arbitrary units (cm^2) with reference to the mean control curve value of each of the 6 time points of study. Individual changes were calculated, averaged, and expressed as $\bar{x} \pm 1$ SE. No stimulation occurred when HCG was injected at 0700; a strong stimulation occurred when HCG was given at 2000. The circadian chronergy of HCG was demonstrated both in May–June and October–November. In addition, the relative responsiveness was greater in May–June than in October–November, depicting a circannual modulation in the circadian chronergy of HCG. (From Lagoguey and Reinberg 1980, reproduced with permission.)

results in circadian changes in the serum concentration of ethanol and erythromycin or in the urinary excretion of lithium as well as tetrahydro-11-deoxycortisol in the case of metyrapone.

New Aspects of Chronopharmacology: Time-Qualified Hormone Administration Induces Qualitative Changes

Results presented thus far have dealt with *quantitative changes* in the effects and metabolism of chemical agents as a function of administration time. *Qualitative changes* may result also from time-qualified hormone administrations. The word "hormone" is derived from a Greek verb meaning "to excite." Not only the intensity of excitation, but also the specific action of a natural or synthetic hormone depends on the time structure of the organism.

A straightforward demonstration of qualitative differences due to specific clock hour administrations of a hormone comes from the work of Margules et al. (1972). This group studied the effect of L-noradrenalin on the hypothalamic control of feeding behavior in rats. For research purposes, a device was implanted to deliver to the lateral hypothalamus a precise quantity of L-noradrenaline. Depending on the time of day (with regard to both the animal's synchronization and the time structure of the rat), L-noradrenaline had different effects. It stimulated feeding behavior during the light span, while during the dark span it inhibited it.

Another example of qualitative changes (e.g., stimulation versus inhibition) comes from research by Knobil and his group (1980) who studied the control of gonadotropin secretion in rhesus monkeys. The discovery of an ultradian rhythmicity of about 1 hr (so-called "circhoral") by Dierschke and his colleagues (1970) for plasma LH was a very significant finding.

Knobil and his group (Nakai et al. 1978; Belchetz et al. 1978; Knobil 1980) demonstrated "the functioning of the hypophysiotropic control system, which directs gonodotropic secretion, is obligatorily intermittent." GnRH, a decapeptide produced by the hypothalamus, specifically stimulates pituitary LH secretion. GnRH, LH, and FSH secretion exhibit physiological ultradian rhythmicity of about 60 min. Hypothalamic lesions, which destroy the arcuate nuclei of female monkeys, abolish the endogenous production of GnRH. Continuous GnRH infusion of female monkeys does not reinitiate gonadotropin secretion. On the other hand, the rhythmic infusion (1 pulse/hr) of the decapeptide does reestablish normal pituitary function. Periodic changes in GnRH secretion permit regeneration of the pituitary receptors for this decapeptide, whereas continuous (nonrhythmic) stimulation does not. The ultradian rhythm of stimulation was found to have an optimal period of 60 min in the arcuate-lesioned and ovariectomized rhesus monkey. The most effective mode of GnRH administration for restoring and maintaining both LH and FSH secretion was 1 mg/min for a duration of 6 min/hr. A period of 12 min (5 pulses GnRH/hr) had an effect similar to that of continuous perfusion: it did not restore the abolished secretion of LH and FSH, and it abolished the pituitary secretion previously restored by the circhoral administration of GnRH. A period of 20 min (3 pulses GnRH/hr) as well as a period of 30 min was less effective or had an inhibitory effect in comparison to the optimal period of 60 min.

A GnRH infusion period of 3 hr caused a change in the LH/FSH ratio. Although GnRH infused at this frequency had only slight effect on the mean plasma LH levels, it did induce elevated FSH plasma titers. In other words, the manipulation of the ultradian period of the rhythmic GnRH infusion not only stimulated or inhibited the LH and FSH secretion by the pituitary but also influenced the respective bioavailability of

these hormones. Emphasis must be given to the role played by the *periodicity,* rather than to the *quantity,* of GnRH delivered, since varying the amplitude (or conventionally speaking, the dose) of the GnRH pulses has little regulatory effect (Wildt et al. 1979). Possible chronotherapeutic uses of these findings have already been illustrated by Naftolin (1978) and Valk et al. (1981) in controlling abnormal (both hypo- and hyper-) secretions of LH in certain specified gynecological diseases.

A third example of a time-dependent change in the specificity of hormones is provided by human chronopharmacologic studies with ACTH 1–17. As indicated earlier, this compound of 17 amino acids was tested by Reinberg et al. (1981a) in 8 healthy human males in a January experiment. Either 100 μg of ACTH or an equal volume of saline (control) was injected IM at different clock times at weekly intervals, either at 0700, 1400, or 2100. Venous blood was sampled before and 20, 40, 60, 90, 120, 150, and 180 min after ACTH or saline injections at each of the aforementioned time points. Radioimmunoassay methods were used for plasma cortisol, testosterone, and aldosterone determinations.

The injection of ACTH 1–17 at 0700 was followed by a clear and statistically significant rise of plasma testosterone. To the contrary, no change was observed, relative to the control spans, when ACTH was injected at 1400 or 2100. The Cosinor method was used to quantify circadian rhythm parameters of plasma testosterone data from both the control and ACTH study spans. The acrophase, corresponding to an injection time inducing the strongest testosterone response measured between 20 and 180 min after ACTH injection, was 0510 (95% CL = 0416–0604). This acrophase was comparable to that for the unstimulated (non-ACTH-stimulated) circadian rhythm of plasma testosterone, being 0348 (95% CI = 0238–0458). In addition, both the amplitude and mesor of the circadian rhythm of serum testosterone were lower in control than in

ACTH-stimulated plasma testosterone studies.

In summary, the data from the ACTH 1-17 study reveal *quantitatively* different effects on both plasma cortisol and testosterone levels depending on the (biological) time of administration. Both are maximally increased following the 0700 injection of ACTH. Very interestingly, the ACTH effect also varies *qualitatively* with respect to administration time. An ACTH injection given at any time will stimulate aldosterone secretion relative to the control values (Fig. 19). However, the data clearly reveal a maximum effect upon plasma aldosterone secretion when given at 1400. Cosinor analysis of control (saline injections) and ACTH-stimulated plasma aldosterone data reveal similar circadian acrophases of around 1400. That is, under usual condi-

tions, the ϕ in aldosterone is about 1400 and the elevation in aldosterone secretion as a response of the adrenal to ACTH is maximum around the time of the maximum basal secretion, at 1400. Considered together, the findings indicate that ACTH has its major effect on plasma cortisol and testosterone when injected at 0700, around the time of the circadian acrophase for each. Its major effect on plasma aldosterone occurs when injected at 1400, around the time of the circadian acrophase of aldosterone under usual circumstances. Such qualitative chronopharmacologic changes are likely to be related to a programed difference in the timing of cortisol, testosterone, and aldosterone secretion by the adrenal cortex. Apart from physiological interest, these experimental findings can be used to optimize ACTH injections, since in most cases it is

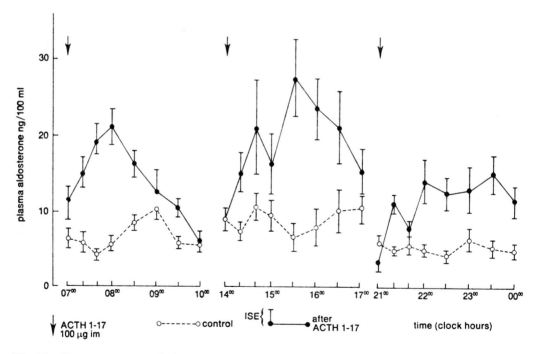

Fig. 19. Response curves of plasma aldosterone to ACTH 1-17 when injected at different times of the day. Changes in plasma aldosterone levels (ng/100 ml) prior to saline (*control*) and ACTH injections at, respectively, 0700, 1400, or 2100 and 20, 40, 60, 90, 120, 150, and 180 min thereafter. Control values varied according to the predictable circadian rhythm of healty subjects. A response to the 100 μg ACTH injection was obtained regardless of the time of day. However, highest aldosterone levels were obtained for the ACTH injection at 1400; the lowest were obtained when ACTH was given at 2100. (From Reinberg et al. 1981a.)

the increase of plasma cortisol which is desired rather than that of aldosterone.

Conclusions

Chronopharmacology involves both the investigation of drug effects as a function of the biological timing as well as the investigation of medications upon temporal structure. The occurrence of regular and thus predictable changes over the span of 24 hr in biological susceptibility and responsiveness to a large variety of physical as well as chemical agents is rather common.

In this chapter, a large number of illustrative examples of human chronopharmacologies has been presented. A wide variety of medicines and chemical agents has been studied in man from a chronopharmacologic point of view. These include reserpine, antihistaminics (cyproheptadine, terfenadine, clemastine, and mequitazine), synthetic ACTH and steroids (dexamethasone, flumethasone, triamcinolone, cortisol, prednisone, and methylprednisolone), and others such as ethanol, [(3-alkyl pyrazolyl) piperazine, Quiadon—a tranquilizer], insulin, chlorothiazide, halothane, prostaglandin, lithium, clofibrate, indomethacin, theophylline, digoxin, and cis-DDP, for example. Although the major focus has been placed upon quantitative and qualitative aspects of circadian chronopharmacology in human beings, it must be pointed out that chronopharmacology is not restricted to the 24-hr domain only; it can be extended to rhythms with periods both greater and shorter than 24 hr. For example, a circamensual chronopharmacology in women requires consideration of changing responsiveness to chemical and physical agents during the menstrual cycle as well as to drug-induced circamensual rhythm alteration. The major reason that emphasis is placed upon circadian chronopharmacology herein is because only this aspect has been well documented thus far.

In this chapter new concepts have been introduced to precisely describe rhythm-dependent effects and activities of medications. These concepts include the following.

1. The *chronokinetics* of a drug refers both to rhythmic changes in drug bioavailability (or pharmacokinetics) and excretion (urinary, among others). The chronokinetics of sodium salicylate, indomethacin, ethanol, ampicillin, erythromycin, digoxin, digitalis, benzodiazepam, theophylline, mequitazine, acetaminophen, phenacetin, propranolol, lithium, diphenylhydantoin, nortriptylin, cis-DDP, ferrous sulfate, and potassium chloride have been demonstrated in man.

2. The *chronesthesy* of a biosystem to a drug refers to changes in the susceptibility of any biosystem (organ systems, parasites, etc.) to medications and other chemically active substances, in general. The chronesthesy of the skin and bronchi for various agents has been shown in man.

3. The *chronergy* of a drug takes into consideration the chronokinetics and the chronesthesies of involved biosystems resulting from exposure to medications or other agents. The term chronergy includes rhythmic changes in the overall general as well as specific effectiveness of medications.

Concepts and findings from investigative chronobiology and clinical chronopharmacology are pertinent and, in certain instances, indispensible for solving problems of drug optimization—enhancement of desired efficiency and/or reduction of undesired effects. This is exemplified most dramatically by the chronocorticotherapy of various steroid-dependent disorders. The chronopharmacologic approach seeks not only to improve the utilization of currently available medications, but to influence the formulation and evaluation of future chemotherapeutic agents. It is fully recognized that additional research is required to evaluate the potential of chronopharmacology in the clinic. To achieve this end additional scientists, well trained in the methods of chronobiology, are required. Currently, advances in chronopharmacology are occurring through the untiring efforts of a relatively small group of investigators. It is anticipated that the teaching of chronobiology to an increasing number of young scientists and physicians will encourage continued research into the potential of chronopharmacology. Nonetheless, the optimization of therapeutic agents based on chronopharmacologic findings is already being applied. This is the case for the administration of corticosteroids and ACTH. This could well be the case for the chronochemotherapy of cancers, since impressive results obtained from laboratory animal experiments (Chap. 4) are now being extended to the treatment of human cancers by clinical investigations performed on small groups of patients (Hrushesky et al. 1980; Lévi et al. 1980).

The development of chronotherapy is also related to the diffusion of methods of data gathering and time series analysis. A set of physiological and/or pathological phenomena can be self-measured and/or self-rated by hospitalized patients educated in these procedures for subsequent use when at work and at home. It is thus possible to attain two major goals with regard to the chronotherapy of a given medication: (1) achieving large-scale trials involving, say, 250 patients or more and (2) learning how chronotherapy can be individualized, taking into account differences between patients.

Acknowledgments

The author is grateful for the many stimulating discussions about chronopharmacokinetics provided by Lawrence Scheving (University of Arkansas), Frank M. Sturtevant (Searle Laboratory), RuthAnn P. Sturtevant (Loyola University, Illinois), David Minors (University of Manchester, U.K.), Alberto Angeli (University of Torino, Italy), Gaston Labrecque (Université Laval, Québec), and Yvan Touitou Francis Lévi (Université de Paris).

References

Altmayer, P, Mayer, D, von Mayersbach, H Lucker, P, Rindt, W, and Wetzelsberger, F (1979) Circadian variations in pharmacokinetic parameters after oral application of hexobarbital. Chronobiologia 6:73.

Andersen, E, and Hellström, K (1982) Diurnal variation in biliary lipids and serum VLDL before and during treatment with clofibrate. Atherosclerosis 41:87–97.

Andlauer, P, Reinberg, A, Fourre, L, Battle, W, and Duverneuil, G (1979) Amplitude of the oral temperature circadian rhythm and the tolerance to shift-work. J Physiol 75:507–512.

Angeli, A, Fonzo, D, Frajria, R, Bertello, PD, Giadano, GP, and Ceresa, F (1975) Independence of the circadian rhythm in metyrapone-induced ACTH release from variations in adrenal 11-β-hydroxylase inhibition. Chronobiologia 2(Suppl 1):3.

Angeli, A, Frajria, R, De Paoli, R, Fonzo, D, and Ceresa, F (1978) Diurnal variation of prednisolone binding to serum corticosteroid binding globulin in man. Clin Pharmacol Ther 23:47–53.

Angeli, A, Agrimonti, F, Frajria, R, Vioino, PL, Barbadoro, E, and Ceresa, F (1981) Circadian patterns of plasma cortisol and testosterone in chronic male alcoholics. Int J Chronobiol 7:199.

Akerstedt, T, and Gillberg, M (1981) Sleep disturbances and shift-work. In: Reinberg, A, Vieux, N, and Andlauer, P (eds), Night and Shiftwork: Biological and Social Aspects. Oxford: Pergamon Press.

Apfelbaum, M, Reinberg, A, Assn, R, and Lacatis, D (1972) Hormonal and metabolic circadian rhythms before and during a low protein diet. Isr J Med Sci 8:867–873.

Aschoff, J, Hoffman, K, Pohl, H, and Wever, R (1975) Re-entrainment of circadian rhythms after phase-shifts of the Zeitgeber. Chronobiologia 2:23–78.

Avlisi, V, Degli, UE, Longini, C, Ruina, M, Pavani, F, Tralli, M, and Bagni, B (1980) Evidence of circadian rhythm of digoxin bioavailability. In: Int. Symp. Clinical Chronopharmacy, Chronopharmacology and Chronotherapeutics. Tallahassee, Florida: Florida A&M Univ.

Axelrod, J (1968) Control of catecholamine metabolism. In: Gual, C, and Ebling, FJG (eds), *Progress in Endocrinology*, Proceedings of the 3rd International Congress of Endocrinology, Mexico DF. Amsterdam: Excerpta Med Int Congress Series No. 184, pp. 286–293.

Aymard, N, and Soulairac, A (1979) Chronobiological changes in pharmacokinetics of dipotassic clorazepate, a benzodiazepine. In: Reinberg, A, and Halberg, F (eds), *Chronopharmacology*. Oxford: Pergamon Press, pp. 111–116.

Bélanger, PM, Labrecque, G, and Dore, F (1981) Rate limiting steps in the temporal variations in the metabolism of selected drugs. Int J Chronobiol 7:208.

Belchetz, PE, Plant, TM, Nakai, Y, Keogh, EJ, and Knobil, E (1978) Hypophysial response to continuous and intermittent delivery of hypothalamic gonadotropin-releasing hormone. Science 202:631–633.

Bouyard, P, Bruguerolle, B, Jadot, G, Mesdjian, E, and Valli, M (1974) Mise en évidence d'un rythme nycthéméral dans le phénomène de la curarisation chez le rat. CR Soc Biol 168:1005–1007.

Bruguerolle, B, Valli, M, Rakoto, JC, Jadot, G, Bouyard, P, and Reinberg, A (1979) Chronopharmacology of pancuronium in the rat: Anesthesia or seasonal influences? In: Reinberg, A, and Halberg, F (eds), *Chronopharmacology*. Oxford: Pergamon Press, pp. 117–123.

Bruinvels, J (1979) Norepinephrine. In: Lommax, P, and Schönbaum, E (eds), *Body Temperature. Regulation, Drug Effects and Therapeutic Implications*. New York: Marcel Dekker, Inc., pp. 257–288.

Carosella, L, Di Nardo, P, Bernabei, R, Cocchi, A, and Carbonin, P (1979) Chronopharmacokinetics of digitalis. Circadian variations of beta-methyl-digoxin serum levels after oral administration. In: Reinberg, A, and Halberg, F (eds), *Chronopharmacology*. Oxford: Pergamon Press, pp. 125–134.

Ceresa, F, and Angeli, A (1977) Chronotherapy corticoide. In: *14th Int. Cong. Therapeutics, Montpellier, 1977*. Paris: Expansion Scientifique, pp. 211–224.

Ceresa, F, Angeli, A, Boccuzzi, G, and Molino, G (1969) Once-a-day neurally stimulated and basal ACTH secretion phases in man and their response to corticoid inhibition. J Clin Endocrinol 29:1074–1082.

Clench, J, Reinberg, A, Ghata, J, and Dupont, J (1975) Chronopharmacological effects of indomethacin in healthy young human subjects. Chronobiologia 2(Suppl 1):14–15.

Clench, J, Reinberg, A, Dziewanowska, Z, Ghata, J, and Dupont, J (1977) Chronopharmacokinetics of indomethacin in 9 healthy young human adults. Chronobiologia 4:105.

Clench, J, Reinberg, A, Dziewanowska, Z, Ghata, J, and Smolensky, M (1981) Circadian changes in the bioavailability and effects of indomethacin in healthy subjects. Eur J Clin Pharmacol 20:359–369.

Colquhoun, WP (1971) *Biological Rhythms and Human Performance*. London: Academic Press.

Crepaldi, G, and Muggeo, M (1974) Plurichronocorticoid treatment of bronchial asthma and chronic bronchitis. Clinical and endocrinometabolic evaluation. Chronobiologia 1(Suppl 1):407–427.

D'Agata, R, Di Stefano, C, Furno, C, and Mughini, L (1968) Sulle variazioni del ritmo circadiano surrenalico dopo somministrazione orale di glicorticoidi. Riv Crit Clin Med 68:652–657.

Del Ponte, A, Capani, F, and Sensi, S (1979) Circadian variation of digoxin effects in healthy subjects. In: Reinberg, A, and Halberg, F (eds), *Chronopharmacology*. Oxford: Pergamon Press, pp. 135–136.

Dettli, L, and Spring, P (1966) Diurnal variations in the elimination rate of a sulfonamide in man. Helvetica Medica Acta 33:291–306.

De Vries, G, Goei, JT, Booy-Noord, H, and Orie, NG (1962) Changes during 24-hours in the lung function and histamine hyperreactivity of the bronchial tree in asthmatic and bronchitic patients. Int Arch Allergy 20:93–101.

Dierschke, DJ, Bhattacharya, AN, Atkinson, LE, and Knobil, E (1970) Circhoral oscillations of plasma LH levels in the ovariectomized Rhesus monkey. Endocrinology 87:850–853.

Di Santo, A, Chodos, D, and Halberg, F (1975) Chronobioavailability of three erythromycin test preparations assessed by each of four indices: time to peak, peak, nadir and area. Chronobiologia 2(Suppl 1):17.

Engelmann, W (1973) A slowing down of circadian rhythms by lithium ions. Zeitschr Naturforsch 28c:733–736.

English, J, and Marks, V (1981) Diurnal variations in methylprednisolone metabolism in the rat. IRCS Medical Science 9:721.

Fournier, A, and Gaultier, M (1955) Alcoolisme. Etude biologique et médicolégale. Actualités Biologiques 2:135–255.

Fukami, N, Kotani, T, Shimoji, K, Moriaka, T, and Isa, T (1970) Circadian rhythm and anesthesia. Jpn J Anesthesiol 19:1235–1240.

Furuya, S, and Yugari, Y (1974) Daily rhythmic change of L-histidine and glucose absorptions in rat small intestine in vivo. Biochem Biophy Acta 343:558–564.

Garrettson, LK, and Jusko, WJ (1975) Diphenylhydantoin elimination kinetics in overdosed children. Clin Pharmacol Ther 17:481–491.

Gaultier, C, Reinberg, A, and Girard, F (1975) Etude circadienne de la resistance pulmonaire totale et de la compliance dynamique chez l'enfant sain. CR Acad Sci 280:1253–1255.

Gaultier, C, Reinberg, A, and Girard, F (1977) Circadian rhythms in lung resistance and dynamic lung compliance of healthy children. Effects of 2 bronchodilators. Respir Physiol 31:169–182.

Gervais, P (1966) Les intoxications alcooliques aiguës. Presse Méd 74:1253–1254.

Gervais, P, Reinberg, A, Gervais, C, Smolensky, M, and DeFrance, O (1977) Twenty-four-hour rhythm in the bronchial hyperreactivity to house dust in asthmatics. J Allergy Clin Immunol 59:207–213.

Gibson, T, Stimmler, L, Jarrett, RJ, Rutland, P, and Shiu, M (1974) Diurnal variations in the effects of insulin on blood glucose, plasma non-esterified fatty acids and growth hormone. Diabetologia 11:83–88.

Gillespie, JA (1967) Vasodilator properties of alcohol. Br Med J 2:274–277.

Goetz, F, Bishop, J, Halberg, F, Sothern, R, Brúnning, R, Senske, B, Greenberg, G, Minors, D, Stoney, P, Smith, I, Rosen, G, Cressey, D, Haus, E, and Apfelbaum, M (1976) Timing of single daily meal influences relations among human circadian rhythms in urinary cyclic AMP, hemic glucagon, insulin and iron. Experientia 32:1081–1084.

Grant, SD, Forsham, PH, and Di Raimondo, VC (1965) Suppression of 17-hydroxycorticosteroids in plasma and urine after single and divided doses of triamcinolone. N Engl J Med 273:1115–1118.

Halberg, F (1960) Temporal coordination of physiologic function. Cold Spr Harb Symp Quant Biol 25:289–310.

Halberg, F (1962) Physiologic 24-hour rhythms. A determinant of response to environmental agents. In: Schaffer, KE (ed), Man's Dependence on the Earthly Atmosphere. New York: Macmillan, pp. 48–49.

Halberg, F (1967) Ritmos y corteza suprarenal. IV: Simposio Panamerican de Farmacolige y Terapeutica, Mexico, 1967. Excerpta Med Int Cong Ser 7:39.

Halberg, F (1969) Chronobiology. Ann Rev Physiol 31:675–725.

Halberg, F (1974) Protection by timing treatment according to bodily rhythms—an analogy to protection by scrubbing before surgery. In: Aschoff, J, Ceresa, F, and Halberg, F (eds), Chronobiological Aspects of Endocrinology. Chronobiologia 1 (Suppl. 1): 17–68.

Halberg, F (1975) When to treat? Indian J Cancer 12:1–20.

Halberg, F, and Reinberg, A (1967) Rythmes circadiens et rythmes de basses frequences en physiologie humaine. J Physiol (Paris) 59: 177–200.

Halberg, F, Tong, YL, and Johnson, EA (1967) Circadian system: an aspect of temporal morphology: procedure and illustrative examples. In: von Mayersbach, H (ed), The Cellular Aspects of Biorhythms. Berlin: Springer-Verlag, pp. 20–48.

Halberg, F, Bartter, FC, Nelson, W, Doe, P, and Reinberg, A (1969a) Chronobiologie. Europ J Toxicol 6:311–318.

Halberg, F, Halberg, E, and Montalbetti, N (1969b) Premesse e svilluppi della cronofarmacologia. Quad Med Quant Sperim Clin Contr 7:7–54.

Halberg, F, Johnson, EA, Nelson, W, Runge, W, and Sothern, R (1972) Autorhythmometry procedures for physiologic self-measurements and their analysis. Physiol Teacher 1:1–11.

Halberg, F, Carandente, F, Cornelissen, G, and Katinas, GS (1977a) Glossary of chronobiology. Chronobiologia 4(Suppl 1):1–190.

Halberg, F, Gupta, BD, Haus, E, Halberg, E, Deka, AC, Nelson, W, Sothern, RB, Cornelissen, G, Klee, J, Lakatua, DJ, Scheving, LE, and Burns, ER (1977b) Steps toward a cancer chronopolytherapy. In: 14th Int. Cong. Therapeutics, Montpellier, 1977. Paris: Expansion Scientifique, pp. 151–196.

Hardeland, R, Hoffman, D, and Resing, L (1973) The rhythmic organization of rodent liver; a review. J Interdiscipl Cycle Res 4:89–118.

Haus, E, and Halberg, F (1959) 24-hour rhythm in susceptibility of C-mice to toxic dose of ethanol. J Appl Physiol 14:878–883.

Haus, E, Halberg, F, Scheving, L, Cardoso, S, Kuhl, J, Sothern, R, Shiotsuka, R, Hwang, DS, and Pauly, JE (1972) Increased tolerance of leukemic mice to arabinosyl cytosine given on schedule adjusted to circadian system. Science 177:80–82.

Haus, E, Halberg, F, Kuhl, JFW, and Lakatua, DJ (1974) Chronopharmacology in animals. In: Aschoff, J, Ceresa, F, and Halberg, F (eds), Chronobiological Aspects of Endocrinology. Chronobiologia 1(Suppl 1):122–156.

Hofmann, K, Günderoth-Palmowski, M, Wiedenmann, G, and Engelmann, W (1978) Further evidence for period lengthening effect of Li$^+$ on circadian rhythms. Z Naturforsch 32c:231–234.

Hrushesky, W, Lévi, F, and Kennedy, BJ (1980) Cis-diamminedichloroplatinum (DDP) toxicity to the human kidney reduced by circadian timing. Proceedings of the American Society for Clinical Oncology 21:C45.

Hughes, A, Jacobon, HI, Wagner, RK, and Jungblut, PW (1976) Ovarian independent fluctuations of estradiol receptor levels in mammalian tissues. Mol Cell Endocrinol 5:379–388.

Job, C, Reinberg, A, and Delbarre, F (1981) Chronoeffectiveness of indomethacin in four patients suffering from evolutive coxarthrosis or ganarthrosis. Int J Chronobiol 7:258.

Johnsson, A, Pflug, B, Engelmann, W, and Klemke, W (1979) Effect of lithium carbonate on circadian periodicity in humans. Pharmakopsychiatr Neuropsychopharmakol 12:423–425.

Jones, BM, and Jones, MK (1975) Effects of a moderate dose of alcohol on female social drinkers at different times in the menstrual cycle. Chronobiologia 2(Suppl 1):34.

Jöres, A (1938) Rhythmus-forschung. Dtsch Med Wochenschr 21:737.

Kafka, MS, Wirz-Justice, A, Naber, D, Marangos, PJ, O'Donohue, TL, and Wehr, TL (1982) Effect of lithium on circadian neurotransmitter receptor rhythms. Neuropsychobiology 8:41–50.

Knobil, G (1980) The role of signal pattern in the hypothalamic control of gonadotropin secretion. In: Ortavant, R, and Reinberg, A (eds), Rythmes et Reproduction. Paris: Masson, pp. 73–80.

Kripke, DF (1982) Phase advance theories for effective illnesses. In: Goodwin, FK, and Wehr, TA (eds), Circadian Rhythms in Psychiatry. Los Angeles: Boxwood Press (in press).

Kripke, DF, and Wyborney, VG (1980) Lithium slows rat circadian activity rhythms. Life Sci 26:1319–1321.

Kyle, GM, Smolensky, MH, and McGovern, JP (1979) Circadian variation in the susceptibility of rodents to the toxic effects of theophylline. In: Reinberg, A, and Halberg, F, (eds), Chronopharmacology. Oxford: Pergamon Press, pp. 239–244.

Kyle, GM, Smolensky, MH, Thorne, LG, Hsi, B, Robinson, A, and McGovern, JP (1980a) Circadian rhythm in the pharmacokinetics of orally administered theophylline. In: Smolensky, MH, Reinberg, A, and McGovern, JP (eds), Recent Advances in the Chronobiology of Allergy and Immunology. Oxford: Pergamon Press, pp. 95–111.

Kyle, GM, Smolensky, MH, Thorne, LG, and McGovern, JP (1980b) Indirect monitoring of theophylline blood levels utilizing saliva: a practical non-invasive approach to verifying dosage and understanding temporal variability in pharmacokinetics. In: Smolensky, MH, Reinberg, A, and McGovern, JP (eds), Recent Advances in the Chronobiology of Allergy and Immunology. Oxford: Pergamon Press, pp. 123–128.

Labrecque, G, Doré, F, Laperrière, A, Pérusse, F, and Bélanger, PM (1979) Chronopharmacology II. Variations in the carrageenin-induced edema, in the action and the plasma levels of indomethacin. In: Reinberg, A, and Halberg, F (eds), Chronopharmacology. Oxford, Pergamon Press, pp. 231–238.

Lagoguey, M, and Reinberg, A (1981) Circadian and circannual changes of pituitary hormones in healthy human males. In: Van Cauter, E, and Copinschi, G (eds), Human Pituitary Hormones. The Hague: Martinus Nijhoff Publ., pp. 261–285.

Lagoguey, M, Reinberg, A, and Legrand, JC (1980) Variations chronobiologiques de la réponse testiculaire a l'HCG chez l'homme adulte sain. Ann Endocrinol 41:59–60.

Lambinet, I, Aymard, N, Soulairac, A, and Reinberg, A (1981) Chronoptimization of lithium administration in five manic depressive patients: reduction of nephrotoxicity. Int J Chronobiol 7:274.

Lee, RE, Smolensky, MH, Leach, C, and McGovern, JP (1977) Circadian rhythms in the cutaneous sensitivity to histamine and selected antigens including phase relationship to urinary cortisol excretion. Ann Allergy 38(4):231–236.

Lesko, LJ, Brousseau, D, Canada, AT, and Eastwood, G (1980) Temporal variations in trough serum theophylline concentrations at steady state. J Pharm Sci 69:358–359.

Lévi, F, Lakatua, D, Haus, E, Hrushesky, W, Halberg, F, Schwartz, S, and Kennedy, BJ (1980) Circadian urinary n-acetyl glucose amidinase (NAG) excretion gauges murine cis-diamine dichloroplatinum (DDP) nephrotoxicity. American Association Cancer Research, San Diego, May.

Lévi, F (1982) Chronopharmacologie de trois agents doués d'activité anticancéreuse chez le rat et la souris. Chronoefficacité et chronotolérance. Thèse de Doctorat ès-Sciences (Paris VI).

Levine, H, and Halberg, F (1972) Circadian Rhythms of the Circulatory System. Brooks Air Force Base, Texas: USAF School of Aerospace Medicine (AFSC), 64 pp.

McAllister, WAC, Mitchell, DM and Collins, JV (1981) Prednisolone pharmacokinetics compared between night and day in asthmatic and normal subjects. Br J Clin Pharmacol 11:303–304.

Margules, DL, Lewis, MJ, Dragovitch, JA, and Margules, A (1972) Hypothalamic norepinephrine: circadian rhythm and the control of feeding behavior. Science 178:640–643.

Markewicz, A, and Semenowicz, K (1979a) Chronokinetics of intestinal absorption and urinary excretion of xylose. Chronobiologia 6:129.

Markewicz, A, and Semenowicz, K (1979b) Time dependent changes in the pharmacokinetics of aspirin. Int J Clin Pharmacol Biopharm 17:409–411.

Markiewicz, A, Semenowicz, K, Korczynaka, J, and Boldys, H (1980) Temporal variations in the response of ventilatory and circulatory functions to propranolol in healthy men. In: Smolensky, MH, Reinberg, A, and McGovern, JP (eds), Recent Advances in the Chronobiology of Allergy and Immunology. Oxford: Pergamon Press, pp. 185–193.

Martin, MM, and Hellman, D (1964) Temporal variation in SU-4885 responsiveness in man; evidence in support of circadian variation in ACTH secretion. J Clin Endocrinol 24:253–260.

Martin, MM, and Mintz, DH (1965) Effect of altered thyroid function upon adrenocortical ACTH and methopyrapone (SU-4885) responsiveness in man. J Clin Endocrinol 25:20–27.

Mattok, GL, and McGilveray, J (1973) The effect of food intake and sleep on the absorption of acetaminophen. Rev Can Biol 32(Suppl autome):77–84.

von Mayersbach, H, Philippens, KMH, and Poesche, WW (1977) Seasonal influences; a reason for non-reproducibility of circadian rhythms in highly standardized rats. In: Int. Soc. Chronobiol. XII Int. Conf., Washington, 1975. Milano: II Ponte, pp. 511–524.

Melani, F, Verrillo, A, Marasco, M, Rivellese, A, Osorio, J, and Bertolini, MG (1975) Diurnal variation of blood sugar and serum insulin in response to glucose and glucagon in healthy subjects. Chronobiologia 2(Suppl 1):45.

Menzel, W (1955) Therapie unter dem Gesichtspunkt biologischer Rhythmen. Ergebn phys diät Ther 5:1.

Mills, JN, Waterhouse, JM, Minors, DS, and Dziewanoska, ZE (1975) A chronotherapeutic trial of hydrochlorothiazide. Chronobiologia 2(Suppl 1):47.

Minors, DS, and Waterhouse, JM (1979) Aspects of chronopharmacokinetics of ethanol in healthy man. Chronobiologia 7:465–480.

Mirouze, J, and Selam, JL (1977) Diurnal rhythm or exogenous insulin efficiency assessed by the artificial pancreas. Chronobiologia 4:133.

Möllerström, J (1953) Rhythmus, Diabetes, und Behandlung. Verhandlungen der 3. [Konferenz der Intern. Gesellsch. für biologische Rhythmusforschung (Hamburg, 1949).] Acta Med Scand Suppl. 278:110–114.

Montalbetti, N (1974) Non-interference in circadian rhythm during clinical use of corticoids. In: Aschoff, J, Ceresa, R, and Halberg, F (eds), Chronobiological Aspects of Endocrinology. Chronobiologia 1(Suppl 1):281–288.

Moore–Ede, MC (1973) Circadian rhythms of drug effectiveness and toxicity. Clin Pharmacol Ther 14:925–935.

Moore–Ede, MC, and Burr, RG (1973) Circadian rhythm of therapeutic effectiveness of oxymetholone in paraplegic patients. Clin Pharmacol Ther 14:448–454.

Moore–Ede, MC, Meguid, MM, Fitzpatrick GF, Boyden, CM, and Ball, MR (1978) Circadian variation in response to potassium infusion. Clin Pharmacol Ther 23:218–227.

Morselli, PL, Marc, V, Garattini, S, and Zaccala, M (1970) Metabolism of exogenous cortisol in humans—diurnal variations in plasma disappearance rate. Biochem Pharmacol 19:1643–1647.

Müller, O (1974) Circadian rhythmicity in response to barbiturate. In: Scheving, LE, Halberg, F, and Pauly, J (eds), Chronobiology. Tokyo: Igaku Shoin, pp. 187–190.

Naftolin, F, and Tolis, G (1978) Neuroendocrine regulation of the menstrual cycle. Clin Obstet Gynecol 21:17–29.

Nair, V (1974) Circadian rhythm in drug action: a pharmacologic biochemical and electromicroscopic study. In: Scheving, LE, Halberg, F, and Pauly, J (eds), Chronobiology. Tokyo: Igaku Shoin, pp. 182–186.

Nakai, Y, Plant, TM, Hess, DL, Keoch, EJ, and Knobil, E (1978) On the sites of negative and positive feedback action of estradiol in the control of gonadotropin secretion in the Rhesus monkey. Endocrinology 102:1008–1014.

Nakano, S, and Hollister, LE (1978) No circadian effect on nortriptyline kinetics in man. Clin Pharmacol Ther 23:199–203.

Nichols, T, Nugent, CA, and Tyler, FH (1965) Diurnal variations in suppression of adrenal function by glucocorticoids. J Clin Endocrinol 25:343–349.

Nicholson, AN, and Stone, BM (1977) Effectiveness of diazepan and its metabolite, 3-hydroxydiazepan. J Physiol 270:29–30.

Nicholson, AN, and Stone, BM (1979) Hypnotic activity during the day of diazepam and its hydroxylated metabolites, 3-hydroxydiazepam (Temazepam) and 3-hydroxy, N-desmethyldiazepam (oxazepam). In: Reinberg, A, and Halberg, F (eds), Chronopharmacology. Oxford: Pergamon Press, pp. 159–169.

Pauly, JE, Burns, ER, Halberg, F, Tsai, S, Betterton, HO, and Scheving, LE (1975) Meal-timing dominates lighting regimen as a synchronizer of the eosinophil rhythm in mice. Acta Anat 93:60–68.

Philippens, KMH (1974) Circadian variation in rat liver mitochondrial activity. In: Scheving, LE, Halberg, F, and Pauly, JE (eds), Chronobiology. Tokyo: Igaku Shoin Ltd., pp. 23–28.

Philippens, KMH, von Mayersbach, H, and

Scheving, LE (1977) Effects of the scheduling of meal-feeding at different phases of the circadian system in rats. J Nutr 107:176–193.

Pöllmann, L (1980) Der Zahnschmerz. Chronobiologie, Beurteilung und Behandlung. München Wien: Carl Hanser Verlag.

Pöllmann, L (1981) Circadian changes in the duration of local anaesthesia. J. Interdispl Cyclic Res 12:187–192.

Procacci, P, Moretti, R, Zoppi, M, Cappelletti, C, and Voegelin, MR (1973) Rythmes circadiens et circatrigintidiens du seuil de la douleur cutanee chez l'homme. Bull Groupe d'Etude Rythmes Biol 5:65–75; and Chronobiologia 1:77–96, 1974.

Radzialowski, FM, and Bousquet, WF (1968) Daily rhythmic variation in hepatic drug metabolism in the rat and mouse. J Pharmacol Exp Ther 163:229–238.

Reinberg, A (1965) Hours of changing responsiveness in relation to allergy and the circadian adrenal cycle. In: Aschoff, J (ed), Circadian Clocks. Amsterdam: North-Holland Publ. Co., pp. 214–218.

Reinberg, A (1967) The hours of changing responsiveness or susceptibility. Perspect Biol Med 11:111–128.

Reinberg, A (1971) Methodologic considerations for human chronobiology. J Interdiscpl Cycle Res 2:1–15.

Reinberg, A (1973) Chronopharmacology. In: Mills, JN (ed), Biological Aspects of Circadian Rhythms. London: Plenum Press, pp. 121–152.

Reinberg, A (1974a) Aspects of circannual rhythms in man. In: Pengelley, ET (ed), Circannual Clocks. AAAS meeting on circannual rhythms, San Francisco, Feb. 1974. New York: Academic Press, pp. 423–505.

Reinberg, A (1974b) Chronobiology and nutrition. Chronobiologia 1:22–27.

Reinberg, A (1974c) Chronopharmacology in man. In: Aschoff, J, Ceresa, F, and Halberg, F (eds), Chronobiological Aspects of Endocrinology. Chronobiologia 1 (Suppl. 1):157–185.

Reinberg, A (1975) Chronosusceptibility, chronopharmacology (with special reference to corticosteroids). Folia Allergol Immunol Clin 22:559–569.

Reinberg, A (1976a) Advances in human chronopharmacology. Chronobiologia 3:151–166.

Reinberg, A (1976b) New aspects of human

chronopharmacology. Arch Toxicol 36:327–339.

Reinberg, A (1977a) Bases experimentales pour la chronotherapie. *14th Int. Cong. Therapeutics, Montpellier, 1977.* Paris: Expansion Scientifique, pp. 127–150.

Reinberg, A (1977b) *Des Rythmes Biologiques a la Chronobiologie* (2éme èd). Paris: Gauthier-Villars.

Reinberg, A (ed) (1979) Chronobiological field studies of oil refinery shift-workers. Chronobiologia 6 (Suppl. 1).

Reinberg, A (1981) Clinical chronopharmacology, including drug effects on sleep and related processes. In: Wheatley, D, and Nicholson, AN (eds), *Psychopharmacology of Sleep.* New York: Raven Press, pp. 73–93.

Reinberg, A, Gervais, P, Chaussade, M, Fraboulet, G, and Duburque, B (1983) Circadian changes in effectiveness of corticosteroids in eight patients with allergic asthma. J Allergy Clin Immunol (in press).

Reinberg, A, and Ghata, J (1977) *Les Rythmes Biologiques* (3ème ed). Paris: Presses Universitaires de France.

Reinberg, A, and Halberg, F (1971) Circadian chronopharmacology. Ann Rev Pharmacol 11:455–492.

Reinberg, A, and Lagoguey, M (1980) Annual endocrine rhythms in healthy young adult men: their implication in human biology and medicine. In: Assenmacher, I, and Farner, D (eds), *Environmental Endocrinology.* New York: Springer, pp. 113–121.

Reinberg, A, and Reinberg, M (1977) Circadian changes of the duration of action of local anaesthetics agent. Naunyn Schmiedebergs Arch Pharmacol 297:149–159.

Reinberg, A, and Sidi, E (1966) Circadian changes in the inhibitory effects of an antihistaminic drug in man. J Invest Dermatol 46:415–419.

Reinberg, A, and Smolensky, M (1974) Circatrigintan secondary rhythms related to hormonal changes in the menstrual cycle: general consideration. In: Ferin, M, Vande Wiele, RL, and Halberg, F (eds), *Biorhythms and Human Reproduction.* London: John Wiley and Sons, pp. 241–258.

Reinberg, A, and Smolensky, M (1982) Circadian changes of drug disposition in man. J Clin Pharmacokinetics 7:401–420.

Reinberg, A, Sidi, E, and Ghata, J (1965) Circadian rhythms of human skin to histamine or allergen and the adrenal cycle. J Allergy 36:273–283.

Reinberg, A, Zagula-Mally, Z, Ghata, J, and Halberg, F (1967) Circadian rhythms in duration of salicylate excretion referred to phase of excretory rhythms and routine. Proc Soc Exp Biol 124:826–832.

Reinberg, A, Zagulla-Mally, Z, Ghata, J, and Halberg, F (1969) Circadian reactivity rhythms of human skin to house dust, penicillin and histamine. J Allergy 44:292–306.

Reinberg, A, Gervais, P, Morin, and Abulker, C (1971a) Rythme circadien humain du seuil de la reponse bronchique a l'acetylcholine. CR Acad Sci 272:1879–1881.

Reinberg, A, Ghata, J, Halberg, F, Apfelbaum, M, Gervais, P, Boudon, P, Abulker, C, and Dupont, J (1971b) Distribution temporelle du traitement de l'insuffisance corticosurrenalienne. Essai de chronotherapeutique. Ann Endocrinol 32:566–573.

Reinberg, A, Chaumont, AJ, Chambon, P, Vincendon, G, Skoulios, G, Bauchart, M, Nicolaï, A, Abulker, C, and Dupont, J (1973) Etude chronobiologique des effets des changements d'horaires de travail (autométrie de 20 sujets postés: système des 3 × 8 à rotation hebdomadiare. Arch Mal Prof et Méd Trav 35:373–394.

Reinberg, A, Clench, J, Aymard, N, Gaillot, M, Bourdon, R, Gervais, P, Abulker, C, and Dupont, J (1974a) Rythmes circadiens des parametres de l'"ethanolemie provoquee chez 6 hommes adultes jeunes et sains. CR Acad Sci 278:1503–1505.

Reinberg, A, Gervais, P, Morin, M, and Abulker, C (1974b) Circadian rhythms in the threshold of bronchial response to acetylcholine in healthy and asthmatic subjects. In: Scheving, LE, Halberg, F, and Pauly, JE (eds), *Chronobiology.* Tokyo: Igaku Shoin Ltd, pp. 174–177.

Reinberg, A, Ghata, J, Halberg, F, Apfelbaum, M, Gervais, P, Abulker, C, and Dupont, J (1974c) Treatment schedules modify circadian timing in human adrenocortical insufficiency. In: Scheving, LE, Halberg, F, and Pauly, JE (eds), *Chronobiology.* Tokyo: Igaku Shoin Ltd., pp. 168–173.

Reinberg, A, Halberg, F, and Falliers, C (1974d) Circadian timing of methylprednisolone effects in asthmatic boys. Chronobiologia 1:333–347.

Reinberg, A, Clench, J, Aymard, N, Gaillot, M,

Bourdon, R, Gervais, P, Abulker, C, and Dupont, J (1975a) Variations circadiennes des effets de l'éthanol et de l'éthanolémie chez l'homme adulte sain (étude chronopharmacolgique). J Physiol (Paris) 70:435–456.

Reinberg, A, Clench, J, Ghata, J, Halberg, F, Abulker, C, Dupont, J, and Zagula-Mally, Z (1975b) Rythmes circadiens des paramètres de l'excrétion urinaire du salicylate (chronopharmacocinétique) chez l'homme adulte sain. CR Acad Sci 280:1697–1700.

Reinberg, A, Guillet, P, Gervais, P, Ghata, J, Vignaud, D, and Abulker, C (1977) One month chronocorticotherapy (Dutimelan 8 15® mite). Control of the asthmatic condition without adrenal suppression and circadian rhythm alteration. Chronobiologia 4:295–312.

Reinberg, A, Lévi, F, Guillet, P, Burke, JT, and Nicolaï, A (1978) Chronopharmacological study of antihistamines in man with special references to terfenadine. Eur J Clin Pharmacol 14:245–252.

Reinberg, A, Ghata, J, and Abulker, C (1979) Chronic (5 to 24 years) chronocorticotherapy in adrenocortical insufficiency: comparison between two treatment schedules. In: Reinberg, A, and Halberg, F (eds), Chronopharmacology. Oxford: Pergamon Press, pp. 77–84.

Reinberg, A, Andlauer, P, Guillet, P, Nicolaï, A, Vieux, N, and Laporte, A (1980a) Oral temperature, circadian rhythm amplitude, aging, and tolerance to shift-work. Ergonomics 23:55–64.

Reinberg, A, Guillemant, S, Ghata, N, Guillemant, J, Touitou, Y, Dupont, W, Lagoguey, M, Bourgeois, P, Briere, L, Fraboulet, G, and Guillet, P (1980b) Clinical chronopharmacology of ACTH 1–17. I. Effects on plasma cortisol and urinary 17-hydroxycorticosteroids. Chronobiologia 7:527–538.

Reinberg, A, Dupont, W, Touitou, Y, Lagoguey, M, Bourgeois, P, Touitou, C, Muriaux, G, Przyrowsky, D, Guillemant, S, Guillemant, J, Briere, L, and Zeau, B (1981a) Clinical chronopharmacology of ACTH 1–17. II. Effects on plasma testosterone, plasma aldosterone, plasma and on urinary electrolytes (K, Na, Ca and Mg). Chronobiologia 8:11–31.

Reinberg, A, Briere, L. Fraboulet, G, Guillemant, S, Touitou, Y, Lagoguey, M, Guillemant, J. DuPont, W, Guillet, P, and Nicolaï, A (1981b) Clinical chronopharmacology of ACTH 1–17. III. Effects on fatigue, oral temperature, heart rate, grip strength and bronchial patency. Chronobiologia 8:101–115.

Reindl, K, Falliers, C, Halberg, F, Chai, H, Hillman, D, and Nelson, W (1969) Circadian acrophase in peak expiratory flow rate and urinary electrolyte excretion of asthmatic children: phase shifting of rhythms by prednisone given at different circadian system phases. Rass Neurol Veg 23:5–26.

Rutenfranz, J (1978) Schichtarbeit und biologische Rhythmik. Arzneim Forsch 28(11):1867–1872.

Rutenfranz, J, and Singer, R (1967) Untersuchungen zur Frage einer Abhängigkeit der Alkoholwirkung von der Tageszeit. Int Z angew Physiol 24:1–17.

Scherrer, J (ed) (1980) Physiologie du Travail (Ergonomie). Paris: Masson.

Scheving, LE, Cardoso, SS, Pauly, JE, Halberg, F, and Haus, E (1974) Variation in susceptibility of mice to the carcinostatic agent arabinosyl cytosine. In: Scheving, LE, Halberg, F, and Pauly, JE (eds), Chronobiology. Tokyo: Igaku Shoin Ltd., pp. 213–217.

Scheving, LE, Donald, F, Vedral, DF, and Pauly, JE (1968) A circadian susceptibility rhythm in rats to pentobarbital sodium. Anat Rec 160:741–750.

Scheving, LE, Sohal, GS, Enna, D, and Pauly, JE (1973) The persistence of a circadian rhythm in histamine response in guinea pigs maintained under continuous illumination. Anat Rec 175:1–7.

Scheving, LE, von Mayersbach, H, and Pauly, JE (1974) An overview of chronopharmacology. Eur J Toxicol 7:203–227.

Scheving, LE, Enna, CE, Jacobson, RR, and Halberg, F (1981) Circadian susceptibility rhythms in response to histamine in innervated and denervated skin of leprosy patients undergoing different treatment protocols. In: Walker, CA, Winget, CM, and Soliman, KFA (eds), Int. Symp. Chronopharmacology and Chronotherapeutics. Tallahassee: Florida A&M Univ Foundation.

Scott, PH, Tabachnik, E, MacLeod, S, Correia, J, Newth, C, and Levison, H (1981) Sustained-release theophylline for childhood asthma: evidence for circadian variation of theophylline pharmacokinetics. J Pediatr 99:476–479.

Segre, EJ, and Klaiber, EL (1966) Therapeutic utilization of the diurnal variation in pituitary-adrenocortical activity. Calif. Med. 104:363–365.

Sensi, S, Capani, F, Tezzi, M, and Del Ponte, A (1975) Further observations on time-related insulin effectiveness of glucose metabolism. Chronobiologia 2(Suppl 1):62–63.

Serafini, U, and Bonini, S (1974) Corticoid therapy in allergic diseases. Clinical evaluation of a chronopharmacological attempt. In: Aschoff, J, Ceresa, F, and Halberg, F (eds), *Chronobiological Aspects of Endocrinology*. Chronobiologia 1(Suppl 1):399–406.

Serio, M, Della Corte, M, Piolanti, P, Romano, S, Giglioli, L, and Giusti, G (1971) Transverse circadian rhythmometry of plasma cortisol in diabetic subjects in relation to therapy. Ann Endocrinol 32:403–408.

Sharma, SD, Deshpande, VA, Samuel, MR, and Vakil, BJ (1979) Chronobioavailability of ampicillin. Chronobiologia 6:156.

Shively, CA, and Vesell, ES (1975) Temporal variations in acetaminophen and phenacetin half-life in man. Clin Pharmacol Ther 18:413–424.

Shively, CA, Simons, RJ, Passananti, GT, Dvorchik, BH, and Vesell, ES (1981) Dietary patterns and diurnal variations in aminopyrine disposition. Clin Pharmacol Ther 29:65–73.

Simmons, DJ, Lesker, PA, and Sherman, NE (1974) Induction of sodium pentobarbital anaesthesia. A circadian rhythm. J Interdiscipl Cycle Res 5:71–75.

Simpson, HW (1977) Aspects of cancer chronotherapy: mammary chronothermography and its perspective for the treatment of breast carcinoma. In: *14th Int. Cong. Therapeutics, Montpellier, 1977*. Paris: Expansion Scientifique, pp. 197–210.

Simpson, HW, Bellamy, N, Bohlen, J, and Halberg, F (1973) Double blind trial of a possible chronobiotic (Quiadon®). Int J Chronobiol 1:287–311.

Smith, ID, Shearman, RP, and Korda, AR (1973) Chronoperiodicity in the response to intraamniotic injection of prostaglandin F2α in the human. Nature 241:279.

Smolensky, M (1974) Rationale for circadian-system phased glucocorticoid management. In: Scheving, LE, Halberg, F, and Pauly, JE (eds), *Chronobiology*. Tokyo: Igaku Shoin, Ltd, pp. 197–201.

Smolensky, MH, and Reinberg, A (1976) The chronotherapy of corticosteroids: Practical application of chronobiologic findings to nursing. Nurs Clin N Am 11:609–620.

Smolensky, MH, Reinberg, A, Lee, R, and McGovern, JP (1974) Secondary rhythms related to hormonal changes in the menstrual cycle: special reference to allergology. In: Ferin, M, Vande Wiele, RL, and Halberg, F (eds), *Biorhythms and Human Reproduction*. London: John Wiley & Sons, pp. 287–306.

Smolensky, MH, Maxy-Kyle, G, and McGovern, JP (1979) Circadian variation in the susceptibility of rodents to the toxic effects of theophylline. In: Reinberg, A, and Halberg, F (eds), *Chronopharmacology*. Oxford: Pergamon Press, pp. 239–244.

Smolensky, MH, Reinberg, A, and McGovern, JP (eds) (1980) *Recent Advances in the Chronobiology of Allergy and Immunology*. Oxford: Pergamon Press.

Smolensky, MH, Reinberg, A, and Queng, JT (1981) The chronobiology and chronopharmacology of allergy. Ann Allergy 47:234–252.

Smolensky, MH, Harrist, R, Scott, PH, MacLeod, S, Newth, C, Levison, H, and Reinberg, A (1982) A chronobiologic evaluation of a sustained-release theophylline compound. In: Takahashi, H, and Halberg, F (eds), *Toward Chronopharmacology*. Oxford: Pergamon Press, pp. 225–233.

Spelsberg, TC, Boyd, PO, and Halberg, F (1979) Circannual rhythms in chick oviduct progesterone receptor and nuclear acceptor. In: Reinberg, A, and Halberg, F (eds), *Chronopharmacology*. Oxford: Pergamon Press, pp. 85–88.

Strumwasser, F, and Viele, DP (1980) Lithium increases the period of the neuronal oscillator. Abstract 241.5, *Proceedings, Society for Neuroscience*, 10th Annual Meeting, Cincinnati, Ohio.

Sturtevant, FM (1976) Chronopharmacokinetics of ethanol. 1. Review of the literature and theoretical considerations. Chronobiologia 3:237–262.

Sturtevant, FM, Sturtevant, RP, Scheving, LE, and Pauly, JE (1975) Chronopharmacokinetics of ethanol in man. Chronobiologia 2(Suppl. 1):69.

Sturtevant, FM, Sturtevant, RP, Scheving, LE, and Pauly, JE (1976) Chronopharmacokinetics of ethanol II. Circadian rhythm in rate of blood level decline in a single subject. Arch Pharm 293:203–208.

Sturtevant, RP (1981) Dose-response relationships in ethanol chronopharmaco-kinetic studies in the rat. In Walker, CA, Winget, CM, and Soliman, KFA (eds), *Int. Symp:*

Chronopharmacology and Chronotherapeutics. Tallahassee: Florida A&M Univ. Foundation, pp. 115–118.

Sturtevant, RP, and Garber SL (1979) Changes in ethanol clearance rhythm in rats as affected by light-dark phase shifts and restricted feeding. Chronobiologia 6:160.

Sturtevant, RP, and Garber, SL (1981) Circadian variation in alcohol dehydrogenase activity levels in rats. Int J Chronobiol 7:324.

Swoyer, J, Lakatua, DJ, Haus, E, Warner, T, and Sackett, L (1975) Circadian rhythm in ethanol disappearance rate from human plasma. Chronobiologia 2(Suppl. 1):71.

Tammeling, CJ, De Vries, K, and Kruyt, EW (1977) The circadian pattern of the bronchial reactivity to histamine in healthy subjects and in patients with obstructive lung disease. In: McGovern, JP, Smolensky, MH, and Reinberg, A (eds), *Chronobiology in Allergy and Immunology.* Springfield, Ill.: Charles C Thomas, pp. 139–149.

Tarquini, B, Romano, S, De Scalzi, M, De Leonardis, V, Benvenuti, F, Chegai, E, Comparini, T, Moretti, R, and Cagnoni, M (1979) Circadian variations of iron absorption in healthy human subjects. In: Reinberg, A, and Halberg, F (eds), *Chronopharmacology.* Oxford: Pergamon Press, pp. 347–354.

Tavadia, HB, Fleming, KA, Hume, PD, and Simpson, HW (1975) Circadian rhythmicity of human plasma cortisol and PHA-induced lymphocyte transformation. Clin Exp Immunol 22:190–193.

Touitou, Y, Bogdan, A, and Reinberg, A (1976) Circadian changes in urinary steroid before, during, and after a 36-hr 4-hourly-sustained administration of metyrapone in eight healthy young human males. J Steroid Biochem 7:517–520.

Touitou, Y, Touitou, C, Bogdan, A, Beck, H, and Reinberg, A (1979) Circadian rhythms in total serum proteins: observed differences according to aging and mental health. Chronobiologia 6:164.

Valk, TW, Marshall, JC, and Kelch, RP (1981) Stimulation of the follicular phase of the menstrual cycle by intravenous administration of low-dose pulsatile gonadotropin-releasing hormone. Am J Obstet Gynecol 141:842–843.

Virey, JJ (1814) *Ephémérides de la vie humaine ou recherches sur la révolution journalière et la périodicite de ses phénomènes dans la santé et les maladies.* Paris: Thèse Fac Med, 23 April.

Walker, CA (1974) Implications of biological rhythms in brain amine concentrations and drug toxicity. In: Scheving, LE, Halberg, F, and Pauly, JE (eds), *Chronobiology.* Tokyo: Igaku Shoin, pp. 205–208.

Walker, CA, and Soliman, KFA (1975) Diurnal periodicity for ethanol absorption, tissue levels, and metabolism in the rat. Chronobiologia 2(Suppl. 1):75.

Wehr, TA, Wirz–Justice, A, Goodwin, FK, Duncan, W, and Gillin, JC (1979) Phase advance of the sleep-cycle as an antidepressant. Science 206:710–713.

Wehr, TA, Wirz–Justice, A, and Goodwin, FK (1982) Advanced circadian rhythms and a sleep-sensitive switch mechanism in depression. In: Goodwin, FK, and Wehr, TA (eds), *Circadian Rhythms in Psychiatry.* Los Angeles: Boxwood Press (in press).

Weitzman, ED, Kripke, DF, Goldmacher, D, McGregor, P, and Nogeire, C (1970) Acute reversal of the sleep-waking cycle in man. Arch Neurol 22:483–489.

Wildt, L, Marshall, G, Hausler, A, Plant, TM, Belchetz, PE, and Knobil, E (1979) Amplitude of pulsatile GnRH input and pituitary gonadotropin secretion. Fed Proc 38:978.

Wilkin, JK (1981) Flushing reactions: consequences and mechanisms. Ann Intern Med 95:468–476.

Wilson, JL, Newman, EJ, and Newman, HW (1966) Diurnal variation in rate of alcohol metabolism. J Appl Physiol 8:556–558.

Wirz–Justice, A, and Wehr, TA (1983) Neuropsychopharmacology and biological rhythms. In: Mendlewicz, J (ed), *Advances in Biological Psychiatry.* Basel: S. Karger.

Wirz–Justice, A, Kafka, MS, Naberg, D, and Wehr, TA (1980) Circadian rhythms in rat brain and β-adrenergic receptors are modified by chronic imipramine. Life Sci 27:341–347.

Wirz–Justice, A, Tobler, I, Kafka, MS, Naber, D, Marangos, PJ, Borbely, AA, and Wehr, TA (1981) Sleep deprivation: effects of circadian rhythms of rat brain neurotransmitter receptors. Psychiatr Res 5:67–76.

Yen, SCC, and Tsai, CC (1972) Acute gonadotrophin release induced by exogenous estradiol during the midfollicular phase of menstrual cycle. J Clin Endocrinol 34:298–305.

7

Chronobiology and Nutrition

Alain Reinberg

In this chapter, evidence for biological rhythms in nutrient intake and the manner in which foodstuffs are metabolized is presented. From a chronobiologic perspective, both nutrients and pharmacological agents enter into metabolic pathways which are rhythmic in their efficiency and patency. Therefore, it is not unexpected that both exhibit 24-hr, 1-year, and other time dependencies in their metabolism and effects on bodily functions. Many of the circadian differences in nutrient metabolism result from rhythms in cellular processes, as discussed in Chap. 3; others are due to rhythms at other levels of biological organization.

Introduction

Over the years a great number of investigations on biological rhythms and nutrition have been conducted. When considering the results of the many studies together, there appear to be four different aspects of biological rhythms and nutrition (Reinberg 1974a; Reinberg and Ghata 1978). The findings of all the studies can be succinctly cat-

egorized according to these aspects; they are identified as:

Aspect 1: the occurrence of ultradian, circadian, circannual, and other rhythms in the spontaneous intake of food.

Aspect 2: the persistence of most, if not all, circadian rhythms during fasting or during adherence to a very restricted diet (known as the Chossat phenomenon; Chossat 1843).

Aspect 3: the use of a timed and restricted duration of food availability to synchronize, under certain circumstances and/or in certain animal species, a limited number of circadian rhythms.

Aspect 4: the occurrence of variation in the metabolism of nutrients as a function of their administration time.

These categorizations (Reinberg 1974a) of chronobiologic findings are artificial, since in many respects they are complementary. Nonetheless, this type of categorization is useful for discussing the chronobiology of nutrition and to achieve a better understanding of the experimental findings for both nutrition and chronobiology.

Aspect 1: Circadian and Other Rhythms in Spontaneous Food Intake

Circadian periodicity in the timing of spontaneous food intake was observed in rats and/or mice by several investigators (Collier et al. 1972, 1973; Le Magnen 1971a,b; and Poirel 1968, 1975). In hibernating mammals circannual rhythms were demonstrated by Haberey et al. (1967). In adult human beings circannual rhythmicity in food preferences was reported and analyzed by Sargent and Sargent (1950) and Sargent (1954). More recently, Debry and his colleagues (1977) examined circannual rhythms in the intake of total calories, proteins, lipids, and carbohydrates using a different group of 26–29 children during each season of one year. A subgroup composed of the same eight children also was investigated throughout the identical 12-month span. The children who participated in these studies came from broken homes; they had been abandoned or were orphans; 60% were males. They were comparable in age (4 years ± 1.5 years), body weight, and height. They were residents of either one of two separate institutions in Nancy, France, and were adhering to a similar and rigorously enforced activity–rest schedule, unchanging throughout the year. The socioecologic synchronization involved lights-on at 0700 and lights-off at 1830. Meals were provided daily at 0800, 1100, 1400, and 1800 and were of similar composition (proportion of carbohydrates, lipids, and proteins). Every day there was a similar timing of mental and physical activities. Each child was asked at fixed meal times to select spontaneously and without restriction the kind and amount of foods desired, uninfluenced as far as possible by the choices of others, and to consume them in any order. During a 7-day span of adherence to this protocol, the amounts of protein, lipid, carbohydrate, and total calories

actually consumed at each meal were carefully determined. Time series thus obtained were analyzed by the Mean Cosinor (Chap. 2) to detect and characterize bioperiodic phenomena.

A statistically significant circadian rhythm was detected for each of the four variables, for each day of the week, and for each of the groups. The trough of the rhythms occurred around 1200 in almost all the studied circumstances. In other words, spontaneously larger meals were usually taken at 0800 (breakfast) and at 1800 (supper) than around midday. The trough of both lipid and protein intake was timed around 1800 only on Sunday. The weekly mean-adjusted levels (mesors) obtained by Cosinor analysis exhibited a circannual rhythm for the spontaneous intake of lipids, carbohydrates, and calories (Fig. 1). The peak of lipid intake occurred during the spring, while the peak of carbohydrate and calorie consumption was during the summer.

Circannual rhythms in the spontaneous intake of food by infants in the United States were reported by Sargent (1954). The infants also displayed a temporal variation in weight gain with a peak between late summer and early autumn. Sargent found a tendency for infants to consume more fat during the spring and summer rather than during the autumn and winter. Consumption of carbohydrates also tended to be maximal during the spring and summer, although considerable individual variability was evident. In addition Sargent investigated circannual rhythms of food intake in adult human beings (Table 1). Soldiers in training camps, urban families, and mill workers (Anonymous 1951) were observed to consume significantly more calories in the fall and winter than in the spring and summer. This was found also in studies of both young and adult rats (Campbell 1945). These findings suggest that the timing of peaks and troughs of circannual rhythms in the consumption of carbohydrates, fats, and calories differs between growing children and mature adults.

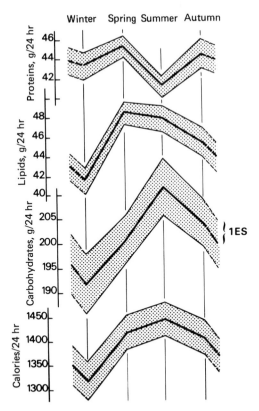

Fig. 1. Circannual changes in the 7-day mean level of spontaneous nutrient and calorie intake in groups of 4-year-old children adhering to a self-selected diet. Statistically significant differences were detected for lipid, carbohydrate, and calorie consumptions when comparing the data of the winter (*trough*) and summer (*peak*) times. The peak in lipids was in the spring. The circannual change in protein intake was not statistically significant. Peak and trough values were t-tested by the student method, being 3.1 for carbohydrates, 2.39 for calories, 2.21 for lipids, and 1.98 (not significant) for proteins. (From Debry et al. 1975, reproduced with permission.)

For every observed biological rhythm, one must consider on the one hand endogenous inherited (genetic) components and on the other hand exogenous components, synchronizers among others, which influence but do not create rhythms. According to Collier and his coworkers (1972, 1973), the study of food consumption has been dominated by a search for those physiological factors, such as the level of circulating metabolites or hormones, the size of the bodily reserves, and the gastrointestinal load, all of which covary with nutritional status and with the initiation and termination of feeding. A major conclusion derived from free-feeding experiments is that the momentary state is irrelevant; more important are those behaviors and functions which pertain to the total food economy of the animal. Thus, the appropriate unit of analysis is the feeding cycle during the 24-hr span rather than the ingestive responses per se. Events which alter metabolic state, such as growth, pregnancy, and environmental conditions, are probably manifested as well as influenced by a modification of the eating pattern, thus affecting the long-term regulation of energy balance.

The circadian rhythm of food intake persists, as do most other rhythms, in man during isolation in a cave without time clue and cue (Migraine et al. 1974). Also relevant are the results obtained by Margules et al. (1972) showing that the (biological) time of the day is a decisive determinant of the effects of L-norepinephrine on feeding behavior in rats. During the dark span a direct application of L-norepinephrine to the hypothalamus *suppresses* feeding behavior, while during the light span it *facilitates* feeding behavior. Also in experiments on rats, Nagai et al. (1982) evaluated the effect of a continuous insulin infusion (0.1 U/hr) into the suprachiasmatic nucleus (SCN) on the circadian rhythm of food intake. Insulin thus administered reduced food intake during the 12-hr dark span and increased it during the 12-hr light span. Saline (1 μl/hr) infused into the SCN as well as insulin (0.1 U/hr) infused into the subcutaneous space did not change the circadian rhythm of food intake. According to Nagai et al. (1982), it is likely that insulin acts directly at the level of the SCN. Again in experiments on rats, Mandenoff and Apfelbaum (1981) demonstrated that two opiate antagonists (Naltrexone and Nalaxone zinc tannate) had a suppressive effect on hyperphagia during the dark span but not during the light span.

Table 1. *Seasonal Change in the Consumption of Total Calories by Rat and Man.*

Type of population	Caloric consumption by season as percent of spring value (= 100%)[a]				Ref.
	Spring (calories)	Summer (%)	Fall (%)	Winter (%)	
Young rats	45.0[b]	*95.0*	100.3	*102.0*	Campbell (1945)
Adult rats	20.5[b]	94.8	101.2	*102.0*	Campbell (1945)
Soldiers	3650[c]	98.3	100.9	*102.7*	Marlin and Hildebrandt (1919)
Soldiers	3570[c]	103.0	*110.3*	103.4	Howe and Berryman (1945)
Mill workers	2680[d]	100.5	*97.3*	*112.8*	Sargent and Sargent (1950)
Urban families	3810[d]	*94.5*	98.1	*104.3*	Dept. of Agriculture (1951)

[a] Italicized values represent timing of maxima and minima.

[b] Calories per 100 g of body weight.

[c] Calories per man per day.

[d] Calories per adult male per day.

Aspect 2: Persistence of Circadian Rhythms During Near-fasting or Dietary Restriction— The Chossat Phenomenon

Persistence of the temperature circadian rhythm of pigeons during total food and water deprivation was first reported by Chossat in 1843. This pioneer work has been widely confirmed since for other animal species, including man, and for other circadian rhythms as summarized in Table 2.

A larger study in terms of both the number of investigated subjects and variables was performed by Apfelbaum et al. (1971, 1972) and Reinberg et al. (1973a, 1974a). A group of 112 healthy obese women, ranging in age from 18 to 25 years, were fed a hypocaloric (220 cal/24 hr), exclusively protein, diet for 3 weeks. The purpose of the diet was to provide sufficient quantities of protein to balance nitrogen loss to protect the lean mass of the body. Proteins were given in the form of calcium caseinate (55 g/24 hr). Although the subjects were deprived of both carbohydrates and lipids, they were provided potassium chloride and vitamins according to their calculated needs (Apfelbaum et al. 1971). The women were synchronized to light-on at 0730 and light-off at 2330. They were provided three (or four) isocaloric meals daily at 0800, 1200 (1600), and 2000. A number of biological variables

were studied: plasma growth hormone, insulin, glucagon, cortisol as well as urinary volume, nitrogen, 17-hydroxycorticosteroids, 17-ketosteroids, potassium, and sodium. Respiratory quotient, oxygen consumption, in addition to rectal temperature, grip strength, tempo, and eye–hand skill were investigated also. Biological sampling and self-measurements of certain skills were done at fixed hours at equal intervals four times daily once or twice weekly, before and during the 3-week adherence to the protein diet. Statistically significant circadian rhythms were detected in all the variables studied before and during the 220 cal/24 hr protein diet (Fig. 2).

A significant decrease in the 24-hr mean level was exhibited by the following variables: respiratory quotient, oxygen consumption, plasma growth hormone, and insulin as well as urinary nitrogen, 17-ketosteroids, and sodium. A rise occurred in plasma cortisol only during the second week of the protein diet. Changes in the mean level of the other variables were not significant (Fig. 3).

In examining the data from some experiments, it appears that every physiological variable need not follow the phenomenon described by Chossat. Plasma gastrin is an exception. There is good agreement between the results of experiments performed on fasted rats (Berard et al. 1976; Accary et

Table 2. *Persistence of Physiological Circadian Rhythms During Food Deprivation or Hypocaloric Diet.*

Subjects	Synchronizer schedule	Type of diet	Studied circadian physiological variations (Δt = sampling interval)	Refs.
Birds (pigeon, etc.)	Natural LD cycle	Complete deprivation of food and water until death	Cloacal temperature (Δt = 12 hr)	Chossat (1843)
766 ♀ C mice 4, 5 months of age	L (0600–1800) D (1800–0600)	No food, no water No food but water (16–76 hr)	Liver glycogen (Δt = 4 hr)	Haus and Halberg (1966)
192 ♀ C mice 3–4 months of age	L (0600–1800) D (1800–0600)	No food, no water during a 36-hr span of time	Rectal temperature, pituitary adrenocorticotropic activity, serum corticosterone, pinnal mitosis (Δt = 4 hr)	Galicich et al. (1963) Halberg et al. (1965)
450 ♂ Wistar rats (200 g)	L (0600–1800) D (1800–0600)	No food, water *ad lib.* during a 5-day span	Plasma and antral gastrin (Δt = 4 hr)	Pansu et al. (1979) Bosshard et al. (1982)
7 ♂ adult Wistar rats	L (0700–1900) D (1900–0700)	No food, water *ad lib.*	Plasma TSH ($\Delta t \cong$ 1 hr by catheter)	Hugues et al. (1982)
7 healthy human adults, 3 ♀ and 4 ♂ 18 to 45 years of age	L (0745–2300) D (2300–0745)	Complete 36-hr bedrest with 4-hourly hypocaloric meals during sampling (336 cal/24 hr as tomato juice)	Heart rate, blood pressure, urinary potassium, 17-hydroxycorticosteroid, adrenaline, noradrenaline, vanillylmandelic acid (Δt = 4 hr)	Reinberg et al. (1970)
8 healthy obese human ♀ 18 to 25 years of age	L (0730–2330) D (2330–0730)	15 to 20 days of caloric restriction (220 cal/24 hr as protein exclusively)	Oxygen consumption ($\dot{V}O_2$) respiratory quotient (RQ = $\dot{V}CO_2/\dot{V}O_2$) (Δt = 0.5 hr)	Apfelbaum, et al. (1971)
6 healthy human ♂ 18 to 25 years of age	L (0700–0000) D (0000–0700)	Low protein diet (30 cal/kg body w/24 hr: egg protein)	Tyrosine and other amino acid concentration in plasma (Δt = 4 hr)	Wurtman et al. (1967, 1968)
104 healthy obese human ♀ 18 to 25 years of age	L (0730–2330) D (2330–0730)	15 to 20 days of caloric restriction (220 cal/24 hr as protein exclusively)	Plasma GH, cortisol insulin, glucagon; urinary water, nitrogen, 17-OHCS, 17-KS, K^+, Na^+; oral temperature; tempo; grip strength; self-rated hunger, fatigue, etc.	Apfelbaum et al. (1972) Reinberg et al. (1973a, 1974)
7 healthy human ♂ 27 ± 1.7 years of age	L (0600–2100) D (2100–0600)	No food, distilled water (48 hr)	Urinary cAMP Δt = 3 hr	Stone et al. (1974)

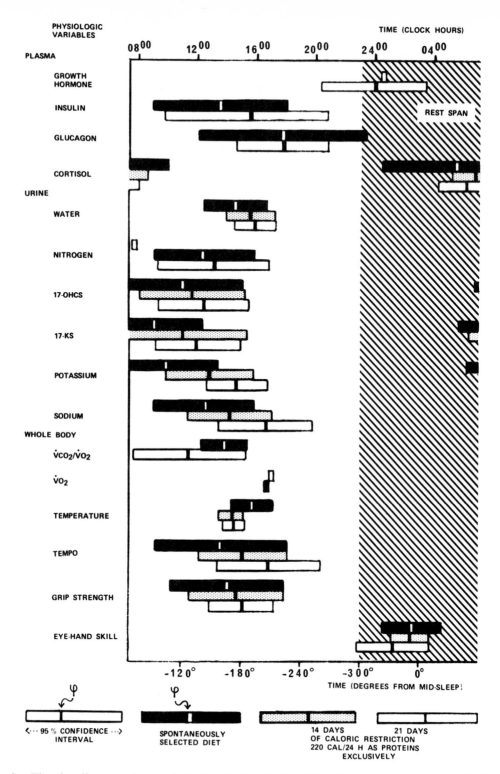

Fig. 2. The circadian acrophases of physiological variables of healthy young obese women before and during adherence to a calorie-restricted protein diet. Results presented pertain only to circadian acrophases referenced to midsleep (φ) and their 95% confidence intervals statistically significant circadian rhythms persisted in the studied physiological variables. A phase shift (Δφ) was detected for urinary potassium and sodium but not for the φ of the other studied circadian rhythms. (From Reinberg et al. 1973a.)

al. 1977b) and fasted human beings (Moor et al. 1974; Accary et al. 1977a). In both, the plasma gastrin circadian rhythm, which was detected when subjects were fed, was rapidly obliterated during fasting. A likely hypothesis is that plasma gastrin reflects the amount of circulating hormone resulting from its liberation rather than from its production. For example, Pansu et al. (1979) studied circadian rhythms of gastrin in the plasma and the gastric antral mucosa—one of the principal sites of gastrin synthesis. The plasma gastrin circadian rhythm was detected in 200-g male rats fed *ad libitum* as well as in animals starved for 2 days. The acrophase coincided approximately with the middle of the activity (dark) span. The plasma gastrin rhythm was obliterated during the next 3 days of fasting and the mesor decreased. The antral gastrin circadian rhythm persisted both in fed and starved animals without a change in the acrophase, which occurred around the beginning of the activity (dark) span.

These findings suggest that the secretion of gastrin is complex. In fed rats, the acrophase of antral gastrin leads in phase that of plasma gastrin. The persistence of a circadian rhythm in gastrin synthesis during fasting favors an endogenous origin for this bioperiodic phenomenon. Differences in the ϕ between the circadian rhythms of plasma and antral gastrin confirm the complex relationship between the synthesis, storage, and secretion of this hormone.

The continued manifestation of human circadian rhythms while adhering to a very restricted protein diet of 220 cal/24 hr without lipid and carbohydrate intake can be considered the equivalent of the Chossat phenomenon. This means that circadian changes in a large number of physiological variables studied in various animal species, including man, are not primarily induced by "fuel" intake. This observation supports the widely accepted hypothesis of most chronobiologists that many circadian rhythms have an endogenous basis. The Chossat phenomenon is one of the experimental arguments, among many others, to

be taken into account demonstrating that the temporal structure, even in man, is genetically inherited rather than acquired by each generation (Pittendrigh 1960; Aschoff 1963).

The continuance of bioperiodic phenomena during fasting and/or while adhering to a diet of very low caloric value is, however, compatible with the fact that the timing of food intake, i.e., the periodicity of meals, is a synchronizer in certain circumstances and for certain animal species (as discussed under Aspect 3). It must be kept in mind that synchronizers (or *Zeitgebers,* Aschoff 1954), while not creating biological rhythms, may affect the rhythm's acrophase and/or period. The synchronizing effect of meal timing whether spontaneous (Aspect 1) or experimentally manipulated (Aspect 3) is a phenomenon complementary to the persistence of circadian rhythmicity during fasting.

The finding of persistence in the circadian rhythms of peripheral blood insulin and glucagon as found in various experiments requires careful interpretation. Since the timing of protein intake is periodic and since protein may induce a rise in insulin (Felig et al. 1973) and glucagon plasma levels (Marliss et al. 1970), it is not possible to conclude solely from the aforementioned study of healthy obese women that the insulin and glucagon circadian rhythms have an exclusively endogenous origin.* Circadian changes in the plasma insulin response to 50 g of glucose taken orally given after a 14-hr fast in separate studies carried out at different times (0800, 1600, and 0000) each on different days have been reported by Sensi et al. (1970) and Capani et al. (1972). Rauline et al. (1981) demonstrated the persistence of the circadian rhythms of plasma insulin, cortisol, gastrin, and testosterone in eight recumbent adult subjects, fed only by venous infusion delivering a constant amount of water, emulsified lipids, 60 g/l amino acids, and carbohydrates over 24 hr.

* Circadian and circannual changes in hormones other than insulin involved in the control of metabolic pathways are not considered in this review.

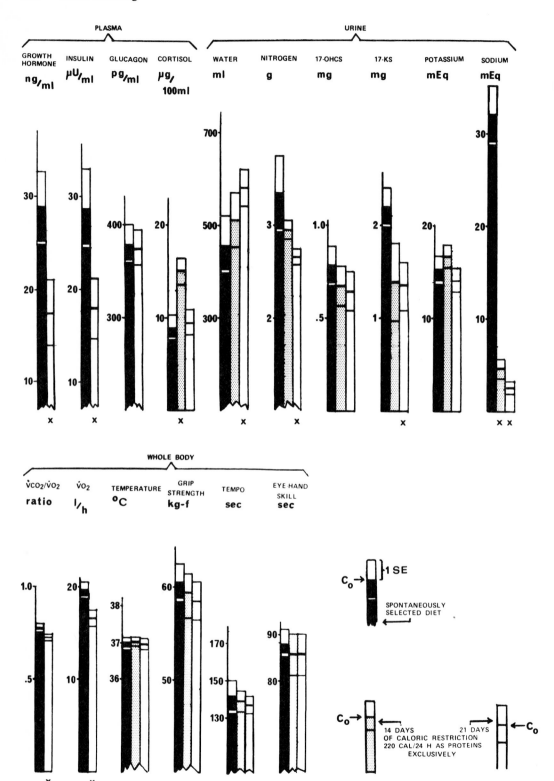

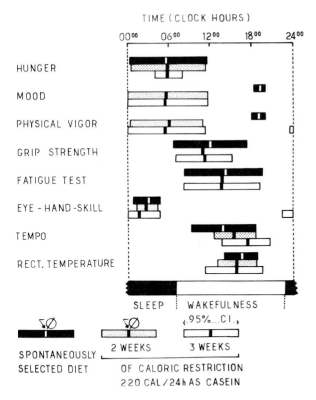

Fig. 4. The circadian ϕ of physiological variables studied in 9 healthy obese young women investigated before and during a 3-week span of adherence to a 220 cal/24 hr protein diet. A statistically significant ϕ shift of about 12 hr occurred only in the circadian rhythms of hunger and mood self-ratings when the subjects were adhering to the restricted protein diet. The ϕs of the other investigated variables showed neither diet-induced shifts nor consistent differences with respect to the timing of the ϕ as found in other types of studies performed on healthy human adults. (From Apfelbaum et al. 1976a, reproduced with permission.)

Thus, an endogenous component of the circadian rhythm of human plasma insulin is probable, even if direct evidence is not as yet available.

From a practical point of view, it is germane to ask whether or not a diet entirely of protein—220 cal/24 hr—is objectively compatible with normal activity. In a group of nine healthy obese women a set of several physiological and psychophysiological variables was studied: self-ratings of hunger, mood, and physical vigor as well as self-recording of grip strength, muscular fatigue, eye–hand skill, tempo, and body temperature. Measurements were performed every 6 hr at fixed times during a 24-hr span once weekly, before (nonrestricted spontaneous food intake) and for 3 weeks during adherence to the 220 cal/24 hr protein diet consisting of 55 g of calcium caseinate supplemented with potassium salts, water, and vitamins (Apfelbaum et al. 1976a,b) (Figs. 4 and 5). The findings indicate that as long as nitrogen balance remains equilibrated a very restricted diet affects neither the grip strength, muscular fatigue, mood, and physical vigor nor their circadian rhythms. The restricted diet does

Fig. 3. The circadian rhythm-adjusted level M (designated in figure as C_o) for a set of physiological variables of healthy young obese women before and during the adherence to a calorie-restricted protein diet. The M equals the 24-hr average ($\bar{x}$) since data were collected at equal intervals. A statistically significant fall (indicated by **x**) in M occurred during calorie restriction for the respiratory quotient, oxygen consumption, plasma growth hormone, and insulin as well as the urinary variables of nitrogen, 17-KS, and sodium. A statistically significant rise in plasma cortisol occurred only during the second week of the protein diet. No change occurred in the M of the other studied variables. (From Reinberg et al. 1973a.)

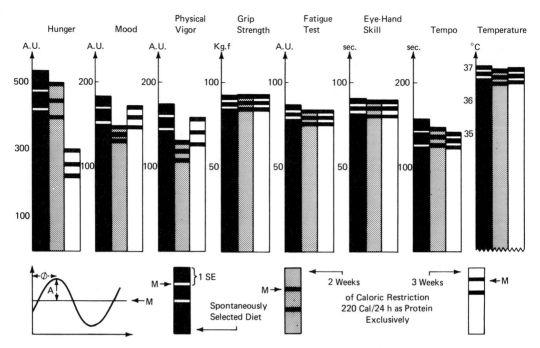

Fig. 5. Circadian-rhythm-adjusted mean (M) for the same study conditions, subjects, and physiological variables as in Fig. 4. A statistically significant diet-induced drop of about 55% occurred during the third week in the hunger self-rating M, apparently related to a change in the "fuel" used by the brain—ketones instead of carbohydrates. A transient drop in both the M of mood and physical vigor self-ratings occurred only during the second week of the diet. The M of the other variables did not exhibit statistically significant changes. As a whole, these results favor the conclusion that the 220 cal/ 24 hr protein diet is not likely to disturb a subject's fitness for nonstrenuous work. (From Apfelbaum et al. 1976a, reproduced with permission.)

induce a statistically significant decrease in hunger as revealed by the self-rating method. Thus, adherence to the calcium caseinate protein diet appears to be compatible with nonstrenuous physical activity and work.

Aspect 3: A Timed and Restricted Duration of Food Availability Is Not a Powerful Synchronizer of Rhythms

In night-active rodents, such as mice, rats, and rabbits, eating occurs mainly, if not exclusively, during the night even if food is available continuously (*ad libitum*) in quantity and in time. In such experimental conditions, the light–dark alternation is

the most powerful synchronizer. When food is provided solely during the light span, with availability restricted to only a few hours such as for 2–4 hr/24 hr, a set of circadian rhythms in certain animal species undergoes phase shifts. This is the case in the rat for the rhythms of rest and activity, brain serotonin (Baker 1953; Mouret and Bobiller 1971; Mouret et al. 1973), certain blood and serum variables, liver temperature (von Mayersbach et al. 1973; Nelson et al. 1973), some liver enzymes (Walker and Potter 1974; Cohn et al. 1970; Fuller 1970), CO_2 emission (Stupfel et al. 1973), plasma corticosterone, and rectal temperature (Krieger 1974; 1979). This is the case also in the rat for the rhythms of intraperitoneal temperature (Ehret et al. 1977, 1978) and blood eosinophil levels (Pauly et al. 1973,

1975). For primates, this is true for the rhythms of body temperature and plasma corticosterone (Sulzman et al. 1977). Experimental results related to rhythm entrainment by a timed and restricted duration of food availability were reported earlier by Shirley (1928), Achelis and Nothdurft (1939), and Kleitman and Engelmann (1947).

Halberg (1974) considering the findings from investigations on rodents proposed as a working hypothesis that a timed and restricted duration of food availability is a powerful synchronizer of circadian rhythms. It seems at present, however, that the results of a limited number of experiments on these animals were overgeneralized. It has to be emphasized that most research on the synchronizing or circadian phase-influencing effect of food intake has utilized as an investigative methodology *competition studies* between (at least) two synchronizers (Aschoff et al. 1975). This type of research results in the simultaneous evaluation of the relative significance or power of various synchronizers, i.e., either meal timing versus the light-dark alternation in studies on rodents or meal timing versus socioecologic synchronization in studies on human beings (Apfelbaum et al. 1969; Aschoff et al. 1971, 1975). In retrospect, it seems that it would have been more pertinent to utilize experimental conditions in which subjects were isolated and insulated from all known synchronizers except the random manipulation of meal times since this would have resulted in more specific findings on the prominence of meal timing as a synchronizer of selected circadian rhythms. Obviously, results of competition studies are more difficult to analyze than studies in which only one major synchronizer is manipulated. Nevertheless, competition studies mimic rather well what may happen in natural conditions.

Some investigators have used sham foods; however, control experiments with sham foods (in terms of taste, palatability, physical properties, and volume, for example) have yet to be conducted. "Intelli-

gent" animals such as mice, rats, and man are able to easily recognize the difference between regular and sham foods; this confounds the purpose of certain control studies. The so-called "artificial feeding" using a catheter inserted into a blood vessel or into the stomach does not satisfactorily solve the problem posed by sham foods since with this approach results might represent changes with regard to the time of the disposition of nutrient(s) rather than the changes in the timing of meals per se. Furthermore, the intake of nutrients by mouth has to be considered as more physiological than is artificial feeding.

It is useful to review the findings of investigations on rats and mice for which the synchronizer effect of scheduled feedings has been documented. In a study involving 360 CDF_1 mice 4 weeks of age, Scheving et al. (1974 a,b) and Pauly et al. (1975) demonstrated that meal timing, achieved by restricting the access to food to a 4-hr span beginning at different clock hours over the 24 hr, dominated the synchronizing effect of the light-dark regimen with regard to the blood eosinophil rhythm. In the same animals, however, the mitotic rhythm of corneal epithelium remained synchronized to the light-dark cycle; only minor changes in the phasing of the rhythms resulted from the timed-restricted feedings. Studies performed by Philippens et al. (1977) on 270 male (specific-pathogen-free) Wistar rats (130 ± 12 g) indicated also that rhythms of this species cannot be entrained by meal timing. For example, the circadian rhythm of mitotic activity in the corneal epithelium exhibited synchronization to the light-dark cycle only. Phase shifts in the timing of the restricted food availability induced an alteration in the serum corticosterone rhythm manifested as a polyphasic pattern with two to three peaks of more or less equal amplitude. However, there was no consistent and predictable synchronizing effect. Cohn et al. (1970) also reported that the circadian pattern of adrenal corticosterone concentration in rats is not related to the cyclicity of food intake, while Krieger (1974, 1979) found in adult female Sprague-Dawley rats that the plasma corticosterone rhythm could be entrained by shifting the timing of food presentation. Nelson et al. (1973b, 1975) reported that plasma corticosterone levels of mice do synchronize to restricted feeding schedules. With regard to this variable, it could be that the synchronizing effect of meal timing differs between strains of rats and/or is sex related. One has to consider that the difference in findings between investigations may represent specific characteristics of the laboratory setting in which studies were conducted. Perhaps extraneous time-dependent alterations in the laboratory environment result in important synchronizing signals. Thus, aspects of human activity related to animal care and other laboratory functions associated with the timing of food to some extent may be responsible for inducing alteration of certain circadian systems. Since experimental facilities differ widely between laboratories, the possibility of extraneous influences acting as synchronizers cannot be dismissed without appropriate control studies.

For other circadian rhythms of male rats (e.g., serum protein, serum lactic dehydrogenase, serum α-hydroxybutiric dehydrogenase), Philippens et al. (1977) demonstrated, as in the case of serum corticosterone, that although meal timing influences the rhythmic pattern, the synchronizing effect of the light-dark cycle still persists. The circadian rhythm of liver glycogen and protein concentration as well as serum glucose was controlled mainly by the timing of food intake. It is a matter of interest that in contrast to all other variables studied by these authors, the circadian rhythm of liver α-hydroxybutiric dehydrogenase appeared to be completely independent of both the light-dark cycle and the feeding schedule.

The suprachiasmatic nucleus (SCN) appears to be one of the oscillators which governs a set of neuroendocrine circadian rhythms (Rietveld and Gross 1980; Szafarczyc et al. 1981; Assenmacher 1982) and also has been studied for the synchronizing effect of cyclic food intakes. Krieger et al. (1977) have demonstrated in the rat that lesioning of the SCN does not abolish rhythms of food intake, adrenal activity, or body temperature. Using implanted electrodes, Inouye (1982) recorded the neural activity of the SCN in male albino rats to investigate the effects of both free feeding and restricted daily feeding schedules (e.g., a 3-hr span of food availability at fixed clock hours for 10–19 days). When rats were kept in LD 12:12 with free access to food, motor activity predominated during D while the neural activity of the SCN predominated during L. When the rats were housed in constant darkness, the circadian rhythm of neural activity in the SCN became free running, despite the fact that food presentation, restricted to a specified 3-hr span, occurred daily at the same fixed clock time. Under these experimental conditions, the motor activity rhythm, however, was synchronized by the timing of food presentation. Manipulation of the timing of the restricted food presentation did not produce a phase shift in the SCN circadian rhythm. These findings indicate that in the rat the circadian rhythms of SCN are not synchronized by the 24-hr rhythm of food intake.

From these experiments, as well as others on rodents, it can be concluded that food availability when restricted only to a few hours during each 24 hr has a prominent and more powerful synchronizing effect than the light-dark cycle (1) only on a restricted set of rhythms and (2) with regard to certain circumstances which are related to strain and/or sex, for example, the corticosterone rhythm of rats and mice. With respect to the findings on rodents, it was premature to propose a "diet plan for shiftworkers and transmeridian travellers" (Ehret et al. 1978) based on the assumption that properly timed specifically formulated meals, which induce a shift in the temperature rhythm of rats, can phase shift the entire temporal structure of man. In fact, in human beings the situation is somewhat different or at least more complex.

In human beings it also appears that only a limited number of circadian rhythms can be entrained by meal timing. Circadian rhythms of heart rate, plasma cortisol, as well as urinary volume, nitrogen, creatinine, 17-hydroxycorticosteroids, 17-ketosteroids, potassium, and sodium were studied in 36 healthy, overweight young women, 18–25 years of age (Apfelbaum 1975). They were investigated while adhering to an unrestricted spontaneous diet with meals at 0800, 1200, and 2000 and also while adhering to a protein diet consisting of 220 cal/24 hr calcium caseinate for 3 weeks. The timing of food consumption was changed weekly according to the following schedule: A = four isocaloric meals at 0800, 1200, 1600, and 2000; B = one meal daily at 0800 (breakfast) and C = one meal daily at 2000 (supper). The subjects were randomized for the sequential order of these meal programs. All subjects were synchronized with light-on at 0730 and light-off at 2330 before and throughout the study span. At the end of each of the study weeks, the selected variables were investigated for circadian rhythms during 24-hr or 48-hr spans. Data were collected every 6 hr at fixed times and analyzed for circadian rhythms using the Cosinor method. Statistically significant circadian rhythms were detected ($p < 0.05$) for practically every variable and experimental circumstance (Fig. 6) with only the acrophase of the circadian rhythm of urinary nitrogen exhibiting a shift (week B). The other investigated variables exhibited neither alterations in acrophase nor amplitude.

In this experiment, apart from the urinary nitrogen and maybe the urinary K^+ and Na^+ rhythms, the timed consumption of the protein diet with respect to the 24-hr scale did not influence the temporal structure. This finding does not agree with the results of studies on rats, mice, and rabbits in which a synchronizing effect of meal timing has been demonstrable at least for certain circadian systems. To understand the

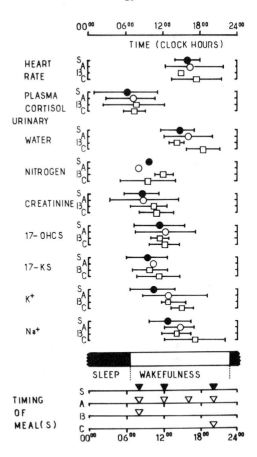

Fig. 6. Acrophase of human circadian rhythms with respect to various meal timings: S = spontaneous diet; A,B,C = protein diet with caloric restriction (220 cal/24 hr as casein, exclusively) as indicated. Subjects were healthy, obese women tested before and during 3 weeks of a protein diet with calorie restriction. (From Apfelbaum et al. 1976b, reproduced with permission.)

discrepancy in the chronobiologic findings between humans and rodents, three possible explanations must be examined:

Duration of Experimental Food Restriction. The experimental duration of study of human beings for each meal timing pattern was only one week. A phase shift

278   Alain Reinberg

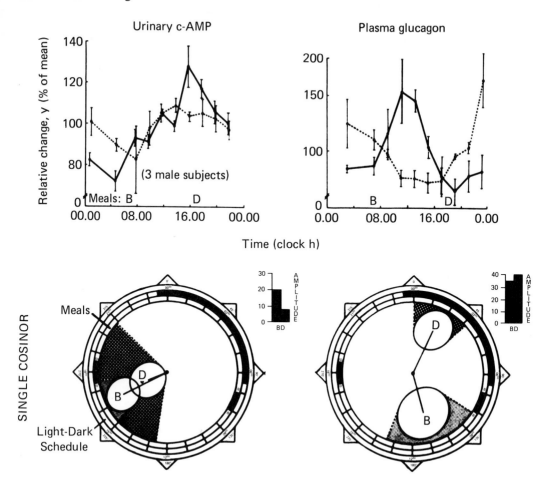

Fig. 7. Circadian rhythms are differently influenced by a single daily 2000-calorie meal given for 7-day spans. Blood and urine samples were obtained every 2 hr during waking and once in the middle of the sleep span from each of 14 young male volunteers during the last 24 hr of one 7-day span while eating breakfast only (B) and another 7-day span while eating dinner only (D). Each data series on plasma glucagon, insulin, serum iron, and urinary cAMP (nmol/hr) was converted to a percentage of the respective 24-hr mean. In the chronograms (**top**) the x̄ ± 1 SE of these converted values across all 14 subjects is plotted against the sampling time, each chronogram presenting results for a given variable on B (*solid line*) and D (*dotted line*). The Cosinor plots (**bottom**) depict the results of fitting a single 24-hr cosine curve to all the data on each variable and meal schedule. The length and direction of each radial line (vector) indicate the amplitude A and acrophase φ, respectively, of the fitted cosine. The ellipse at the tip of each vector represents the 95% confidence region for A and φ. Statistically significant rhythms in all variables are indicated by the fact that none of these confidence regions overlap the "pole" (*center of plot*). Whereas the φ of insulin, glucagon, and iron rhythms are different for B and D; that of cAMP is similar through the different meal schedules. (From Goetz et al. 1976, reproduced with permission.)

(Δφ) of many physical variables usually requires longer than 7 days, but this is not a rule since the possibility of fast adjustment of circadian rhythms has been demonstrated in certain subjects, e.g., shift workers and students phase shifted by a syn-

chronizer manipulation (Reinberg et al. 1973b, 1979b,c).

Physiological Factors. When food is not available *ad libitum*, in both time and quantity, an alteration of the circadian pattern of

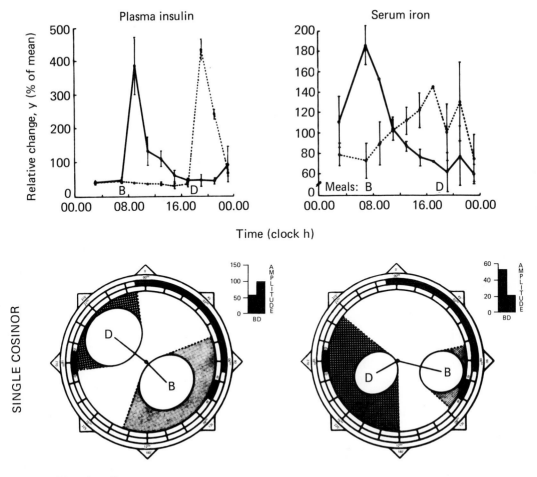

Fig. 7. (*Continued*)

behavior and activity in rodents is obligatory to meet nutritional needs. In contrast, for human beings involved in this type of study, there is the implication, whether direct or indirect (via human rights committees or others), that they eventually will receive their meal(s).

Meal Composition. The findings on human beings pertaining to the effects of meal timing as a synchronizer of circadian rhythms relate only to a protein diet. The effect of meal timing, with the meal not restricted to protein, could be different. This latter possibility has been studied by Goetz et al. (1976). Healthy young adults were provided a 2000 cal/24 hr diet given as a single meal daily, either at 0800 (breakfast)

or at 2000 (supper). A statistically significant change in the ϕ of 8 hr to 12 hr was exhibited by the circadian rhythms of plasma insulin and glucagon as well as serum iron (Fig. 7). Smaller $\Delta\phi$'s amounting to only 2–3 hr, but still statistically significant, occurred in the rhythms of plasma cortisol and growth hormone as well as those of the white blood cells and lymphocytes. The other studied variables did not show a $\Delta\phi$ in this "once-a-day" meal timing study.

Another study was performed by Bazin et al. (1979) with experimental conditions more resembling a "normal" pattern of food consumption. With respect to the control span during which the spontaneous diet was allowed, 14 clinically healthy men,

20–22 years of age, ate three meals daily throughout two spans of 3 weeks' duration. During the "big breakfast" weeks, the subjects consumed 60% of their total daily calories at breakfast, 30% at lunch, and 10% at dinner. During still another span of 3 weeks, the "big dinner" weeks, the situation was reversed; the men consumed 10% of their total daily calories at breakfast, 30% at lunch, and 60% at dinner. Throughout, the subjects were diurnally active with rest from 2200 to 0700.

The circadian rhythm of plasma cortisol was not altered. However, for both serum nonesterified fatty acids (NEFA) and ketone bodies, two peaks within each 24 hr appeared in the chronogram on a "big breakfast," but not on a "big dinner" schedule, with one of the peaks occurring around 0200, a time quite delayed from the ingestion of the major meal. According to this change in waveform and/or in frequency, the ϕ of these rhythms seemed to have advanced rather than delayed in timing with a change from the "big breakfast" to "big dinner" schedule.

Thus, the selected timed consumption of the large daily meal can phase shift some of the investigated circadian rhythms in healthy young adults. According to Halberg (1974), the manipulation of meal timing might serve to phase shift, at least partially, some human circadian rhythms. In rodents such phase changes of physiological rhythms have been associated with phase alterations in the organism's susceptibility to various therapeutic agents, including medications, antimitotic agents, and X rays. Phase shifting of physiochemical circadian rhythms in human beings may provide a means to achieve chronoptimization of certain therapeutic agents, including cytostatic ones (Halberg 1960, 1969; Halberg and Reinberg 1976; Haus et al. 1974; Reinberg 1967, 1974b; Reinberg and Halberg 1971). However, the evidence on hand today reveals that changes in meal timing in human subjects influence mainly, if not exclusively, the acrophase of certain circadian rhythms of plasma hormones, such as insulin and glucagon, and that of the circadian rhythms of certain nutrient metabolites, such as nitrogen, ketones, and NEFA. There is as yet no experimental evidence that in healthy adult human beings meal timing is a powerful synchronizer of circadian rhythms. Results of studies on shift workers, discussed later in the chapter, also favor this conclusion for Aspect 3.

Aspect 4: Bioperiodic Changes in Nutrient Metabolism

Changes in the metabolism of a given nutrient are related to hormonal and other chronophysiological phenomena in much the same manner as are bioperiodic changes in the chronopharmacologic effects of a given drug (Reinberg 1973a,b) (see Chap. 6). As in the case of timed drug administrations, one must consider two possible effects when scheduling timed food intake: (1) alteration of the temporal structure as noted by phase shifts and (2) metabolic changes resulting from the timed absorption of a nutrient. Both effects have been investigated and substantiated experimentally.

Evidence for the alteration of the temporal structure comes from Peret et al. (1972) and Nelson et al. (1973a,b), who showed for the rat a phase shift in the liver glycogen circadian rhythm induced by a timed protein intake. Another study by Zigmond et al. (1969), also on rats, showed a phase shift in some circadian rhythms of enzyme activity induced by a timed food administration. Such phase shifts resulting from the timing of nutrients seem to be restricted, however, to a rather specific set of physiological variables. Because of this, an internal dissociation of rhythms results, rather than an internal desynchronization. Phase shifts in rodents due to the timed intake of nutrients should be differentiated from the possible synchronizer effects that the timing of nutrients can induce in certain circumstances and certain animal species (Aspect 3). These differences in effects upon rhythms, phase alteration versus synchronization [or dissociation versus desynchronization (Aschoff et al. 1975)], must be kept in mind even if the chronophysiological bases of these two phenomena are yet unknown and are apparently similar or closely related.

It is useful to consider some illustrative examples of the second effect—biological rhythms and the induction of metabolic changes by timing the intake of nutrients. The metabolism of nutrients is not constant; instead, it varies as a function of their timing. This is best exemplified by the blood glucose tolerance test (GTT), whether carried out by "loading" glucose orally or intravenously. When the GTT is performed under carefully standardized conditions, different findings result from tests done in the morning as compared to ones done in the afternoon or evening (Bowen and Reeves 1967; Campbell et al. 1975; Capani 1972; Gibson et al. 1975; Jarrett 1972; Jarrett and Keen 1972; Lestradet et al. 1970; Sensi et al. 1970; Whichelow et al. 1974; Zimmet et al. 1974). The oral GTT is both sex and age dependent; nevertheless, temporal differences have been found for the oral GTT in groups matched for age and sex as demonstrated by Zimmet et al. (1974). The mean blood sugar levels at 120 and 150 min vary between males and females, being higher in women than in men in both morning and afternoon tests. Moreover, the swing in the mean blood sugar level when comparing the responses of the morning and afternoon tests is greater in older than in younger subjects (Fig. 8).

Differences in the plasma insulin and growth hormone responses to GTTs when performed in the morning versus the afternoon have been reported by Whichelow et al. (1974). Plasma insulin levels were lower following afternoon as compared to morning intravenous GTT studies. As expected, blood sugar levels were lower when the intravenous GTT was performed during the morning rather than during the afternoon. This finding is in agreement with that obtained from research conducted using an oral GTT (Jarrett and Keen 1970, 1972). It should be noted that time-related differences observed in oral and intravenous GTTs could be at least partially related to circadian changes in the plasma insulin responsiveness (Fig. 9) and the absorption of glucose from the gastrointestinal tract demonstrated both by in vivo and in vitro experiments (Furuya and Yugari 1974; Fisher and Garner 1976).

Related to the temporal differences in the GTT response are findings indicating

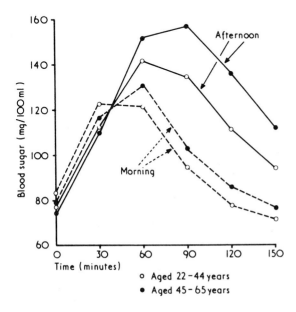

Fig. 8. Mean blood sugar levels in subjects ranging in age from 22 to 44 (○) and 45 to 65 (●) years. Both young and older age groups exhibited greater glucose levels following the afternoon GTT. The older persons exhibited greatest blood sugar levels independent of the time when the GTT was conducted. (From Zimmet et al. 1974, reproduced with permission.)

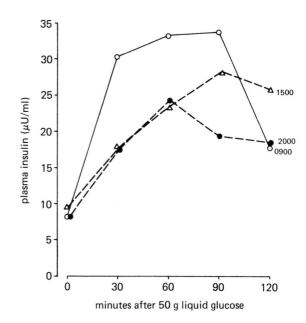

Fig. 9. Mean plasma insulin levels of 24 human subjects following a 50 g oral GTT. Three different test times, each on a separate day, revealed the insulin response to glucose loading was greatest and most rapid in the morning, 0900. (From Jarrett 1972, reproduced with permission.)

that insulin is more effective in reducing blood glucose levels when tests are done in the morning than in the afternoon (Fig. 10). In one investigation (Gibson et al. 1975), insulin (0.05 units/kg body weight) was given intravenously to 14 subjects, both at 0800 and 1700, in random order 8 hr after a 50 g glucose meal. Fasting glucose levels prior to insulin administration were similar at 0800 and 1700, but the 48 ± 10% fall in blood glucose in the morning test was significantly greater (p < 0.001) than the 34 ± 7% dip found in the afternoon test.

Complementary findings were reported by Mirouze et al. (1976) using an "artificial pancreas" in insulin-dependent diabetic subjects. With the artificial pancreas, blood sugar is monitored continuously. When the glucose level rises to a predetermined set point, a controlled amount of insulin is injected intravenously through a catheter. When the glucose level decreases beyond a predetermined level, a flux of glucose is delivered. In this manner, the artificial pancreas maintains the blood glucose level oscillating between fixed limits with both the quantity and timing of the injected insulin recorded. Records of diabetic patients using the artificial pancreas reveal the need

for insulin varies temporally; it is greatest between late morning and early afternoon and least during the night.

In addition to these circadian changes, seasonal variations in the level of blood glucose and the plasma insulin response to orally administered glucose have been observed (Campbell et al. 1975a,b; Méjean et al. 1977; Debry et al. 1977). In one study by Campbell et al. (1975a,b), oral GTTs were performed on 12 young men in the Antarctic. Tests were conducted in the morning and afternoon at 3-month intervals—in March, June, September, and December. The characteristic diurnal variation in glucose tolerance described above was found to persist throughout the year; however, the magnitude of difference between the morning and afternoon tests was greater during the warmer Antarctic months of December and March. There were significant seasonal differences in glucose tolerance; blood glucose values were lowest, both in the morning and afternoon, during the Antarctic midsummer (in December). The highest insulin levels and the greatest diurnal variation occurred in March (autumn). In subsequent tests, there was a progressive decline in insulin levels, so that in De-

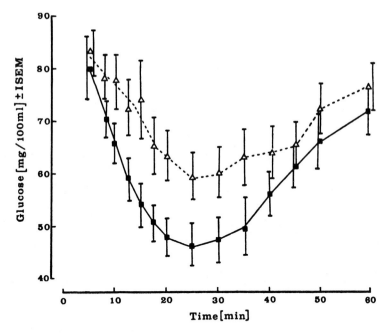

Fig. 10. Mean blood glucose levels following a single timed IV insulin infusion (0.05 units/kg body weight) in 14 healthy subjects. A different test day was used for the morning and evening studies. At 8 hr prior to each infusion, at either 0800 or 1700, a 50 g glucose meal was given at, respectively, 0000 and 0900. Thereafter, subjects fasted until sampled for blood glucose. The effect of insulin on blood glucose was considerably greater when administered at 0800 (*solid line*) as compared to 1700 (*dotted line*). (From Gibson et al. 1975, reproduced with permission.)

cember both the absolute level and the diurnal variation were less than those observed in tests carried out during the other seasons. Complementary studies revealed no diurnal or seasonal differences in the growth hormone (GH) response to the oral GTT.

In Nancy, France, Méjean et al. (1977) conducted GTTs on 60 healthy young males (20–30 years of age), giving each an oral GTT at 0800 every month throughout a 1-year span. The plasma insulin response was analyzed in terms of the usual pharmacokinetic parameters, such as peak height, time to peak, and area under the time-concentration curve (Fig. 11). The insulin peak height was greatest and the time to peak shortest in September (autumn). It was the reverse in April (spring). Such physiological seasonal rhythms must be kept in mind to achieve a better understanding of circan-

nual changes in food consumption as manifested by eating behavior (Aspect 1), insulin effectiveness (Chrometzka 1949; Hommel and Fisher 1971), the incidence of diabetes (Gamble and Taylor 1969), and other metabolic events (David 1967; Haberey et al. 1967; Hughes 1931; Kayser 1961; Krulin and Sealander 1972; Mirouse et al. 1976a,b; Pengelley 1974; Reinberg 1974c; Scheving et al. 1974b; Smolensky et al. 1974).

Circadian and Ultradian Rhythms in the Eating Behavior and Nutrient Intake of Shift Workers

Ultradian, circadian, and circannual rhythms in food intake have been detected and quantified through the study of various animal species (Ardisson et al. 1975; Baker 1953; Campbell 1945; Collier et al. 1972; Haberey et al. 1967; Le Magnen 1971a,b;

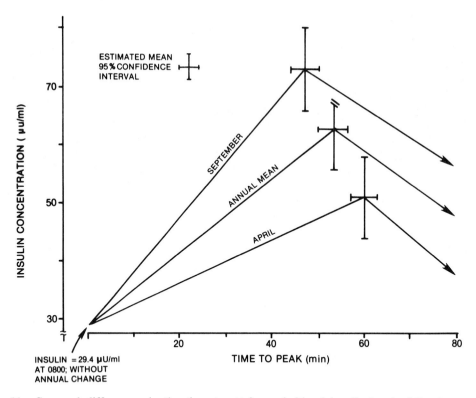

Fig. 11. Seasonal differences in the time to attain peak blood insulin levels following an oral ingestion of 50 g glucose at 0800 in diurnally active subjects dwelling in the Northern Hemisphere (Nancy, France). Studies were conducted at monthly intervals. Major differences occurred between April and September. The span of time for insulin to reach its peak height and the level attained at the peak varied. The peak insulin height for the September as compared to the April test was approximately 1.5 times higher. The time to reach the peak insulin level was longer in April than in September. (From Méjean et al. 1977, reproduced with permission.)

Margules et al. 1972), including human beings (Debry et al. 1973, 1977; Halberg and Reinberg 1967; Hellbrügge et al. 1964; Howe and Berrymann 1945; Reinberg 1971a,b; Sargent 1954; Sargent and Sargent 1950). The respective importance of rhythmic alterations in the environment acting as synchronizers and in endogenous factors, with respect to genetic constitution, has been evaluated in two types of experiments: suppression of known synchronizers and manipulation of work/rest schedules, without changes in meal timing.

Studies of food consumption have been conducted on infants raised under so-called self-demand conditions (Halberg and Reinberg 1967; Hellbrügge et al. 1964; Martin du Pan 1973). Children raised in this manner initiate on their own accord, by self-demand, eating and rest–activity patterns, while as much as possible many aspects of the environment, such as temperature and light, are maintained constant. In the *newborn* raised in this manner, feeding rhythms of approximately 90 min are characteristic. In *older infants* the self-demand schedule results, by the second and third month of life, in four to five meals per day. In isolated healthy young human *adults* (Migraine et al. 1974; Nillus 1967) maintained in the constant environmental conditions of an underground cave for 15 days without time cue and clue, a circadian rhythm with about three meals every 24 hr occurs. The usual pattern persists with modification neither in the timing and number of meals nor the quantity (calories) and quality—proportion of proteins, lipids, and carbohydrates—of food consumption.

As reported in an earlier section of this chapter (Aspect 3), manipulation of meal timing (e.g., one meal daily as a "big breakfast" only or as a "big dinner" only) results in a shift of the circadian acrophase of certain variables only—plasma insulin, glucagon, ketone bodies, NEFA, triglycerides, and urinary nitrogen. Other variables such as plasma cortisol and energy expenditure exhibit only very small acrophase shifts, if any (Apfelbaum et al. 1976a,b; Bazin et al. 1979; Goetz et al. 1976).

Another approach besides "isolation" to assess the respective role of environmental and endogenous factors on eating patterns is to study the effects of competition between several synchronizers as experienced, for example, by shift workers. New methods have been developed and applied to field studies (Reinberg et al. 1971b, 1979; Halberg et al. 1972; Reinberg et al. 1973a,b) to investigate the effects of changes in the synchronizer schedule on food consumption (including the timing, number, and composition of meals) and also on other physiological circadian rhythms of shift workers. In these investigations, a rapid rotation of shifts—every 3 to 4 days rather than the conventional every 7 days—was chosen for study since it is better tolerated by employees from a psychological and physiological point of view (Andlauer 1971; Foret and Benoit 1977; Vieux et al. 1979; Reinberg et al. 1979a–c). The purpose of the research (Reinberg et al. 1979a,c) was to answer the following questions related to the nutrition of shift workers: (1) Is there a change in eating habits in terms of meal timing and number, on the one hand, and in terms of quality and quantity of food intake on the other hand? (2) Does the timing of major meals play a role in the rate of adjustment after changes in the work–rest schedule?

Seven healthy adult male oil refinery operators, ranging in age from 21 to 36 years of age (mean, 26.4 years), all working in the same department, volunteered to record precisely what and when anything was eaten. This was done at work and at home each day during 8 consecutive weeks between late October and early December 1974. Five subjects were shift workers. Two others worked the usual daytime hours and did not participate in shift work. At any time, both at work and at home, all subjects had free access to a large choice of cold and hot meals and beverages in unrestricted quantities. The participants were given specially prepared data sheets—one per 24 hr—to facilitate and standardize the self-recording of food intake and the self-measurements of selected physiological variables performed 5 times/24 hr every 4 hr, except during sleep, at fixed clock hours. Subjects were instructed to adhere to their usual life style and to record each ingested item, including snacks, biscuits, soft and alcoholic beverages, etc., with relevant particulars such as clock time and the nature (trivial but precise name) as well as quantity of food intake. Ambiguities or imprecisions sometimes encountered in the self-reported data were cleared verbally.

Five of the employees had been engaged in shift work for an average of 2 years, with the range being 7 months to 3 years. None had experienced medical or psychological problems, and none had experienced body weight changes, and could be considered tolerant of shift work according to both clinical and chronobiologic criteria (Reinberg et al. 1979b,c). The timing of work given in the order of shift rotation was: "normal day" from 0745 to 1630; night shift from 2100 to 0600; morning shift from 0600 to 1300; and evening shift from 1300 to 2100. The shift duration was 3 to 4 days long. Off days, amounting to as many as 29 days per 100, were scheduled between shifts, mainly after night and morning shift transitions. The timing of work for the two non-shift workers was that of a normal day—from 0745 to 1630—with time off during weekends and special holidays. From a statistical point of view, the small number of subjects is balanced by the large mass of data gathered from each individual, which varied from 180 to 250 recorded food intakes. Since the timing of meals and the corresponding intake of nutrients were recorded continuously, data could be analyzed at 1-hr intervals in the 24-hr scale. Hourly values were presented as a mean ($\bar{x} \pm 1$ SE) for the group of five shift workers and as a mean for the control group (two non-shift workers). Thus, eating behavior was summarized in a set of chronograms showing the number of meals, total calories, proteins, lipids, and carbohydrates consumed in each situation—during normal days, off days, night shifts, etc. Food intake was expressed as 24-hr means for each variable, situation, and group of subjects. For certain variables interindividual differences were minimized by expressing each hourly value as a percentage of the total/24 hr for each variable, type of shift, and subject. The average values obtained for protein, lipid, and carbohydrate intake were examined both as a percentage of the total calorie intake and as absolute values (calories).

Total Calories Ingested During 24-hr Spans

Approximately 2000 cal/24 hr were ingested by the shift workers. Small but statistically significant differences were detected between shifts. Reduced intake occurred while working night shifts (1827 ± 64 cal) and during off days (1849 ± 47 cal). Increased intake occurred while working morning (2090 ± 50 cal) and evening (2013 ± 49 cal) shifts.

Relative Nutrient Intake

Proteins. The ingestion of proteins was approximately 17% of the total calorie intake/24 hr. There was little variance in protein consumption by shifts; the relative amount of proteins consumed while working each of the shifts as well as the off days was similar.

Lipids. The intake of lipids amounted to about 43% of the total calorie intake/24 hr. Nonstatistically significant alterations, with a slight decrease during the night shift and a slight increase during the normal day work, were observed.

Carbohydrates. The consumption of carbohydrates represented about 40% of the total calorie intake/24 hr. Variation between shifts was not significant. Highest intake occurred while working night shifts; lowest ingestion occurred during off days.

In summary, during the night shift employees ate less fat, more sugar, and an identical amount of protein as compared to when working other shifts. The relative amount of dietary proteins, lipids, and carbohydrates was similar in shift workers and non-shift workers.

Ethanol. The consumption of alcoholic beverages (beer, cider, wine, etc.) amounted to about 10% of the overall caloric intake of shift workers. This amount was smaller than that of the non-shift workers.

Number and Timing of Food Intakes

Non-shift workers. Both during normal work and during off days the non-shift workers consumed the main meals of lunch and supper at fixed times, around 1200 and 2000, respectively. Breakfasts were eaten early in the morning around 0600 on normal days and later about 0900 on off days. Snacks were consumed during and after work. Major protein, lipid, and carbohydrate intakes occurred during breakfast, lunch, and supper. However, carbohydrates were eaten between these main meals during the off days. Overall, about 80% of the total calories/24 hr were taken at the times of the main meals.

Shift workers. The number of meals varied from four during the evening shift to many more manifested as what can be best described as nibbling behavior during the night shift (Fig. 12). However, the main

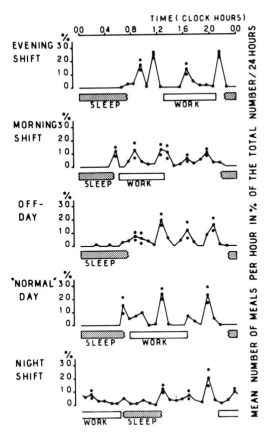

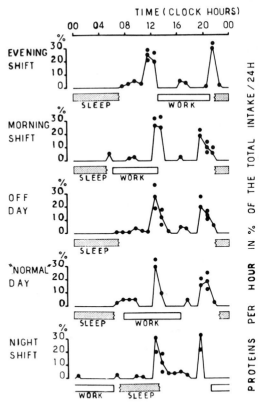

Fig. 12. Changes of the meal timings and of the number of meals in 5 shift workers. Data recorded by each subject during a 57-day span of time. 100% = total number of meals/24 hr. Data were calculated on an hourly basis for each subject and each shift. Resulting percentages were averaged. A dot on the curves represents x̄ (with ±1 SE shown as black dots under and/or above the line). Prominent peaks are significantly different from zero. Large food intakes occurred around 1200 and 2000. Nibbling behavior surfaced during the night shift (**bottom**). (From Reinberg et al. 1979a.)

Fig. 13. Changes of ingested proteins in 5 shift workers. Duration of individual data gathering = 57 days. 100% = total protein intake/24 hr. Data were calculated on an hourly basis for each subject and each shift. Resulting percentages were averaged. A dot on the curves represents x̄ (with ±1 SE shown as black dots above and/or under the line). Statistically significant prominent peaks occurred around 1200 (lunch) and 2000 (supper) with only minor changes from shift to shift. (From Reinberg et al. 1979a.)

meals of lunch and supper were maintained with their usual timing, around 1200 and 2000, in all work conditions. Other food intakes took place during breakfast as well as morning and afternoon snacks, with nibbling during night work.

Striking differences were seen in the quality and relative quantity of calories ingested at each meal. Proteins (Fig. 13) and lipids (Fig. 14) were ingested mainly during lunch and supper, even during the night shift. Two prominent peaks occurred around 1200 and 2000 for both lipid and protein ingestion. More than 70% of the total daily consumption of these nutrients occurred during lunch and supper. Breakfast and snacks were relatively poor in protein and lipid; however these latter were eaten during night work. In contrast, during the night shift nutrients as carbohydrates were consumed at short intervals, there being

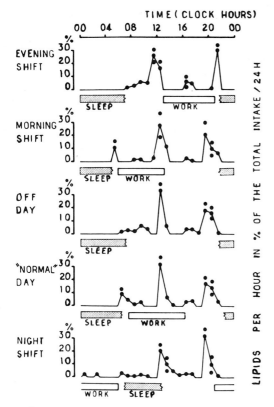

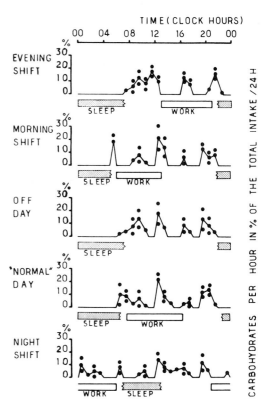

Fig. 14. Changes of ingested lipids in 5 shift workers. (See the legends for Figs. 12 and 13.) Statistically significant prominent peaks were exhibited around 1200 (lunch) and 2000 (supper), with only minor differences between shifts. (From Reinberg et al. 1979a.)

Fig. 15. Changes of ingested carbohydrates in 5 shift workers. (See the legends for Figs. 12 and 13.) Statistically significant prominent peaks occurred around 1200 (lunch) and 2000 (supper). However, during the night shift, carbohydrates were consumed frequently, giving rise to nibbling behavior (7–8 carbohydrate intakes/24 hr, with some occurring during the span allotted for day-sleep, when the subject was transiently awake). (From Reinberg et al. 1979a.)

about eight peaks in the 24-hr scale as shown in Fig. 15. Night work and even day sleep, on the occasion of a brief awakening, were associated with frequent carbohydrate intakes in the form of biscuits, soft drinks, and sandwiches. During the other shifts, a relatively large amount of carbohydrate was ingested at breakfast and/or in the morning. However, in all situations, including the night shift, peaks of carbohydrate intake (10–20% of the 24-hr total) occurred during lunch and supper.

The temporal patterns of calorie consumption are depicted in Fig. 16. Two prominent peaks occurred around 1200 and 2000 when working shifts, including the night and morning ones, as well as during the off days. Work during the morning shift was associated with an additional large intake of calories at breakfast, while that during the night shift was associated with a number of brief intakes of carbohydrate-rich snacks.

Effects of Work Shifts on Physiological Variables

Time series of the self-measurements of biological functions as well as the analyses of the urinary samples were examined using the Single Cosinor method (Chap. 2). End point and confidence interval estimates for

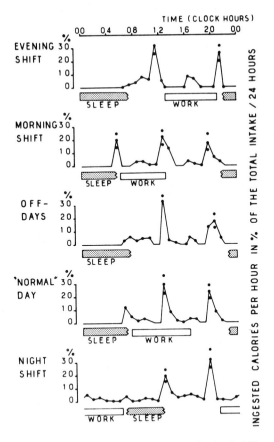

Fig. 16. Changes of ingested calories in 5 shift workers. (See the legends for Figs. 12 and 13.) Statistically significant prominent peaks were found around 1200 (lunch) and 2000 (supper), with only minor changes between shifts, including the night shift, despite the fact that nibbling behavior for carbohydrates was displayed. (From Reinberg et al. 1979a.)

ranging from approximately 4.40 hr for the rhythms of urinary K^+ (P < 0.001), 17-hydroxycorticosteroids—17-OHCS (P < 0.0005), and vanillylmandelic acid—VMA (P < 0.005) to about 6 hr for urinary Na^+ and 5-hydroxyindole acetic acid—5-HIAA (P < 0.002). A phase advance in the work schedule of about 8.50 hr when going from the night to morning shift was followed on the second or the third day by a $\Delta\phi$ ranging from approximately 4 hr for the rhythm of urinary K^+ (P < 0.0005), 17-OHCS (P < 0.01), and 5-HIAA (P < 0.005) to approximately 6 hr for urinary VMA and Na^+ (P < 0.0005). These $\Delta\phi$'s in the urinary variables were similar to the $\Delta\phi$'s of the physical variables. For all the variables, the adjustment was rapid. However, the $\Delta\phi$'s remained smaller than the changes in the synchronizer (work–rest) shifts.

Changes in the Eating Patterns of Shift Workers

Based upon earlier studies of workers of the same oil refinery, the consumption of carbohydrates was found to be lower when studied in 1974 than it was when studied in 1963. On the other hand, fat consumption seemed to be higher (Vieux et al. 1963). Shift workers, like many others nowadays, prefer having their meals at the company cafeteria instead of bringing homemade sandwiches. The observed changes over the 11-year span in the consumption of nutrients might be due to many things such as socioeconomic factors, the type of work, the nature of the sample, as well as geographic influences. These must be considered when comparing nutrition data of different studies. The shift workers studied by Debry et al. (1967) consumed on the average, 2809 cal/24 hr, with 13.6% proteins, 39.4% lipids, and 46.9% carbohydrates. Despite minor differences between the recent and earlier studies, the results of the two seem to be similar: (1) protein ingestion was not influenced by shift work; it remained constant, at least when expressed as a percentage of the total calorie intake/24 hr and (2) major food intakes occurred with the

circadian acrophases, amplitudes, and 24-hr rhythm-adjusted means were derived for each day and each variable. A phase shift in the work–rest schedule was followed in all cases by an acrophase shift, $\Delta\phi$, of the studied variables (Reinberg et al. 1973b; Vieux et al. 1979).

In this group of five selected shift workers, a rapid $\Delta\phi$ followed after either a phase advance or a phase delay of the subjects' synchronization. A phase delay of 7.25 hr in synchronizer schedule when changing from the normal day to the night shift was followed on the second or third day by a $\Delta\phi$

main meals: 37–42% at lunch and 33–33.5% at supper (Debry et al. 1967; Reinberg et al. 1979a).

In our chronobiologic study, the most striking observation was the manifestation of a "nibbling" behavior during the night shift. In fact, this ultradian rhythm (with $\tau \cong 3$ hr) resembles that of infants raised on self-demand schedules (Halberg and Reinberg 1967; Hellbrügge et al. 1964; Martin du Pan 1973). However, this nocturnal intake of food consisted mainly, if not exclusively, of carbohydrates. Moreover, shift work and particularly the occurrence of such nibbling behavior did not result in a major change in either the mean 24-hr calorie intake or in the percentage of calories as proteins. This constitutes an argument in favor of precise physiological control of food intake for both the total amount of calories and the percentage consumption of calories as protein by man, since nutritional balance continued to persist even when environmental factors, in this case those associated with shift work, were manipulated. In connection with this, the duration of sleep was similar during the night and morning shifts (~6 hr) on the one hand, and during the evening shift, normal day, and off day on the other (~8.5 hr) (Andlauer 1971; Foret and Benoit 1977; Reinberg et al. 1973b; Vieux et al. 1979). Therefore, it seems logical to consider that the "nibbling" behavior which occurred doing the night shifts was related to the odd hours of sleep and wakefulness rather than to a change in the duration of sleep. Neither the timing nor the duration of the hours of work at the refinery per se exhibited a synchronizing effect on the rhythm of food consumption or the other studied rhythms (Reinberg et al. 1973b, 1979a–c).

Timing of Major Meals Does Not Play a Role in the Adjustment of the Shift Worker

Other experiments have shown that in human beings a change in the timing of food intake, without an alteration in the activi-ty–rest schedule, is able to shift the acrophases of a limited number of explored variables, such as urinary nitrogen (Apfelbaum et al. 1976) as well as plasma insulin and glucagon (Goetz et al. 1976). Under the conditions of our reported study, shift work represented an alteration in the timing of rest and activity in the 24-hr scale but not in the timing of lunch and supper. Nevertheless, shift work was associated with the occurrence of rapidly accomplished acrophase shifts in the following circadian rhythms: sleep onset and termination, mood and fatigue self-ratings, random number addition test, heart rate, peak expiratory flow, grip strength, and systolic blood pressure as well as the urinary excretions of water, K^+, Na^+, 17-OHCS, catecholamines (VMA), and 5-HIAA.

The constancy in the timing of the major meals, around 1200 and 2000, coexisting with $\Delta\phi$'s resulting from shift work leads one to conclude that meal timing had a minor synchronizing effect, if any, on the studied physiological variables. In other words, the alternation of the activity–rest schedule in the 24-hr scale as well as corresponding changes in the social routine related to shift work appear to be a more powerful and effective synchronizer of biological rhythms than meal timing (Reinberg et al. 1979a).

Chronobiological Aspects of Ethanol Metabolism Related to Nutrition

When addressing chronobiologic aspects of nutrition, it is pertinent to discuss the metabolism and effects of ethanol when given at different times. Ethanol can be considered either a drug or a nutrient. Circadian variations in the blood level and the effect of ethanol on healthy adult men have been investigated (Reinberg et al. 1975a). Six healthy adult male volunteers, 22 to 26 years of age, synchronized to diurnal activity from 0700 to 0000 and nocturnal rest, were given a set dosage of ethanol (0.67 g/ kg body weight) in a series of four tests scheduled at weekly intervals to evaluate the effects of alcohol ingestion at different times—0700, 1100, 1900, and 2300. Prior to being given ethanol, each subject was fasted for 12 hr. Tests for assessing psychological state and performance (self-rating of mood, physical vigor, and inebriety; tempo and random number addition test), physical state (heart rate, systolic and diastolic blood pressure, peak expiratory flow, oral temperature, and grip strength), blood constituents (plasma ethanol, cortisol, lactic acid, pyruvic acid, glucose, and erythrocyte K^+), and urinary variables (volume, epinephrine, norepinephrine, and 5-HIAA) were conducted at 4-hr intervals during work and at home during the waking span.

The parameters characterizing the ethanol pharmacokinetics (chronopharmacokinetics) varied in a circadian manner ($P < 0.05$). The peak height of ethanolemia as well as the time to peak were greater when ethanol was ingested at 0700 than at any other time. Also, a circadian rhythm in the biosystem's susceptibility (*chronesthesy*, see Chap. 6) was demonstrated ($P < 0.05$)

with the peak corresponding neither to the clock-hour administration of greatest ethanolemia nor to that of the peak of other chronopharmacokinetic variations. This infers the sensitivity of the brain to ethanol is not phase related to its metabolism.

Endogenicity of the Circadian Periodicity of Metabolic Processes

The endogenicity of the circadian rhythms of metabolic and hormonal processes must be considered as important background when attempting to understand the bioperiodic changes of nutrient metabolism (Aspect 4). Apfelbaum and his colleagues (1971), as well as Reinberg (1973b), viewed the persistence of circadian rhythmicity in respiratory quotient (RQ = $\dot{V}CO_2/\dot{V}O_2$) of subjects adhering to a 220 cal/24 hr protein diet a result of the predominance of gluconeogenesis at certain times of the day and glycolysis at others. The existence of such alternation in "fuel" production and utilization over time (24 hr) constitutes another demonstration that cell functions are pro-

Table 3. *Circannual Rhythm in the Respiratory Quotient $\dot{V}CO_2/\dot{V}O_2$ of Five Healthy Young Subjects.*

Sex	Age (years)	Weight (kg)	Height (cm)	Rhythm detection P value	Mesor M[b] ±1 SE	Amplitude A[b,c]	Acrophase ϕ[c]
M	34	52.9	161	<0.022	0.850 ±0.004	0.015 (0.005 to 0.025)	16 September (21 Aug. to 23 Sept.)
M	28	60.1	170	>0.05	0.833 ±0.004	—	12 July
F	30	53.4	163	<0.05	0.836 ±0.006	0.021 (0.006 to 0.036)	25 October (12 Sept. to 7 Dec.)
F	19	55.6	163	<0.006	0.832 ±0.004	0.020 (0.010 to 0.030)	27 August (31 July to 24 Sept.)
F	24	55.5	158	>0.05	0.764 ±0.003	—	2 August
Pooled data of all subjects. M and A as % of the individual monthly mean/yr				<0.0001	100 ±0.2	1.4 (0.8 to 2)	8 September (15 Aug. to 2 Oct.)

[a] American citizens living in Buffalo, N.Y., adhering to a controlled diet. Measurements were performed between 0800 and 1000 under strictly basal conditions after a ~12-hr fast. There were 2–20 measurements/subject/month during, respectively, 24, 24, 13, 13, and 12 consecutive months.

[b] M and A as RQ = $\dot{V}CO_2/\dot{V}O_2$ except for the bottom row.

[c] Information in parentheses is 95% Confidence Limit (CL); when rhythms not detected, A and CL not given.

Source: Reanalysis (Single Cosinor) of data published by F.R. Griffith et al. (1929).

gramed, by the very nature of their temporal morphology, for different activities at different times (see Chap. 3). The acrophase of the RQ circadian rhythm, meaning a timing of values closer to 1.0, occurs when the organism uses predominantly carbohydrate as fuel. Under the experimental conditions of the protein-restricted diet study previously described in this chapter, the RQ ϕ occurs at 1147 with the 95% confidence internal ranging between 0748 and 1546. At the ϕ, the RQ is approximately 0.746, while at the trough 12 hr later it is about 0.724. The difference between the RQ peak and trough values is statistically significant, $P < 0.04$ (Table 3 and Figs. 2 and 3). This finding is consistent with the persistence in fasting mice of the circadian rhythm of liver glycogen (Haus and Halberg 1966).

Conclusion

It is likely that circadian and circannual rhythms in general represent adaptive phenomena when considered from the perspective of the reproduction and survival of species. From a nutritional point of view, this hypothesis was suggested by Sargent in 1954. Circannual changes in the eating behavior of children (presumably as yet not altered by either social or educational influences) are considered the expression of adaptive phenomena by our species to annual changes in food availability, e.g., carbohydrates and fat. The implicit mechanism is metabolic in nature. Seasonal variations are envisioned as being governed by nutritional demands and "expectations" of tissues, which are signaled by annual changes in the daily photoperiod and/or other environmental factor(s) serving as stimuli. From an evolutionary perspective, Sargent perceived the annual rhythm to be biphasic, consisting of an anaphase (from the beginning of spring until the end of summer) corresponding to the duration of activity and preparation for inactivity, and a cataphase (from the beginning of autumn until the end of winter) cor-

responding to the reverse. During the anaphase (summer), tissues and organs "expect" to use carbohydrate, available in large amount, as the chief source of fuel and to store fat for the anticipated span of inactivity. During the cataphase (winter) the metabolism of stored fat occurs either by direct utilization or by gluconeogenesis.

In spite of some qualifications (Reinberg 1974c), Sargent's hypothesis concerning the alternation of lipid and carbohydrate metabolism during the course of the year is a very stimulating one. In fact, indirect evidence supports it. First, circannual changes of body weight have been found in North American infants (Sargent 1954) as well as in school aged German children (Hildebrandt 1962) with the peak between late summer and early fall. In nonobese healthy human males living in France (Lagoguey and Reinberg 1981), the circannual crest of body weight was found in September-October, at a time when the annual acrophase of plasma testosterone occurred (Lagoguey et al. 1976; Reinberg and Lagoguey 1980). Second, the existence of a circannual rhythm in respiratory quotient (RQ) demonstrated by Griffith et al. (1929) constitutes additional evidence for Sargent's hypothesis. Time series published by Griffin and his colleagues (1929) reanalyzed using the Single Cosinor revealed that the circannual acrophase occurred between midsummer and midfall (Table 3). It seems that at this time of year the human organism uses carbohydrates as a major source of energy; this is not the case during winter. Third, the circannual rhythmicity in insulin responsiveness to the oral glucose tolerance test is also supportive (Campbell et al. 1975; Méjean et al. 1977). The quickest and greatest response of plasma insulin seems to occur during the fall, September (Fig. 11), when the availability of carbohydrate apparently was greatest for our ancestors. The similarity in results obtained by Campbell et al. (1975) and Méjean et al. (1977) in both the Northern and Southern Hemispheres with regard to actual season rather than calendar month suggests that day length (photoperiod) may serve as an appropriate signal for these circannual rhythms.

Obviously, circannual changes in the eating behavior of children (Sargent 1954; Debry et al. 1973, 1975) and in their weight gain, with a peak between late summer and early autumn, cannot be explained only by the circannual change in insulin responsiveness and related effects. Nevertheless, a coherent body of knowledge suggests that autumn corresponds in time to the peak of carbohydrate consumption in young children, plasma insulin response to oral GTT, as well as RQ in young adults. Moreover, many other physiological functions change over the year. This includes, for example, circannual rhythms in levels of hormones such as plasma testosterone, growth hormone, thyroid stimulating hormone, thyroxin, cortisol, catecholamines, aldosterone, and others (Lagoguey and Reinberg 1976, 1981). These as well as other temporal variabilities over the year have to be taken into account for a better understanding of circannual changes in metabolic and nutritional processes. In addition, the fact that the annual peak time of a set of anabolizing factors occurs around autumn has to be kept in mind when tentatively viewing biological rhythmicity as an adaptive phenomenon serving to enable (physiological) preparedness for environmental alteration (Reinberg and Lagoguey 1980).

The findings put forward in this chapter, along with knowledge of the circadian organization of human physiochemical functions, favor the conclusion that bioperiodic changes in energy metabolism are presumably related to circadian rhythms in growth hormone, insulin, glucagon, and cortisol secretion, among others (Apfelbaum et al. 1975). Such component circadian rhythms are in turn phase dependent on metabolic circadian rhythms. Even after significant restriction in nutrient intake, the temporal structure persists with circadian changes in both metabolic and metabolically active hormones. As a consequence of circadian variability in metabolic pathways, *when* food is consumed appears to be an almost equally important consideration as *what* is consumed. Since metabolic activities display circadian rhythms to such a great extent, as exemplified by the relative predominance of glycolysis in the morning in diurnally active human beings, one can expect that food as fuel might to some extent be "wasted" when taken in the morning and "stored" when taken in the evening. In experiments by Halberg, "breakfast-only" versus "supper-only" once-a-day meal schedules were compared for body weight maintenance. A trend toward weight gain occurred when the single daily meal of 2000 calories was consumed at 2000. A trend toward weight loss was observed when the single daily meal was consumed at 0800. In conclusion, we agree with Halberg (1969, 1974), who reemphasized that "we are not only *what* we eat but *when* we eat."

The possible implications of circadian and circannual rhythms in nutrient effects and metabolism require further study with regard to long-term effects, such as one's risk of diabetes and cardiovascular disease. Similarly, the implication of a once-a-day chronobiologically scheduled "big breakfast" or "big supper" meal timing for people dwelling in countries where the supply of food is highly restricted is intriguing, yet requiring evaluation.

References

Achelis, JD, and Nothdurft, H (1939) Über Ernährung und motorische Aktivität. Pflügers Arch 241:651–673.

Accary, JP, Brigant, L, Bonfils, S, Reinberg, A, and Apfelbaum, M (1977a) Circadian rhythm in plasma gastrin, studied in 11 moderately obese women on spontaneous diet and after a very restricted diet (200 cal/day as casein exclusively). Abstract for *International Society for Chronobiology, XIII International Conference,* Pavia.

Accary, JP, Dubrasquet, JM, and Bonfils, S (1977b) Chronobiological studies on blood gastrin level and gastric acid secretion in pylorus ligated rats. Abstract for *International Society for Chronobiology, XIII International Conference,* Pavia.

Andlauer, P (1971) Différentes modalités du travail en équipes alternantes. Arch Mal Prof Méd Travail 32:393–395.

Anonymous (1951) *Seasonal Patterns of Food Consumption: City Families.* Washington, D.C.: Bureau of Human Nutrition and Home Economics, U.S. Dept. Agricul., Special Report, No. 3, p. 16.

Apfelbaum, M., Reinberg, A., Nillus, P., and Halberg, F (1969) Rythmes circadiens de l'alternance veille-sommeil pendant l'isolement souterrain de sept jeunes femmes. Presse Med 77:879–882.

Apfelbaum, M, Reinberg, A, Lacatis, D, Abulker, C, Bostsarron, J, and Riou, F (1971) Rythmes circadiens de la consommation d'oxygène et du quotient respiratoire de femmes adultes jeunes en alimentation spontanèe et après restriction colorique. Rev Eur Etud Clin Biol 16:135–143.

Apfelbaum, M, Reinberg, A, Assan, R, and Lacatis, D (1972) Hormonal and metabolic circadian rhythms before and during a low protein diet. Isr J Med Sci 8(6):867–873.

Apfelbaum, M, Reinberg, A, and Lacatis, D (1975) Effects of meal timing on circadian rhythms in 9 physiologic variables of young healthy but obese women during a caloric restriction. In: Jéquier, E (ed), *2nd Internat. Congress: Energy Balance in Man.* Genève: Médicine et Hygiène, pp. 22–26.

Apfelbaum, M, Reinberg, A, and Duret, F (1976a) Chronobiological study of the human fitness for working during a 220 cal/24 h diet as protein exclusively. Int J Chronobiol 4:51–62.

Apfelbaum, M, Reinberg, A, and Lacatis, D (1976b) Effects of meal timing on circadian rhythms in nine physiological variables of young healthy but obese women on a calorie restricted diet. Int J Chronobiol 4:29–37.

Ardisson, JL, Dolisi, C, Camous, JP, and Gastaud, M (1975) Rythmes spontanés des prises alimentaires et hydriques chez le chien: étude préliminaire. Physiol Behav 14:47–52.

Aschoff, J (1954) Zeitgeber der tierischen Tagesperiodik. Naturwissenschaften 41:59–56.

Aschoff, J (1963) Comparative physiology; diurnal rhythms. Ann Rev Physiol 25:581–600.

Aschoff, J, Fatranska, M, Gieke, H, Doerr, P, Stamm, D, and Wisser, H (1971) Human circadian rhythms in continuous darkness. Entrainment by social cues. Science 171:213–215.

Aschoff, J, Hoffmann, K, Pohl, H, and Wever, R (1975) Re-entrainment of circadian rhythms after phase-shifts of the Zeitgeber. Chronobiologia 2:23–78.

Assenmacher, I (1982) CNS structures controlling circadian neuroendocrine and activity rhythms in rats. In: Aschoff, J, Daan, S, and Groos, G (eds), *Vertebrate Circadian Systems.* Berlin, Heidelberg: Springer-Verlag, pp. 85–95.

Baker, RA (1953) A periodic feeding behavior in the albino rat. J Comp Physiol Psychol 46:422–426.

Bazin, R, Apfelbaum, M, Assan, R, Brigant, L, de Gasquet, L, Griglio, S, Halberg, F, Leliepvre, X, Longchampt, J, Malewiak, MI, Planche, E, Rozen, R, and Tonnu, NT (1979) Circadian rhythms related to energy metabolism modified by food redistribution at conventional mealtimes—big breakfast versus big dinner. In: Reinberg, A, and Halberg, F (eds), *Chronopharmacology.* Oxford: Pergamon Press, pp. 303–309.

Bérard, A, Pansu, D, and Chayvialle, JA (1976) Variations nycthmérales de la gastrinémie et du renouvellement cellulaire intestinal au cours du jeûne chez le rat. Biol Gastroentérol 9:314.

Bobillier, P, and Mouret, JR (1971) The alterations of the diurnal variations of brain tryptophan, biogenic amines and 5-hydroxyindole acetic acid in the rat under limited time feeding. Int J Neurosci 2:271–282.

Bosshard, A, Pansu, D, Chayvialle, JA, and Reinberg, A (1982) Effect of fasting and Somatostatin administration on circadian rhythms of jejunal cell renewal and plasma gastrin level in rats. Digestion 23:245–252.

Bowen, AJ, and Reeves, RL (1967) Diurnal variation in glucose tolerance. Arch Intern Med 119:261–264.

Campbell, HL (1945) Seasonal changes in food consumption and rate of growth of the albino rat. Am J Physiol 143:428–433.

Campbell, IT, Jarrett, RJ, and Kleen, A (1975a) Diurnal and seasonal variation in oral glucose tolerance: studies in the Antarctic. Diabetologia 11:139–145.

Campbell, IT, Jarrett, RJ, Rutland, P, and Stimmer, L (1975b) The plasma insulin and growth hormone response to oral glucose: diurnal and seasonal observations in the Antarctic. Diabetologia 11:147–150.

Capani, F, Caradonna, P, Carotenuto, M,

Camilli, G, and Sensi, S (1972) Circadian rhythm of immunoreactive insulin under glycemic stimulus. Biochim Biol Sper 10:115–124.

Chossat, C (1843) Recherches expérimentales sur l'inanition. Mem Acad R Sci Inst Fr 8:438–640.

Chrometzka, F (1940) Sommer-Interrhythmus im menschlichen Stoffwechsel des Sommer-Winterrhythmus des diabetes. Stoffwechsels, Klin, Wochnenshchr 19:972–976.

Cohn, C, Joseph, D, Larin, F, Shoomaker, WJ, and Wurtman, RJ (1970) Influence of feeding habits and adrenal cortex on diurnal rhythm of hepatic tyrosine transminase activity. Proc. Soc Exp Biol Med 133:460–462.

Collier, G, Hirsch, E, and Hamlin, PH (1972) The ecological determinants of reinforcement in the rat. Physiol Behav 9:705–726.

Collier, G, Hirsch, E, Kanarek, R, and Marwine, A (1973) Environmental determinants of patterns of feeding. Int J Chronobiol 1:322 (abstract).

David, DE (1967) The annual rhythm of fat deposition in woodchucks (*Marmota monax*). Physiol Zool 40:391–403.

Debry, F, Girault, P, Lefort, J, and Thiebault, J (1967) Enquête sur les habitudes alimentaires des travailleurs "à feu continu." Bulletin de l'INSERM 22:1169–1202.

Debry, G, Bleyer, R, and Reinberg, A (1973) Circadian, circaseptan and circannual rhythms in spontaneous nutrient and calorie intake of 4 ± 1.5 year old healthy children. Int J Chronobiol 1:323–324.

Debry, G, Bleyer, R, and Reinberg, A (1975) Circadian, circannual and other rhythms in spontaneous nutrient and caloric intake of healthy four year olds. Diabète Metabol 1:91.

Debry, G, Méjean, L, Villaume, C, Drouin, P, Martin, JM, Pointel, JP, and Gay, G (1977) Chronobiologie et nutrition humaine. In: Mirouze, J, (ed), *XIV Congrès International de Thérapeutique*. Montpellier, 1977. Paris: L'Expansion Scientifique, pp. 225–245.

Ehret, CF, and Dobra, KW (1977) The oncogenic implications of chronobiotics in the synchronization of mammalian circadian rhythms: barbiturates and methylated xanthines. In Nieburgs, HE (ed), *Proc. Third International Symposium on the Detection and Prevention of Cancer*. New York: Marcel Dekker, pp. 1101–1114.

Ehret, CF, Groh, KR, and Meinert, JC (1978)

Circadian dyschronism and chronotypic ecophilia as factors in aging and longevity. In: Samis, HV Jr, and Capobianco, S (eds), *Aging and Biological Rhythms*. London, New York: Plenum Publishing Corporation, pp. 185–213.

Felig, P, Cahill, GF, and Marliss, EB (1973) Metabolic pathways in starvation. In: Apfelbaum, M (ed), *Energy Balance in Man*. Paris: Masson, pp. 83–94.

Fisher, RB, and Garner, MLG (1976) A diurnal rhythm in the absorption of glucose and water by isolated rat small intestine. J Physiol (London) 254:821–825.

Foret, J, and Benoit, O (1977) Shift-work and sleep. In: *3rd Europ. Congr. Sleep Res,* Montpellier, 1976. Basel: Karger, pp. 81–86.

Freinkel, N, Mager, M, and Vinnick, L (1968) Cyclicity in the interrelationships between plasma insulin and glucose during starvation in normal young man. J Lab Clin Med 71:171–178.

Fuller, RW (1970) Daily variation in liver tryptophan, tryptophan pyrolase and tyrosine transaminase in rats fed ad libitum or single daily meals. Proc Soc Exp Biol Med 133:620–622.

Furuya, S, and Yugari, Y (1976) Daily rhythmic changes of L-histidine and glucose absorptions in rat small intestine in vivo. Biochem Biophy Acta 343:558–564.

Galicich, JH, Halberg, F, and French, LA (1963) Circadian adrenal cycle in C mice kept without food and water for a day and half. Nature 197:811–813.

Gamble, DR, and Taylor, KW (1969) Seasonal incidence of diabetes mellitus. Br Med J 3:631–633.

Ghata, J, Halberg, F, Reinberg, A, and Siffre, M (1969) Rythmes circadiens desynchronisés (17-hydroxycorticostéroides, température rectale, veille-sommeil) chez deux sujets adultes sains. Ann Endocrinol 30:245–260.

Gibson, T, Stimmler, L, Jarrett, RJ, Rutland, P, and Shiu, M (1975) Diurnal variation in the effects of insulin in blood glucose, plasma non-esterified fatty acids and growth hormone. Diabetologia 11:83–88.

Goetz, F, Bishop, J, Halberg, F, Sothern, RB, Brünning, R, Senske, B, Greenberg, B, Minors, D, Stoney, P, Smith, ID, Rozen, GD, Cressey, D, Haus, E, and Apfelbaum, M (1976) Timing of single daily meal influences relations among human circadian rhythms in urinary cyclic AMP and hemic glucagon, insulin and iron. Experientia 32:1081–1084.

Griffith, FR Jr, Pucher, GW, Brownell, KA, Klein, JD, and Carmer, ME (1929) Studies in human physiology I. The metabolism and body temperature (oral) under basal conditions. Am J Physiol 87:602–632.

Haberey, P, Dantlo, C, and Kayser, C (1967) Evolution saisonnière des voies métaboliques du glucose et du choix alimentaire spontané chez un hibernant, le Lérot (Eliomys quercinus). Arch Sci Physiol 21:59–66.

Halberg, F (1960) Temporal coordination of physiologic function. Cold Spring Harbor Symp Quant Biol 25:289–310.

Halberg, F (1969) Chronobiology. Ann Rev. Physiol 31:675–725.

Halberg, F (1974) Protection by timing treatment according to bodily rhythms. An analogy to protection by scrubbing before surgery. Chronobiologia 1(Suppl. 1):23–68.

Halberg, F, and Reinberg, A (1967) Rythmes circadiens et rythmes de basses fréquences en physiologie humaine. J Physiol Paris 59:117–200.

Halberg, E, Nelson, W, Scheving, LE, Stupfel, M, Halberg, F, Mouquot, JE, Vickers, RA, and Gorlin, RJ (1973) Interactions of meal scheduling, lighting and housing influence the timing of circadian rhythms to a different extent at different levels of murine organization. Int J Chronobiol 1:317–328.

Haus, E, and Halberg, F (1966) Persisting circadian rhythms in hepatic glycogen of mice during inanition and dehydration. Experientia 22:113–115.

Haus, E, Halberg, F, Kühl, JFW, and Lakatua, DJ (1974) Chronopharmacology in animals. Chronobiologia 1 (Supp. 1):122–156.

Hellbrügge, T, Ehrengut–Langei, J, Rutenfranz, J, and Stehr, K (1964) Circadian periodicity of physiological functions in different stages of infancy and childhood. NY Acad Sci 117:361–373.

Hildebrandt, G (1962) Biologische Rhythmen und ihre Bedeutung für die Bäder- und Klimaheilkunde. In: Amelung, W, and Evers, A (ed), Handbuch der Bäder- und Klimaheilkunde. Stuttgart: F.K. Schattauerverlag, pp. 730–785.

Hommel, H, and Fisher, U (1971) Jahresperiodik der Insulinwirkung am eviszerierten Kaninchen und am isolierten perfundierten Rattenherzen. Diabetologia 7:6–9.

Howe, PE, and Berrymann, GH (1945) Average food consumption in the training camps of the United States Army (1941–1943). Am J Physiol 144:588–594.

Hughes, E (1931) Seasonal Variation in Man. London: H.K. Lewis, p. 126.

Hugues, JN, Reinberg, A, Jordan, D, Sebaoun, J, Modigliani, E, and Burger, AG (1982) Effects of starvation on circadian variations of plasma TSH in rats. Acta Endocrinol 101:403–407.

Inouye, ST (1982) Restricted daily feeding does not entrain circadian rhythms of the suprachiasmatic nucleus in the rat. Brain Research 232:194–199.

Jarrett, RJ (1972) Circadian variations in blood glucose levels, in glucose tolerance and in plasma immunoreactive insulin levels. Acta Diabetol Lat 9:263–275.

Jarrett, RJ, and Keen, H (1970) Further observations on the diurnal variation in oral glucose tolerance. Br Med J 4:334–337.

Jarrett, RJ, and Keen, H (1972) Diurnal variation in oral glucose tolerance: a possible pointer of the evolution of diabetes mellitus. Br Med J 2:341–345.

Kayser, C (1961) Le sommeil hivernal, problème de thermorégulation. Rev Can Biol 16:303–389.

Kleitman, N (1949) Biological rhythms and cycles. Physiol Rev 29:1–29.

Kleitman, N (1963) Sleep and Wakefulness, 2nd ed. Chicago: University of Chicago Press, p. 552.

Kleitman, N, and Engelmann, TG (1947) Diurnal cycle in activity and body temperature of rabbits. Fed Proc Fed Am Soc Exp Biol 6:143.

Krieger, DT (1974) Food and water restriction shifts corticosterone, temperature, activity and brain amine periodicity. Endocrinology 95:1195–1201.

Krieger, DT (1979) Rhythms in CRF, ACTH and corticosteroids. In: Krieger, DT (ed), Endocrine Rhythms. New York: Raven Press, pp. 123–142.

Krieger, DT, Hauser, H, and Krey, C (1977) Suprachiasmatic nuclear lesions do not abolish food shifted circadian adrenal and temperature rhythmicity. Science 197:398–399.

Krulin, SG, and Sealander, JA (1972) Annual lipid cycle of the gray bat (Myotis grisesceus). Comp Biochem Physiol A 42:537–549.

Lagoguey, M, and Reinberg, A (1976) Circannual rhythms in plasma LH, FSH and testosterone and in the sexual activity of healthy young Parisian males. J Physiol (Lond) 257:19–20.

Lagoguey, M, and Reinberg, A (1981) Circadian and circannual changes of pituitary and other hormones in healthy human males. In: Van Cauter, E, and Copinschi, G (eds), *Human Pituitary Hormones.* The Hague: Martinus Nijhoff Publ., pp. 261–285.

Le Magnen, J (1971a) Advances in studies of the physiological control and regulation of food intake. In: Stellac, E, and Spragues, JM (eds), *Progress in Physiological Psychology,* Vol. 4. New York: Academic Press, pp. 204–261.

Le Magnen, J (1971b) La périodicité spontanée de la prise d'aliment ad libitum du rat blanc. J Physiol (Paris) 58:323–349.

Lestradet, H, Labram, C, and Alcalay, D (1970) Diabète du soir: espoir Ou l'importance de l'horaire dans l'interprétation d'une courbe d'hyperglycémie provoquée. Presse Méd 78:1481–1482.

Mandenoff, A, and Apfelbaum, M (1981) Differential effects of opiate antagonists on food intake according to time of injection. Int J Chronobiol 7:87.

Margules, DL, Lewis, MJ, Dragovitch, JA, and Margules, A (1972) Hypothalamic norepinephrine: circadian rhythms and the control of feeding behavior. Science 178:640–643.

Marliss, EB, Aoki, TT, Unger, RH, Soeldner, JS, and Cahill, G Jr (1970) Glucagon levels and metabolic effects in fasting man. Clin Invest 49:2256–2261.

Martin du Pan, R (1973) Remarques à propos de la régulation des besoins énergétiques du nourrisson. In: Apfelbaum, M. (ed), *Energy Balance in Man.* Paris: Masson, pp. 317–322.

von Mayersbach, H, Muller, O, Philippens, K, Scheving, L, and Brock, E (1973) Effects of restricted feeding schedules on various parameters of blood serum and liver of rats. Int J Chronobiol 1:342.

Méjean, L, Reinberg, A, Guy, G, and Debry, G (1977) Circannual changes of the plasma insulin response to glucose tolerance test of healthy young human males. In: *Proc. XXVIIth Internat. Congress Physiological Sciences,* Paris, 18–23 July. No. 1475, p. 498 (abstract).

Migraine, C, and Reinberg, A (1974) Persistance des rythmes circadiens de l'alternance veille-sommeil et du comportement alimentaire d'un homme de 20 ans pendant son isolement souterrain, avec et sans montre. C R Acad Sci 279:331–334.

Mirouze, J, Monnier, L, Selam, JL, and Phan Than Chi, F (1976a) Evaluation of exogenous homeostasis by the artificial pancreas in insulin-dependent diabetics. Diabetologia 12:375–478.

Mirouze, J, Selam, JL, and Phan, TC (1976b) Infusion insulinique par débit asservi á l'enregistrement glycémique continu. *Journée Annuelle de Diabétologie Hôtel-Dieu,* 13, 15 mai 1976. Paris: Flammarion Med. Sciences, pp. 303–312.

Mirouze, J, Selam, JL, Pham, TC, and Orsetti, A (1977) Le pancréas artificiel extracorporel: nouvelle orientation du traitement insulinique. *XIVeme Congrés International de Thérapeutique,* Montpellier, France. Paris: Expansion Scientifique, pp. 79–91.

Moore, JG, and Wolfe, M (1974) Circadian plasma gastrin patterns in feeding and fasting man. Digestion 11:226–231.

Mouret, JR, and Bobiller, P (1971) Diurnal rhythms of sleep in the rat: augmentation of paradoxical sleep following alterations of the feeding schedule. Int J Neurosci 2:265–270.

Mouret, J, Coindet, J, and Chouvet, G (1973) Circadian rhythms of sleep in the rat: importance of the feeding schedule. Int J Chronobiol 1(4):345.

Murlin, JR, and Hilderbrandt, FN (1919) Average food consumption in the training camps of the United States Army. Amer J Physiol 49:531–556.

Nagai, K, Mori, T, Nishio, T, and Nakagawa, H (1982) Effect of intracranial insulin infusion on the circadian feeding rhythm of rats. Biomed Res 3:175–180.

Nelson, W, Cadotte, L, and Halberg, F (1973a) Circadian timing of single daily meal affects survival of mice. Proc Soc Exp Biol Med 144(3):766–769.

Nelson, W, Nichols, G, Halberg, F, and Kottke, G (1973b) Interacting effects of lighting LD (12:12) and restricted feeding (4 hrs/24 hrs) on circadian temperature rhythm of mice. Int J Chronobiol 1(4):347.

Nelson, W, Scheving, LE, and Halberg, F (1975) Circadian rhythms in mice fed a single daily meal at different stages of lighting regimen. J Nutrition 105:171–184.

Nillus, P (1967) *Etude de quelques conséquences biophysiologiques de l'isolement souterrain de sept jeunes femmes bien por-tantes.* Paris: Thése Med.

Pansu, D, Chayvialle, JA, Bosshard, A, Descos, F, and Reinberg, A (1979) Circadian rhythms in plasma and antral gastrin of rats. Effects of fasting versus feeding. In: Reinberg, A, and Halberg, F (eds), *Chronopharmacology.* Oxford: Pergamon Press, pp. 331–335.

Pauly, JE, Burns, ER, Beterton, H, Tsai, S, Halberg, F, and Scheving, LE (1973) Effect of restricted feeding schedules on blood eosinophil levels and mitotic activity as well as other parameters in mice. Int J Chronobiol 1(4):348–349.

Pauly, JE, Burns, ER, Halberg, F, Tsai, S, Betterton, HO, and Scheving, LE (1975) Meal timing dominates the lighting regimen as a synchronizer of the eosinophil rhythm in mice. Acta Anat 93:60–68.

Pengelley, ET (ed) (1974) *Circannual Clocks.* New York: Academic Press, p. 523.

Peret, J (1973) Bioperiodic changes of nutrient metabolism. Int J Chronobiol 1:349 (abstract).

Peret, J, Chanez, M, and Macaire, I (1972) Consommation de proteines et rythmes circadiens du glycogéne hépatique chez le rat. C R Acad Sci 274:1562–1565.

Philippens, KMH, von Mayersbach, H, and Scheving, LE (1977) Effects of the scheduling of meal-feeding at different phases of the circadian system in rats. J Nutrition 107:176–193.

Pittendrigh, CS (1960) Circadian rhythms and the circadian organization of living systems. Cold Spring Harbor Symp Quant Biol 25:159–182.

Poirel, C (1968) Variations temporelles du comportement d'exploration chez la souris. C Soc Biol 162(12):2312–2316.

Poirel, C (1975) *Les Rythmes Circadiens en Psychopathologie.* Paris: Masson, p. 113.

Rauline, G, Reinberg, A, Apfelbaum, M, Lagoguey, M, Guillemant, S, Carayon, A, and Studler, JM (1981) Persistence of a set of circadian rhythms in five recumbent subjects continuously fed with infused nutrients. Int J Chronobiol 7:100.

Reinberg, A (1967) The hours of changing responsiveness or susceptibility. Perspect Biol Med 11:111–128.

Reinberg, A (1971a) La chronobiologie. La Recherche 2:242–250.

Reinberg, A (1971b) Methologic consideration for human chronobiology. J Interdispl Cycle Res 2:1–15.

Reinberg, A (1973a) Biological rhythms of potassium metabolism, In: *Potassium. Biochemistry and Physiology,* 8th Colloq. Int. Potash Institute. Berne: International Potash Institute, pp. 160–180.

Reinberg, A (1973b) Biological rhythms and energy balance in man. In: Apfelbaum, M (ed), *Energy Balance in Man.* Paris: Masson, pp. 285–295.

Reinberg, A (1974a) Chronobiology and nutrition. Chronobiologia 1:22–27.

Reinberg, A (1974b) Chronopharmacology in man. In: Aschoff, J, Ceresa, F, and Halberg, F (eds), *Chronobiological Aspects of Endocrinology.* Stuttgart: F.K. Schattauer, pp. 305–337.

Reinberg, A (1974c) Aspects of circannual rhythms in man. In: Pengelley, ET (ed), *Circannual Clocks,* New York: Academic Press, pp. 423–505.

Reinberg, A, and Halberg, F (1971). Circadian chronopharmacology. Ann Rev Pharmacol 11:455–492.

Reinberg, A, and Ghata, J (1978) *Les Rythmes Biologiques,* 3rd ed. Paris: Presses Universitaires de France.

Reinberg, A, and Lagoguey, M (1980) Annual endocrine rhythms in healthy young adult men: their implication in human biology and medicine. In: Assenmacher, I, and Farner, D (eds), *Environmental Endocrinology.* New York: Springer-Verlag, pp. 113–121.

Reinberg, A, Ghata, J, Halberg, F, Gervais, P, Abulker, C, Dupont, J, and Gaudeau, C (1970) Rythmes circadiens du pouls, de la pression artérielle, des excrétions urinaires en 17-hydroxycorticostéroides, catécholamines, et potassium chez l'homme adulte sain et au repos. Ann Endocrinol 31:272–287.

Reinberg, A, Apfelbaum, M, and Assan, R (1973a) Chronophysiologic effects of restricted diet (220 cal/24 h as casein) in young healthy but obese women. Int J Chronobiol 1:391–404.

Reinberg, A, Chaumont, AJ, Laporte, A, Chambon, P, Vincendon, G, Skoulios, G, Bauchart, M, Nicolaï, A, Abulker, C, and Dupont, J (1973b) Etude chronobiologique des effets des changements d'horaires de travail (autométrie de 20 sujets postés: système des 3 × 8 à rotation hebdomadaire). Arch Mal Prof & Méd Trav 35(3):373–394.

Reinberg, A, Apfelbaum, M, Assan, R, and Lacatis, D (1974) Persisting circadian rhythms in insulin, glucagon, cortisol, etc., of healthy young women during caloric restriction (protein diet). In: Scheving, LE, Halberg, F, and Pauly, J (eds), *Chronobiology*. Tokyo: Igaku Shoin, pp. 88–93.

Reinberg, A, Clench, J, Aymard, N, Galliot, M, Bourdon, R, Gervais, P, Abulker, C, and Dupont, J (1975a) Variations circadiennes des effets de l'éthanol et de l'éthanolémie chez l'homme adulte sain. Etude chronopharmacologique. J Physiol (Paris) 70:435–456.

Reinberg, A, Lagoguey, M, Chauffournier, JM, and Cesselin, F (1975b) Circannual and circadian rhythms in plasma testosterone in five healthy young Parisian males. Acta Endocrinol 80:732–743.

Reinberg, A, Migraine, C, Apfelbaum, M, Brigant, L, Ghata, J, Vieux, N, Laporte, A, and Nicolaï, A (1979a) Circadian and ultradian rhythms in the eating behavior and nutrient intake of oil refinery operators. In: Reinberg, A (ed), *Chronobiological Field Studies of Oil Refinery Shift Workers*. Chronobiologia, Suppl. 1:89–102.

Reinberg, A, Vieux, N, Andlauer, P, Smolensky, M, Ghata, J, Laporte, A, and Nicolaï, A (1979b) Shift work tolerance: perspectives based upon findings derived from chronobiologic field studies on oil refinery operators. In: Reinberg, A (ed), *Chronobiological Field Studies on Oil Refinery Shift Workers*. Chronobiologia, Suppl. 1:105–113.

Reinberg, A, Vieux, N, Chaumont, AJ, Laporte, A, Smolensky, M, Nicolaï, A, Abulker, C, and Dupont, J (1979c) Aims and conditions of shift work studies. In: Reinberg, A (ed), *Chronobiological Field Studies of Oil Refinery Shift Workers*. Chronobiologia, Suppl. 1:7–23.

Rietveld, WJ, and Groos, GA (1980) The central neural regulation of circadian rhythms. In: Scheving, LE, and Halberg, F (eds), *Chronobiology: Principles and Applications to Shifts in Schedules*. Alphen aan den Rijn, The Netherlands: Sijthoff and Noordhoff, pp. 189–204.

Sargent, F II (1954) Season and the metabolism of fat and carbohydrate: a study of vestigial physiology. Meteorol Monogr 2:68–80.

Sargent, F II, and Sargent, VW (1950) Season, nutrition and pellagra. N Engl J Med 247:447–453 and 507–514.

Scheving, LE, Pauly, JE, Burns, ER, Halberg, E, Tsai, S, and Betterton, HO (1974a) Lighting regimen dominates interactive meal sched-

ules and synchronizes mitotic rhythm in mouse corneal epithelium. Anat Rec 180:47–52.

Scheving, LE, von Mayersbach, H, and Pauly, JE (1974b) An overview of chronopharmacology. Eur J Toxicol 7:203–227.

Scheving, LE, Burns, ER, Pauly, JE, Tsai, TH, Betterton, HO, and Halberg, F (1976) Meal scheduling, cellular rhythms and the chronotherapy of cancer. In: *Proceedings of the Tenth International Congress of Nutrition*. Kyoto: Victoria-sha Press, pp. 141–142.

Sensi, S, Capani, F, Caradonna, P, Policiccho, D, and Carotenuto, M (1970) Diurnal variation of insulin response to glycemic stimulus. Biochim Biol Sper 9:153–156.

Shirley, M (1928) Studies in activity. J Comp Physiol 8:159–186.

Simpson, HW, Bellamy, N, Bohlen, J, and Halberg, F (1973) Double blind trial of a possible chronobiotic (Quiadon®). Int J Chronobiol 1:287–311.

Smolensky, M, Reinberg, A, Lee, R, and McGovern, JP (1974) Secondary rhythms related to hormonal changes in the menstrual cycle: special reference to allergology. In: Ferin, M, Vande Wiele, RL, and Halberg, F (eds), *Biorhythms and Human Reproduction*. London: John Wiley, pp. 287–306.

Stone, JE, Polk, ML, Dobbs, J, Graham, ME, Scheving, LE, and Kanabrocki, EL (1974) Circadian variation in human urinary cyclic AMP and the effect of different diets on this rhythm. Int J Chronobiol 2:163–170.

Stupfel, M, Halberg, F, Halberg, E, and Lee, JK (1973) Computer prepared displays of feeding time and lighting effects upon circadian rhythms in CO_2 emission by rats. Int J Chronobiol 1:203–221.

Sulzman, FG, Fuller, CA, and Moore-Ede, MC (1977) Feeding time synchronizes primate circadian rhythms. Physiol Behav 18:775–779.

Szafarczyk, A, Ixart, G, Alonso, G, Malaval, F, Nouguier-Soule, J, and Assenmacher, I (1981) Effects of raphe lesions on circadian ACTH, corticosterone and motor activity rhythms in free-running blinded rats. Neuroscience Letters 23:87–92.

Vieux, N, Carre, D, and DeMones, P (1963) Le travail en quarts continus dans une raffinerie de pétrole. Arch Mal Prof Méd Travail 24:139–143.

Vieux, N, Ghata, J, Laporte, A, Migraine, C, Nicolaï, A, and Reinberg, A (1979) Adjustment of shift workers adhering to a three- to four-day rotation. In: Reinberg, A (ed), *Chronobiological Field Studies of Oil Refinery Shift Workers*. Chronobiologia (Suppl 1) 1:37–42.

Walker, PR, and Potter, RV (1974) Diurnal rhythms of hepatic enzymes from rats adapted to controlled feeding schedules. In: Scheving, E, Halberg, F, and Pauly, J (eds), *Chronobiology*. Tokyo: Igaku Shoin, pp. 17–22.

Whichelow, MJ, Sturge, RA, Keen, A, Jarrett, RJ, Stimmler, L, and Grainger, S (1974) Diurnal variation in response to intravenous glucose. Br Med J 2:488–491.

Wurtman, RJ, Chou, C, and Rose, CM (1967) Daily rhythm in tyrosine concentration in human plasma; persistence on low-protein diets. Science 158:660–663.

Wurtman, RJ, Rose, CM, and Larin, FF (1968) Daily rhythms in the concentration of various amino acids in human plasma. N Engl J Med 279:171–175.

Zigmond, MJ, Shoemaker, WJ, Larin, F, and Wurtman, RJ (1969) Hepatic tyrosine transaminase rhythm: interaction of environmental lighting, food consumption and dietary protein content. J Nutr 98:71–75.

Zimmet, PZ, Wall, JR, Rome, R, Stimmler, L, and Jarrett, RJ (1974) Diurnal variation in glucose tolerance: associated changes in plasma insulin, growth hormone and non-esterified fatty acids. Br Med J 2:485–488.

Index